Clinical Ophthalmic Oncology

Bhupendra C. K. Patel • Jacob Pe'er
Arun D. Singh
Editors

Clinical Ophthalmic Oncology

Eyelid Tumors

Springer

Editors
Bhupendra C. K. Patel
Division of Facial Cosmetic
and Reconstructive Surgery
University of Utah
Salt Lake, UT, USA

Jacob Pe'er
Division of Ophthalmology
Hadassah Medical Center
Jerusalem, Israel

Arun D. Singh
Cole Eye Institute
Cleveland Clinic
Cleveland, OH, USA

ISBN 978-3-031-72330-8 ISBN 978-3-031-72328-5 (eBook)
https://doi.org/10.1007/978-3-031-72328-5

This Springer imprint is published by the registered company Springer Nature Switzerland AG
The registered company address is: Gewerbestrasse 11, 6330 Cham, Switzerland

Contents

Eyelid Tumors: Examination Techniques

1

Catherine J. Hwang, Julian D. Perry, and Bhupendra C. K. Patel

1.1 Introduction

Neoplasia may develop within any eyelid structure. Examination of the eyelid is thought to be relatively straightforward, given its anterior location and the ability to visualize its anterior and posterior surfaces. However, examination including structure and function is critical to determine the layers of the eyelid involved and if there might be extension posteriorly into the orbit or medially into the lacrimal system. The examination of an eyelid tumor determines the need for any ancillary tests and the surgical plan.

1.2 History

The history begins with a description of the symptoms: severity, onset, and rate of progression. A targeted review of systems reveals additional clues to the etiology.

1.2.1 Presenting Symptoms

Eyelid neoplasia present with a limited spectrum of symptoms (Box 1.1). Most often, patients notice an abnormal eyelid appearance or asymmetry compared to the contralateral eyelid. The eyelid may harbor a distinct lesion, displaying elevation, ulceration, crusting, bleeding, altered pigmentation, telangiectasia, or other visible cutaneous or conjunctival changes. The patient may complain of loss of eyelashes or an irregularity along the eyelid margin.

C. J. Hwang (✉) · J. D. Perry
Oculofacial Plastic Surgery, Cleveland Clinic, Cole Eye Institute, Cleveland, OH, USA
e-mail: Hwangc2@ccf.org

B. C. K. Patel
Division of Facial Cosmetic and Reconstructive Surgery, University of Utah, Salt Lake, UT, USA

Eyelid neoplasia may produce symptoms that occur with or without visible structural changes. Sensory symptoms such as pain, tenderness, itching, or vision symptoms due to keratopathy, induced astigmatism, or obstruction of vision may develop. Motor symptoms, such as blepharoptosis or lagophthalmos, may develop owing to involvement of the eyelid retractors and protractors, or indirectly from a mass effect. Functional symptoms develop from mechanical keratoconjunctivitis, exposure keratopathy, or decreased lacrimal outflow.

1.2.2 Rate of Onset

Rapidity and progression help characterize the pathology. Most symptoms from eyelid tumors develop over weeks to months, but associated hemorrhage, infection, and inflammation may be acute. Both benign (e.g., angiomas, papillomas) and malignant (e.g., cutaneous malignancies, metastases) eyelid tumors can produce hemorrhage. Any eyelid tumor that blocks lacrimal outflow or causes diminished cutaneous integrity can result in infection. Eyelid tumors may also be associated with a significant inflammatory reactions.

1.2.3 Past Medical History

Because the majority of eyelid neoplasms are epidermal in origin, the past medical history should focus on risk factors for epidermal malignancy. Information should be obtained regarding family history of cutaneous malignancy, skin type, freckle density, eye color, hair color, and prior history of skin cancer. Patients of Celtic or Scandinavian descent with blonde or red hair, blue eyes, and fair skin carry a greater risk for cutaneous malignancy [1, 2]. The history should also

B. C. K. Patel et al. (eds.), *Clinical Ophthalmic Oncology*, https://doi.org/10.1007/978-3-031-72328-5_1

include immunosuppression, tobacco use, prior radiotherapy, sun exposure, and similar growths elsewhere on the skin.

1.3 Examination

The physical examination of an adult with suspected eyelid neoplasia does not end with direct visualization of the lesion. It should include a comprehensive inspection of the eyelid, ocular adnexa and orbit, eye, and other cutaneous lesions described in the history. Underlying conditions that may make reconstruction more challenging should be noted, including prominent globe, midface ptosis, hypoplastic orbital rim, lack of cutaneous or tissue redundancy, previous scarring from cutaneous malignancy repair or other surgery, asymmetry, lymph node enlargement, lagophthalmos, trichiasis, dry eye syndrome, and blepharitis.

1.3.1 Examination of Eyelid and Periocular Lesions

The entire face should be evaluated to note Fitzpatrick skin type and any other cutaneous lesions. The eyelid examination should focus particularly on signs of malignancy, including telangiectasia, nodularity, pearly translucency, ulceration, bleeding, crusting, irregularity of the eyelid margin, meibomian gland effacement, misdirection of lashes or trichiasis, and loss of cilia (Fig. 1.1; Box 1.2). Examination of eyelid and periocular lesions should be undertaken systematically and incorporate all of the following:

1.3.1.1 Site

Anatomical Location

Eyelid lesions are best described in relation to the known structures like the medial canthus, lateral canthus, punctum, and whether involving the eyelid margin or not. Ideally, all lesions should be pointed out to the examiner using a hand mirror.

Relationship to Surrounding Structures

Skin lesions will be mobile while lesions arising from the tarsal plate will be fixed.

1.3.1.2 Size

Size can be measured with a ruler or using the slit-lamp. Size should include the length, width, and height to allow for assessment of change in size over time.

1.3.1.3 Shape

Shapes can be described as round, oval, irregular, etc.

1.3.1.4 Surface

Appearance

Is the surface smooth or rough, is it flat or raised, nodular, regular or irregular?

Evidence of crusting, ulceration, necrosis, bleeding

Is the eyelid margin irregular?

Is there Meibomian gland effacement

Is there misdirection of lashes or presence of trichiasis; loss of lashes

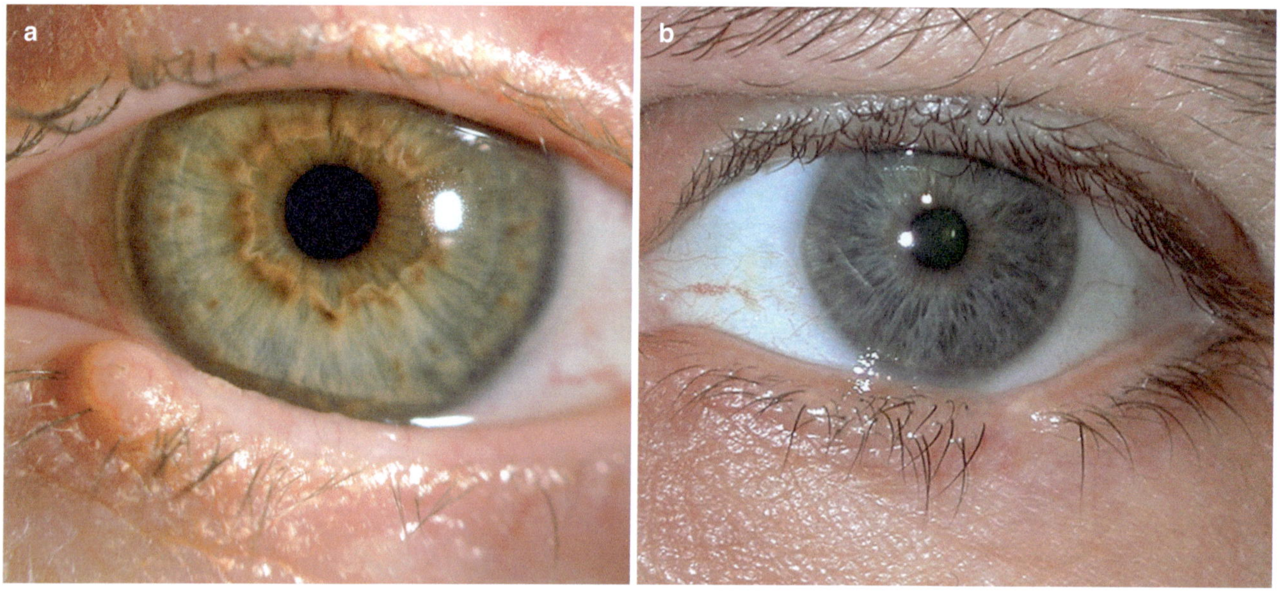

Fig. 1.1 Photograph of lower eyelid shows a benign eyelid nodule without loss of lashes (**a**) and loss of eyelid tissue with cilia loss secondary to a malignant tumor (**b**)

Color

Normal skin-colored, red, dark, black, yellow, white, etc. Look for pearly translucency

1.3.1.5 Consistency

Eyelid lesions can be described as hard, firm or soft. Many malignant lesions become hard over time, especially when they invade surrounding structures like the medial canthus or underlying bone.

1.3.1.6 Pulsatility

Arterio-venous malformations may primarily affect the eyelid and show pulsatility.

1.3.1.7 Compressibility

Venous malformations will be compressible. This is best done with a Q-tip.

1.3.1.8 Fluctuation

With eyelid and adnexal lesions, this is best done with Q-tips. Fluctuation may be seen in hydrocystomas and larger cystic lesions like abscesses.

1.3.1.9 Mobility

The skin may be mobile over the lesion or the lesion may be mobile under the skin and other underlying structures. Chronic chalazia will demonstrate a lump with the skin over the lump being mobile. Basal cell carcinomas that have not invaded the tarsus will be mobile over the tarsal plate. Some benign conditions such as a cyst of Moll or sebaceous collection at the root of an eyelash will be fixed to the eyelid margin and may be soft or firm.

Mobility of lesions of the adnexal region should be assessed to determine deeper fixation as tumors in the medial canthal region in particular may invade the deeper structures and require radiological examination.

1.3.1.10 Transillumination

A pen torch is used to assess transillumination. Hydrocystomas and cysts of Moll will transilluminate brightly while other cystic lesions like sebaceous cysts and lipomas will transilluminate poorly.

1.3.1.11 Auscultation

Arteriovenous malformation may demonstrate a bruit or murmur over the lesion. This is especially so if there is an underlying carotid-cavernous fistula.

1.3.1.12 Palpation

Check for mobility of the lesion on palpation.

Chronically infected lesions will demonstrate induration of surrounding tissues as will slow-growing malignant adnexal tumors with ischemia.

Is the lesion tender to palpation?

1.3.1.13 Eyelid Examination

Function of the eyelid including levator excursion, orbicularis function, lagophthalmos, and lid lag in downgaze should be measured and noted. Horizontal eyelid laxity, blepharoptosis, cutaneous insufficiency, and other preexisting eyelid malpositions, scarring, and conditions should be noted, as they may challenge repair and will affect the reconstruction design.

In addition, patients that relate these preoperative conditions to eyelid tumor surgery in the follow-up period can be reminded of the preoperative findings.

1.3.2 Ocular Adnexal Examination

Eyelid tumors may spread directly to the lacrimal gland, orbit, or lacrimal outflow apparatus. Conversely, primary tumors of these areas may occasionally present with only eyelid signs and symptoms. The structure and function of the orbit and ocular adnexal tissues in proximity to the lesion should be evaluated. In particular, movement of the eyes should be assessed as limitation of the movement of an eye may be related to a tumor that may already have spread posteriorly into the orbit. Globe position (hyperglobus, hypoglobus, esoglobus, exoglobus) should be assessed and exopthalmometry measurements should be made where indicated.

The examiner should palpate for preauricular, submandibular, cervical, and supraclavicular adenopathy. They may be prominent in the presence or malignancy or infection. Most of the upper eyelids and lateral lower eyelids drain to the preauricular lymph nodes, while the medial upper and lower eyelids drain to the submandibular lymph nodes. It has been shown, however, that most eyelid tumors will drain into the preauricular region (TAO) Cranial nerves V and VII should be tested carefully to assess for involvement and possible perineural spread of an eyelid malignancy.

1.3.3 Eye Examination

The ocular examination should focus on detecting findings caused by, or associated with, the eyelid lesion. Slit lamp biomicroscopy may reveal signs of mechanical or exposure keratoconjunctivitis, or it may reveal signs of conjunctival spread of sebaceous cell carcinoma or cutaneous malignancy. During the evaluation of a pigmented eyelid lesion, the sclera and episclera should be observed for pigmentary changes as well. Direct intraocular extension of eyelid tumors is extremely rare, but fundoscopy may reveal signs of ocular or orbital involvement (choroidal folds, venous congestion) in suspected cases.

1.4 Diagnostic Evaluation

1.4.1 Ancillary Laboratory and Imaging Studies

History and physical examination of a suspected eyelid tumor occasionally dictates ancillary testing. In cases of suspected eyelid granulomas, inflammatory labs may be indicated such as antinuclear cytoplasmic antibodies (p-ANCA/c-ANCA), and angiotensin converting enzyme (ACE) to rule out more specific causes of inflammation. If the examination reveals associated orbital or lacrimal outflow signs, computed tomography (CT) or magnetic resonance imaging (MRI) may help to determine the extent of the lesion. Schirmer testing could be considered to document underlying dry eye disease. Lacrimal probing and irrigation should be performed for peri-punctal lesions, for lesions in proximity to the nasolacrimal drainage system, and for patients with preexisting epiphora. Photodocumenation of the lesion and periorbita should also be performed, especially prior to biopsy. Marking the lesion and taking a photograph is helpful in localization if further procedures or monitoring are needed.

1.4.2 Dermatoscopy

Dermatoscopy is an in vivo noninvasive technique that may improve the clinical accuracy in diagnosing melanoma and other pigmented skin lesions [3]. Optical coherence tomography (OCT) may represent a new and promising technique for noninvasive investigation of skin tumors [4, 5]. This modality may not only distinguish tumor tissue from normal tissue, but may also visualize the epidermis, the dermoepidermal junction, and the dermis, as well as hair follicles, blood vessels, and sweat glands [6]. Although noninvasive techniques may improve diagnostic accuracy, the clinical diagnosis of eyelid tumors remains imperfect, and biopsy still represents the gold standard.

1.4.3 Biopsy

Based on clinical examination, the clinician is accurate in diagnoses in a high percent of patients anywhere from 83.7% to 96.9% [7, 8]. When the lesion is clinically misdiagnosed it is often thought the lesion is benign but in fact histologically malignant. Malignant lesions can be clinically misdiagnosed as benign, especially when they are small and have nondescript surface features, thereby emphasizing the need for a confirmatory histology via incisional or excisional biopsy [7, 8].

The goal of biopsy is to determine the pathologic nature of the lesion, while minimizing adverse functional and cosmetic consequences. Tumor location and the presumptive clinical diagnosis largely dictate the approach and technique. Shave biopsy or excisional biopsy can be performed of lesions to determine pathology.

Biopsy-proven epidermal malignancies require margin-controlled excision and repair, with either frozen section control of Moh's micrographic surgery. Melanoma, sebaceous cell carcinoma, and Merkel cell carcinoma require excision with wide margins. Some tumors, such as capillary hemangioma, may resolve spontaneously or require nonsurgical treatment (Chap. 10).

1.5 Treatment Planning

Information gathered from the history and eyelid examination determines the initial surgical plan for biopsy. This information also determines whether any special studies on the biopsy specimen are required. Any testing specific for the suspected diagnosis should be communicated to the pathologist in advance. For example, if sebaceous carcinoma is suspected, then the specimen usually is sent fresh for Oil Red O staining. However, the specimen can be evaluated with immunohistochemistry on paraffin section with adipophilin and androgen receptor depending on the pathologist's preference [9]. If suspicion for lymphoproliferative disease exists, a fresh specimen for immunohistochemistry and cytology may be indicated. Such foresight may avoid inconclusive biopsy results, the need for an additional tissue biopsy, and lost time. When sending fresh specimens and specimens where there is a suspicion of lymphoproliferative disease, the transportation of the specimen should always be accompanied by a conversation with the reading pathologist so that the specimens may be stored in the required manner and the appropriate tests carried out.

A detailed eyelid examination may also increase the efficiency of any anticipated surgery by determining the probable extent of tumor burden. For instance, if examination points to a larger, possibly infiltrating lesion rather than a smaller, localized process, the examination may dictate map biopsies to determine the extent of the lesion. Conversely, if examination shows a small, discreet lesion, then it may call for excisional biopsy to minimize the number of surgical interventions. Shave biopsy is also widely used and allows for examination of the tissue without significant disruption. The downside of shave biopsy is evaluation of the pathology at the depth of the lesion is sometimes inadequate. The examination results can direct the patient discussion to illuminate surgical risks and realities.

1.6 Conclusion

A systematic approach to the evaluation of suspected eyelid neoplasia allows the clinician to diagnose and treat these tumors efficiently and effectively. Current clinical diagnostic techniques remain inaccurate, and the threshold for biopsy should remain quite low. In the future, we hope less invasive diagnostic and therapeutic techniques will be available, as well as for improved preventive options and better early detection to limit the morbidity of these common tumors.

Box 1.1 Symptoms of Eyelid Neoplasia
Sensory: tenderness, itching, visual changes
Motor: ptosis, lagophthalmos
Structural: visible or palpable lesion, change in symmetry, ulceration, bleeding, lash loss
Functional: keratopathy, tearing
Secondary: pigmentation, lymphadenopathy

Box 1.2 Signs of Malignant Eyelid Tumor
Telangiectasia
Nodularity, pearly translucency
Ulceration, bleeding, crusting, margin notch
Misdirection of lashes or trichiasis
Loss of cilia
Effacement of meibomian gland orifice

References

1. Gandini S, Sera F, Cattaruzza MS, et al. Meta-analysis of risk factors for cutaneous melanoma: III. Family history, actinic damage and phenotypic factors. Eur J Cancer. 2005;41:2040–59.
2. Cook BE, Bartley GB. Epidemiologic characteristics and clinical course of patients with malignant eyelid tumors in an incidence cohort in Olmsted County, Minnesota. Ophthalmology. 1999;106:746–50.
3. Lallas A, Apalla Z, Chaidemenos G. New trends in dermatoscopy to minimize the risk of missing melanoma. J Skin Cancer. 2012;2012:820474. https://doi.org/10.1155/2012/820474. Epub 2012 Oct 8
4. Khandwala M, Penmetsa BR, Dey S, et al. Imaging of periocular basal cell carcinoma using en face optical coherence tomography: a pilot study. Br J Ophthalmol. 2010;94:1332–6.
5. Bergeron S, Arthurs B, Sanft D, Mastromonaco C, Burnier M. Optical coherence tomography of peri-ocular skin cancers: an optical biopsy. Ocul Oncol Pathol. 2021;7(2):149–58.
6. Gambichler T, Jaedicke V, Terras S. Optical coherence tomography in dermatology: technical and clinical aspects. Arch Dermatol Res. 2011;303:457–73.
7. Kersten RC, Ewing-Chow D, Kulwin DR, Gallon M. Accuracy of clinical diagnosis of cutaneous eyelid lesions. Ophthalmology. 1997;104:479–84.
8. Margo CE. Eyelid tumors: accuracy of clinical diagnosis. Am J Ophthalmol. 1999;128:635–6.
9. Schmitz EJ, Herwig-Carl MC, Holz RG, Loeffler KU. Sebaceous gland carcinoma of the ocular adnex—variability in clinical and histological appearance with analysis of immunohistochemical staining patterns. Graefes Arch Clin Exp Ophthalmol. 2017;255(11):2277–85.

2 Eyelid Tumors: Classification and Differential Diagnosis

Jacob Pe'er and Shahar Frenkel

2.1 Introduction

In spite of being a small organ, the eyelids contain numerous histological elements that can be the origin of several types of benign or malignant tumors. In this chapter, we review the basic anatomy of the eyelid, outline a clinically relevant classification of eyelid tumors, and briefly discuss their differential diagnosis.

2.2 Anatomical Features

The eyelids are composed of four layers: skin and subcutaneous tissue, striated muscle (orbicularis oculi), tarsus, and conjunctiva [1]. The rest of the orbital entrance, which clinically may be considered part of the eyelids, is covered behind the skin and the orbicularis muscle by the orbital septum that holds back the orbital fat.

2.2.1 Eyelid Skin

The eyelid skin, especially the lower eyelid, is among the most sunlight-exposed anatomical structures. The eye and the eyelids are one of the most observed parts of the face, and therefore, eyelid tumors are usually diagnosed at an early stage. The eyelid skin is the thinnest in the body and lacks subcutaneous fat but otherwise contains all other skin structures. Starting at the eyelid margin, the pretarsal part (10 mm in the superior eyelid and 4 mm in the inferior eyelid), the skin and orbicularis oculi muscle are normally firmly attached to the tarsal plate, whereas in the preseptal part they are more loosely attached. The skin epithelium is keratinized stratified squamous epithelium and is the origin of all types of benign and malignant epidermal tumors. Melanocytes are spread in the basal layer of the epithelium and may give rise to melanocytic cutaneous lesions. The dermis contains fibrous tissue, blood and lymphatic vessels, and nerves that can give rise to many types of fibrous tissue tumors, fibrohistiocytic tumors, vascular tumors, and neural tumors.

2.2.2 Adnexal Glands

The eyelids are rich in glandular tissue that may be the origin of various glandular tumors. Eccrine gland tumors may arise from the sweat glands of the eyelid skin as well as from the accessory lacrimal glands of Krause and Wolfring at the superior fornix and at the internal superior margin of the tarsus, respectively. The glands of Moll can give rise to apocrine tumors at the eyelid skin. The sebaceous glands of Zeiss along the hair follicle (eyelashes) and the meibomian gland are the origin of sebaceous gland tumors at the eyelid margin.

2.2.3 Orbicularis Oculi

The entire orbital entrance is covered by the orbicularis oculi—a striated muscle that is divided into pretarsal and preseptal zones, which are part of the eyelids and are involved in the eyelid movements, and the orbital zone that is located over the external orbital bones.

2.2.4 Tarsus

The tarsi are firm plates composed of dense connective tissue that serve as the skeleton of the eyelids. The upper tar-

J. Pe'er (✉)
Ocular Oncology Service, Division of Ophthalmology, Hadassah Medical Center, Jerusalem, Israel
e-mail: peer@hadassah.org.il

S. Frenkel
Faculty of Medicine, Hebrew University of Jerusalem, Jerusalem, Israel

B. C. K. Patel et al. (eds.), *Clinical Ophthalmic Oncology*, https://doi.org/10.1007/978-3-031-72328-5_2

sal plates are much larger than the lower ones (10 vs. 4 mm, respectively, along the vertical axis). The meibomian glands, large sebaceous glands, are embedded in the connective tissue of the tarsal plates. The superior tarsal muscle (Muller's muscle)—a smooth muscle, is attached to the upper margin of the tarsus. A parallel muscle does not exist in the inferior tarsus, but the aponeurosis of the inferior rectus muscle attaches to the inferior edge of the inferior tarsus. The upper and lower orbital septum, a thin sheet of fibrous tissue, arises from the periosteum in the orbital rim and fuses with the levator aponeurosis superiorly and the lower margin of the lower tarsus inferiorly. All these histological structures can give rise to rare fibrous, striated, and smooth muscular and glandular tumors. The orbital fat behind the septum and the fat under the orbital part of the orbicularis oculi can be the origin of rare lipomatous tumors.

2.2.5 Palpebral Conjunctiva

The posterior eyelid surface is lined by the conjunctiva—a translucent mucous membrane that is composed of epithelium and subepithelial stroma—the substantia propria. The anatomical and histological features of the conjunctiva and the possible tumors that can originate from this tissue are described elsewhere (Volume 4, Chap 2).

2.2.6 Eyelid Margin

The eyelid margin is a flat area on the edge of each eyelid. The anatomical structures that are seen in the margin from the skin backward are the eyelashes and their lash follicles, the gray line which consists of the tips of the pretarsal orbicularis muscle—the muscle of Riolan, the meibomian gland orifices, and the mucocutaneous junction just posterior to them.

2.2.7 Vascular System

The eyelid has extensive arterial vascularity that comes from two main sources—the internal carotid and external carotid arteries with anastomoses between these two systems. The venous and lymphatic drainage is important in understanding the routes of possible eyelid tumor metastases: The venous drainage is into the angular vein medially, the superficial temporal vein laterally, and the orbital veins, anterior facial vein, and the pterygoid plexus posteriorly. The lymphatic drainage of the medial portions of the eyelids is into the submandibular lymph nodes and of the lateral portions into the superficial pre-auricular (parotid) nodes and then into the deeper cervical nodes.

2.2.8 Nerve Supply

The sensory nerve supply to the eyelids is from the fifth cranial nerve, and the motor nerve supply to the striated muscles is from the third and seventh cranial nerves, and to the smooth muscles from sympathetic nerves.

2.3 Classification of Eyelid Tumors

Tumors of the eyelid may be classified, like tumors in other organs, according to their tissue or cell of origin and as benign or malignant. In most groups of tumors, unique histological subtypes behave differently in spite of being of the same cell of origin.

The classification of eyelid tumors that appears in this section is based primarily on the second and fifth editions of the World Health Organization (WHO) International Histological Classification of Tumors (Table 2.1) [2, 3]. The epithelial tumor classification has been modified and divided into groups according to the tumor cell of origin. Some tumors that are missing from the WHO list have been added from other sources [4–6].

Table 2.1 Major types of eyelid tumors

Category	Subtypes
Epidermal tumors	Non-melanocytic tumors
	Melanocytic tumors
Adnexal tumors	Sebaceous gland tumors
	Sweat gland tumors
	Lacrimal gland tumors
	Hair follicle tumors
	Cystic lesions
Stromal tumors	Fibrous tissue tumors
	Fibrohistiocytic tumors
	Lipomatous tumors
	Smooth muscle tumors
	Skeletal muscle tumors
	Vascular tumors
	Perivascular tumors
	Neural tumors
	Lymphoid, plasmacytic, and leukemic tumors
	Cartilage and bone tumors
	Hamartoma and choristoma
	Palpebral conjunctival tumors
Secondary tumors	
Metastatic tumors	
Inflammatory and infectious lesions that simulate neoplasms	

Table 2.2 Classification of epidermal tumors of the eyelid

Category	Subtypes	
Non-melanocytic	Benign	Squamous cell papilloma
		Seborrheic keratosis
		Inverted follicular keratosis
		Reactive hyperplasia (pseudoepitheliomatous hyperplasia)
	Premalignant	Actinic (solar) keratosis
		Intraepithelial neoplasia
		Sebaceous nevus (of Jadassohn)
		Xeroderma pigmentosum
		Keratoacanthoma
	Malignant	Basal cell carcinoma
		Squamous cell carcinoma
		Mucoepidermoid carcinoma
Melanocytic	Epithelial pigmentation	Ephelis or freckles
		Lentigo simplex
		Solar lentigo
	Benign	Junctional nevus
		Intradermal nevus
		Compound nevus
		Spitz nevus
		Balloon cell nevus
		Blue nevus
		Cellular blue nevus
		Oculodermal nevus of Ota
	Premalignant	Congenital dysplastic nevus
		Lentigo maligna (melanotic freckle of Hutchinson)
	Malignant	Melanoma arising from nevi
		Melanoma arising in lentigo maligna
		Melanoma arising de novo

Table 2.3 Classification of adnexal and cystic tumors of the eyelid

Category	Subtypes	
Sebaceous gland tumors	Benign	Sebaceous gland hyperplasia
		Sebaceous gland adenoma
	Malignant	Sebaceous gland carcinoma
Sweat gland and lacrimal gland tumors	Benign	Syringoma
		Papillary syringadenoma
		Eccrine spiradenoma
		Eccrine acrospiroma
		Pleomorphic adenoma (benign mixed tumor)
		Eccrine cylindroma
		Apocrine adenoma
		Other benign tumors
	Malignant	Sweat gland (eccrine) adenocarcinoma
		Mucinous sweat gland adenocarcinoma
		Apocrine gland adenocarcinoma
		Adenoid cystic carcinoma
		Microcystic adnexal carcinoma
		Porocarcinoma
Hair follicle tumors	Benign	Trichoepithelioma
		Trichofolliculoma/trichoadenoma
		Trichilemmoma
		Pilomatrixoma (calcifying epithelioma of Malherbe)
	Malignant	Carcinoma of hair follicles
Other cystic lesions	Benign	Epidermal inclusion cyst
		Sebaceous cyst
		Retention cyst
		Eccrine hidrocystoma
		Apocrine hidrocystoma
		Trichilemmal cyst
		Other benign cystic lesion

The vast majority of the eyelid tumors, benign and malignant, are of cutaneous origin, mostly epidermal. These tumors are divided into non-melanocytic and melanocytic tumors (Table 2.2). Benign epithelial proliferations, basal cell carcinoma, cystic structures, and melanocytic nevi represent about 85% of all eyelid tumors [7–9]. The squamous cell carcinoma and the melanoma are relatively rare [8]. Tumors arising from adnexal structures (Table 2.3), fibrous tissue, fibrohistiocytic and muscular tumors (Table 2.4), and other stromal tumors (Tables 2.5 and 2.6) are less frequent. Lymphoid tumors, hamartomas and choristomas, and inflammatory and infectious lesions that simulate neoplasms are listed in Table 2.7.

Table 2.4 Classification of fibrous, fibroushistiocytic, and muscular tumors of the eyelid

Origin	Type	Tumor
Fibrous	Benign	Fibroma
		Keloid
		Nodular fasciitis
		Proliferative fasciitis
		Fibromatosis
	Malignant	Fibrosarcoma
		Congenital fibrosarcoma
Fibrous histiocytic	Benign	Xanthelasma
		Xanthoma
		Dermatofibroma
		Xanthogranuloma
		Fibrous histiocytoma
		Juvenile xanthogranuloma
		Necrotic xanthogranuloma
		Reticulohistiocytoma
	Intermediate	Atypical fibroxanthoma
		Dermatofibrosarcoma protuberans
		Angiomatoid fibrous histiocytoma
	Malignant	Malignant fibrous histiocytoma
		Malignant giant cell fibrous histiocytoma
		Malignant fibroxanthoma
Smooth muscle	Benign	Leiomyoma
		Angiomyoma
	Malignant	Leiomyosarcoma
Skeletal muscle	Benign	Rhabdomyoma
	Malignant	Rhabdomyosarcoma

Table 2.5 Classification of vascular and perivascular tumors of the eyelid

Category	Subtypes	
Vascular	Benign	Nevus flammeus (port wine stain)
		Papillary endothelial hyperplasia
		Capillary hemangioma
		Cavernous hemangioma
		Venous hemangioma
		Epithelioid hemangioma (angiolymphoid hyperplasia)
		Arteriovenous malformation
		Lymphangioma
	Malignant	Angiosarcoma
		Lymphangiosarcoma
		Kaposi's sarcoma
Perivascular	Benign	Hemangiopericytoma
		Glomus tumor
	Malignant	Malignant hemangiopericytoma
		Malignant glomus tumor

Table 2.6 Classification of neural, lipomatous, cartilage, and bone tumors of the eyelid

Category		Subtypes
Neural	Benign	Traumatic neuroma
		Neurofibroma
		Plexiform neurofibroma
		Schwannoma (neurilemoma)
		Others, e.g., neuroglial choristoma
	Malignant	Malignant peripheral nerve sheath tumor
		Merkel cell tumor
Lipomatous	Benign	Lipoma
		Others, e.g., hibernoma
	Malignant	Liposarcoma
Cartilage and bone	Benign	Chondroma
		Osteoma
	Malignant	Chondrosarcoma
		Mesenchymal chondrosarcoma
		Osteosarcoma

Table 2.7 Classification of lymphoid tumors, hamartomas, choristomas, and inflammatory and infectious lesions that simulate neoplasms

Category	Subtypes
Lymphoid	Benign lymphoid hyperplasia
	Lymphoma
	Plasmacytoma
	Leukemic infiltration
Hamartomas and choristomas	Dermoid cyst
	Phakomatous choristoma
	Ectopic lacrimal gland
Inflammatory and infectious lesions	Chalazion
	Pyogenic granuloma
	Verruca vulgaris
	Molluscum contagiosum
	Others
Others	e.g., myxoma

2.4 Differential Diagnosis

Various characteristics of the tumor and the patient's general health are important in making the correct diagnosis. The important features that should be noted in examining the eyelid tumor are the following: the tumor location—upper or lower eyelid, inner or outer canthus; is it on the eyelid margin; the eyelid layer involved—skin, subcutaneous tissue or palpebral conjunctiva; is the tumor solid or cystic; tumor size; the color of the lesion—pigmented or non-pigmented; skin color—red, pink, yellow, white, or blue; the tumor consistency—hard, soft, or rubbery; its surface—smooth, irregular, papillary, ulcerated, umbilicated, cratered, or keratinized; its shape—flat or raised, pedunculated, papillary; is the tumor thin or thick; is the tumor solitary or are there several or multiple tumors; is there loss of eyelashes (madarosis); the patient's race, age, and gender; is the tumor movable with the skin or is it fixed to the subcutaneous layers; the existence of systemic diseases such as genetic diseases (e.g., neurofibromatosis) or systemic malignancies; and the existence of diseases or malignancies in the surrounding structures—the eyeball, conjunctiva, orbit, lacrimal drainage system, and neighboring skin.

Certain features of the tumor are suggestive of malignancy [5]. Development of a new lesion or changes in size, shape, color, or surface appearance of an existing lesion is suspicious for malignant conversion. Poorly defined borders, palpable induration beyond visible boundaries, loss of fine cutaneous rhytides, hypervascularity, ulceration and destruction of the normal eyelid architecture are all worrisome. Lesions that are not freely mobile due to invasion of underlying structures and those associated with regional lymphadenopathy, hypersthesia, paresthesia, or pain, indicating lymphatic or perineural spread are also suspicious for malignancy. Lesions associated with chronic inflammation that respond partially or temporarily to topical corticosteroids or antibiotics also may harbor malignancies. However, one should keep in mind that on the one hand malignant tumors can appear without any worrisome signs, while totally benign tumors can express some of the above-mentioned features.

2.4.1 Epidermal Non-melanocytic Tumors

The most common benign epithelial tumor is the squamous papilloma that is often sessile or pedunculated with papillary shape and keratinized surface (Table 2.2). Squamous papillomata may be multiple. Other epithelial tumors may look similar to squamous papilloma, including the premalignant actinic keratosis that may be multiple, or small squamous cell carcinoma. Basal cell carcinoma comprises over 90% of all malignant eyelid tumors [7]. Its common location is the lower eyelid and medial canthus; it is usually firm and often has an ulcerated center. Other ulcerated eyelid tumors, such as keratoacanthoma or the more rare papillary syringadenoma, should be differentiated from BCC. Features of keratoacanthoma, such as rapid growth and possible spontaneous regression, can help in its diagnosis. Staging of carcinomas of the eyelid skin and adnexa can be found in the AJCC Cancer Staging Manual [10].

2.4.2 Epidermal Melanocytic Tumors

The most common pigmented eyelid lesions are the nevi, which are usually flat or mildly elevated and can appear anywhere in the eyelid in any size, and when appearing on the eyelid margin can be sessile (Table 2.2). Congenital nevi usually appear at birth and acquired nevi between the ages of 5 and 20 years. Nevi should be differentiated on the one hand from flat epithelial pigmentation such as ephelides (freckles) and, on the other hand, from the flat premalignant lentigo maligna or from malignant melanoma that is relatively rare in the eyelids.

2.4.3 Adnexal and Cystic Tumors

The eyelid adnexa include many different glands that are the origin of various benign and malignant tumors (Table 2.3). These include cystic lesions such as eccrine and apocrine hidrocystoma that are totally benign and may be transparent, or have a distinct color like the blue apocrine hidrocystoma, which gains its color from the deapth of its location and the Tyndall effect. On the other hand, there are very malignant solid sebaceous gland carcinomas that may resemble chalazion, but unlike chalazion cause loss of eyelashes.

2.4.4 Stromal Tumors

The stromal eyelid tumors usually have a smooth surface, being under the skin (Tables 2.4, 2.5, and 2.6). The tumor elevation may have normal skin color, but many of the tumors will have a distinct color. Xanthomatous lesions are usually yellow. Most hemangiomas, diffuse or localized, are red. Subcutaneous varix is soft and blue, and Kaposi's sarcoma is blue or red. Merkel cell tumor is red or violaceous. An eyelid acute myeloblastic leukemic (AML) mass can have a green hue (chloroma or myeloid sarcoma). Eyelid lymphoma can be manifested as a smooth, firm subcutaneous nodule. Sometimes also subcutaneous tumors can be sessile or even ulcerated, so such phenomena, which are usually seen in epidermal tumors, should not exclude them.

2.4.5 Inflammatory and Infective Simulating Conditions

In the differential diagnosis of eyelid tumors, we should include lesions that simulate tumors (Table 2.7). The most common simulating lesions are inflammatory lesions such as chalazion or pyogenic granuloma (a misnomer for granulation tissue) or infectious viral lesions such as molluscum contagiosum or verruca vulgaris that is clinically and histologically similar to squamous papilloma. Many dermatological diseases such as amyloidosis and malakoplakia or connective tissue disease and systemic metabolic diseases such as hemachromatosis may, sometimes, simulate eyelid tumors and should be differentiated from them.

References

1. Bedrossian EH. Embryology and anatomy of the eyelid. In: Tasman W, Jaeger EA, editors. Duane's foundation of clinical ophthalmology, ocular anatomy, embryology and teratology, vol. 1. Philadelphia: Lippincott Williams & Wilkins; 2004. p. 1–24. Chapter 5.
2. Campbell RJ, Sobin LH. Tumours of the eyelid. In: Histological typing of tumours of the eye and its adnexa, World Health Organization international histological classification of tumors. 2nd ed. Berlin: Springer; 1998. p. 3–9.
3. Milman T, Grossniklaus HE, Goldman-Levy G, et al. The 5th edition of the World Health Organization classification of tumours of the eye and orbit. Ocul Oncol Pathol. 2023:1–25. On-line

4. Shields JA, Shields CL. Atlas of eyelid and conjunctival tumors. Philadelphia: Lippincott Williams & Wilkins; 1999. p. 3–189.
5. Hassan AS, Nelson CC. Benign eyelid tumors and skin diseases. Int Ophthalmol Clin. 2002;42:135–49.
6. Soparkar CN, Patrinely JR. Eyelid cancers. Curr Opin Ophthalmol. 1998;9:49–53.
7. Kersten RC, Ewing-Chow D, Kulwin DR, Gallon M. Accuracy of clinical diagnosis of cutaneous eyelid lesions. Ophthalmology. 1997;104:479–84.
8. Cook BE, Bartley GB. Epidemiologic characteristics and clinical course of patients with malignant eyelid tumors in an incidence cohort in Olmsted County, Minnesota. Ophthalmology. 1999;106:746–50.
9. Wang L, Shan Y, Dai X, et al. Clinicopathological analysis of 5146 eyelid tumours and tumour-like lesions in an eye center in South China, 2000-2018: a retrospective cohort study. BMJ Open. 2021;11:e041854.
10. Esmaeli B, Dutton JJ, Graue GF, et al. Eyelid carcinoma. In: Amin MB, et al., editors. AJCC cancer staging manual. 8th ed. Springer; 2017., ch.64. p. 779–85.

Eyelid Tumors: Benign Squamous Tumors

3

Gabrielle Yeaney and Arun D. Singh

3.1 Introduction

The eyelid consists of six layers with epidermis externally and palpebral conjunctiva internally. Between these two (from outer to inner) are dermis, loose subcutaneous layer, orbicularis muscle, and tarsal plate. The epithelium consists of squamous cells and melanocytes primarily with smaller numbers of Langerhans cells and Merkel cells. The presence of Langerhans cells is important to recognize, as they, like melanocytes, are positive for the immunohistochemical stain S100. Benign tumors of the eyelid include a variety of non-pigmented and pigmented epidermal tumors, which arise from squamous and melanocytic cells respectively, adnexal tumors (Chap. 9), stromal tumors (Chap. 10), and benign lymphoid proliferations. Important to note is that not all clinically pigmented lesions are melanocytic, since squamous cell proliferations can include scattered melanocytes or melanin pigment, thus giving a pigmented appearance to a lesion. The benign epidermal tumors of the eyelid are similar to those observed in the other sun-exposed areas of the skin, but they may also include conjunctival tumors as well. Some of these tumors represent manifestations of systemic disease (Chap. 15). A classification of the epidermal eyelid tumors is presented in Table 3.1. Only the descriptions of the most common and frequently observed benign tumors, along with their corresponding premalignant lesions and tumor-like nonneoplastic lesions are included in this chapter.

G. Yeaney (✉)
RT Department of Pathology and Laboratory Medicine, Diagnostics Institute, CC Lerner College of Medicine of CWRU, Cleveland Clinic, Cleveland, OH, USA
e-mail: yeaneyg@ccf.org

A. D. Singh
Cole Eye Institute, Cleveland Clinic, Cleveland, OH, USA
e-mail: Singha@ccf.org

Table 3.1 Classification of epidermal tumors of the eyelid, excluding melanocytic and adnexal tumors

Benign	Squamous cell papilloma
	Seborrheic keratosis
	Inverted follicular keratosis
	Molluscum contagiosum
	Verruca vulgaris
	Reactive hyperplasia (pseudoepitheliomatous hyperplasia)
Potentially premalignant	Actinic (solar) keratosis
	Intraepithelial neoplasia
	Sebaceous nevus (of Jadassohn)
Malignant	Basal cell carcinoma
	Squamous cell carcinoma

3.2 Squamous (Non-melanocytic) Tumors

3.2.1 Squamous Papilloma or Fibroepithelial Polyp

Squamous papilloma is the most common benign tumor typically occurring in middle-aged or older adults. There are several synonyms for squamous papilloma, including skin tag, acrochordon, and fibroepithelial polyp (FEP). The clinical appearance is that of a pedunculated or sessile nodular growth with a variably convoluted surface with or without hyperkeratosis. They are often multiple, present at the lid margin, and are skin-colored (Fig 3.1a) [1].

Microscopically FEP consists of benign normal or hyperplastic (acanthotic) squamous epithelium with variable hyperkeratosis or parakeratosis overlying loose or dense fibrovascular tissue, which creates the exophytic nodule (Fig. 3.1b). They sometimes have overlapping features with seborrheic keratosis. If symptomatic, shave biopsy/excision may be performed.

B. C. K. Patel et al. (eds.), *Clinical Ophthalmic Oncology*, https://doi.org/10.1007/978-3-031-72328-5_3

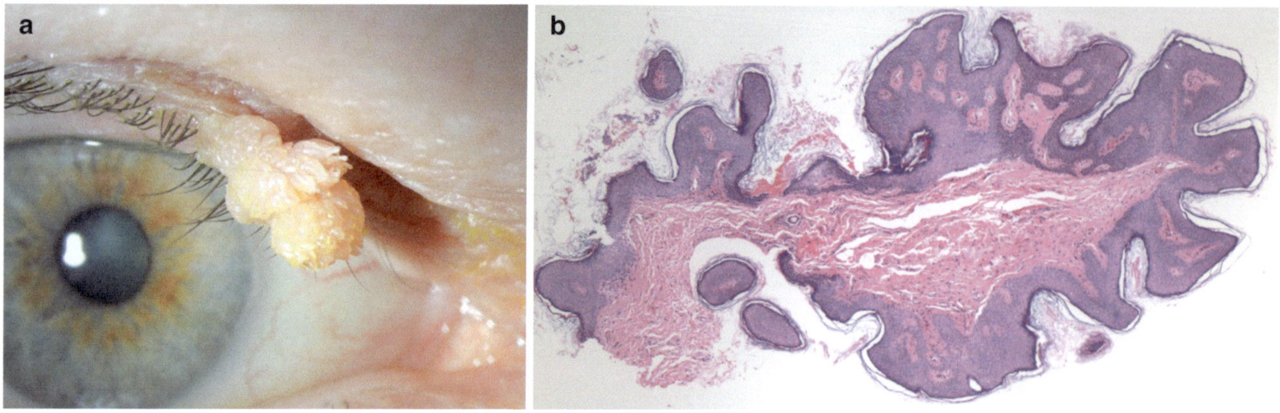

Fig. 3.1 Squamous papilloma. Clinical appearance (**a**). Polypoid lesion consisting of benign squamous epithelium with variable acanthosis and hyperkeratosis overlying a fibrovascular core (**b**. hematoxylin and eosin; magnification 40×)

3.2.2 Seborrheic Keratosis

Seborrheic keratoses (SKs) are commonly acquired skin lesions which can occur on the eyelid affecting middle-aged and elderly patients. The clinical appearance varies considerably in terms of size (few millimeters to several centimeters) and degree of pigmentation making it sometimes difficult to differentiate clinically from nevi, pigmented basal cell carcinomas, and melanoma [1]. They are sharply demarcated warty plaques or dome-shaped growths with a greasy and cerebriform surface, which may become friable with inflamed eczema-like features (Fig. 3.2a).

Seborrheic keratoses show a range of histological patterns according to the predominant histologic features: acanthotic (Fig. 3.2b), adenoid/reticulated (Fig. 3.2c), clonal, irritated, and pigmented. The most common type is the acanthotic, in which there is a proliferation of squamous basaloid cells protruding above the skin surface, which is punctuated by horn pseudocysts. Typically, the basal plane of the lesion is in alignment with the surrounding uninvolved squamous epithelium. Irritated SK shows chronic inflammation. Hyperpigmentation can occur, which is due to transfer of melanin to the keratinocytes. When a patient experiences a sudden appearance of a seborrheic keratosis or an increase in the number or size of these lesions, this may be associated with an internal malignancy, most commonly adenocarcinoma of the stomach, and is referred to as the Leser-Trelat sign [2, 3]. Even in lesions that are large, the growth pattern is superficial with growth predominantly above the epidermal surface. Therefore, deep excision is unnecessary, and these lesions are often removed by shave biopsy.

3.2.3 Inverted Follicular Keratosis

Inverted follicular keratosis is a somewhat controversial entity, as many consider it to be a variant of seborrheic keratosis. It is commonly seen on the face, particularly the cheeks, upper lip, and less often, eyelid [4–7]. It usually occurs in older men. Usually, a solitary lesion of recent onset (less than 3 months), it may be nodular, papillomatous, or cystic in appearance. Inverted follicular keratosis may recur following incomplete excision, and thus be clinically mistaken for squamous cell carcinoma [7].

Histopathologically, there are whorls of squamous epithelium, so called squamous eddies, hyperkeratosis, parakeratosis, acantholysis, generally little if any melanin pigment, and dermal chronic inflammation. There may be mitotic activity (Fig. 3.3) [6, 7]. Rarely recurs after excision, and re-excision is curative.

3.2.4 Molluscum Contagiosum

Molluscum contagiosum is a nonneoplastic skin infection caused by a virus from the poxvirus group. This entity occurs frequently in children but may also occur in adults anywhere on the body except the palms and soles. It appears as papules that are white or flesh colored measuring 2–5 mm, often with a central dimple or plug containing cheesy or waxy material (Fig. 3.4).

Molluscum contagiosum is characterized by downward growth of hyperplastic epidermis, sometimes forming multiple lobules. The keratinocytes contain large eosinophilic intracytoplasmic inclusion bodies (“molluscum bodies”),

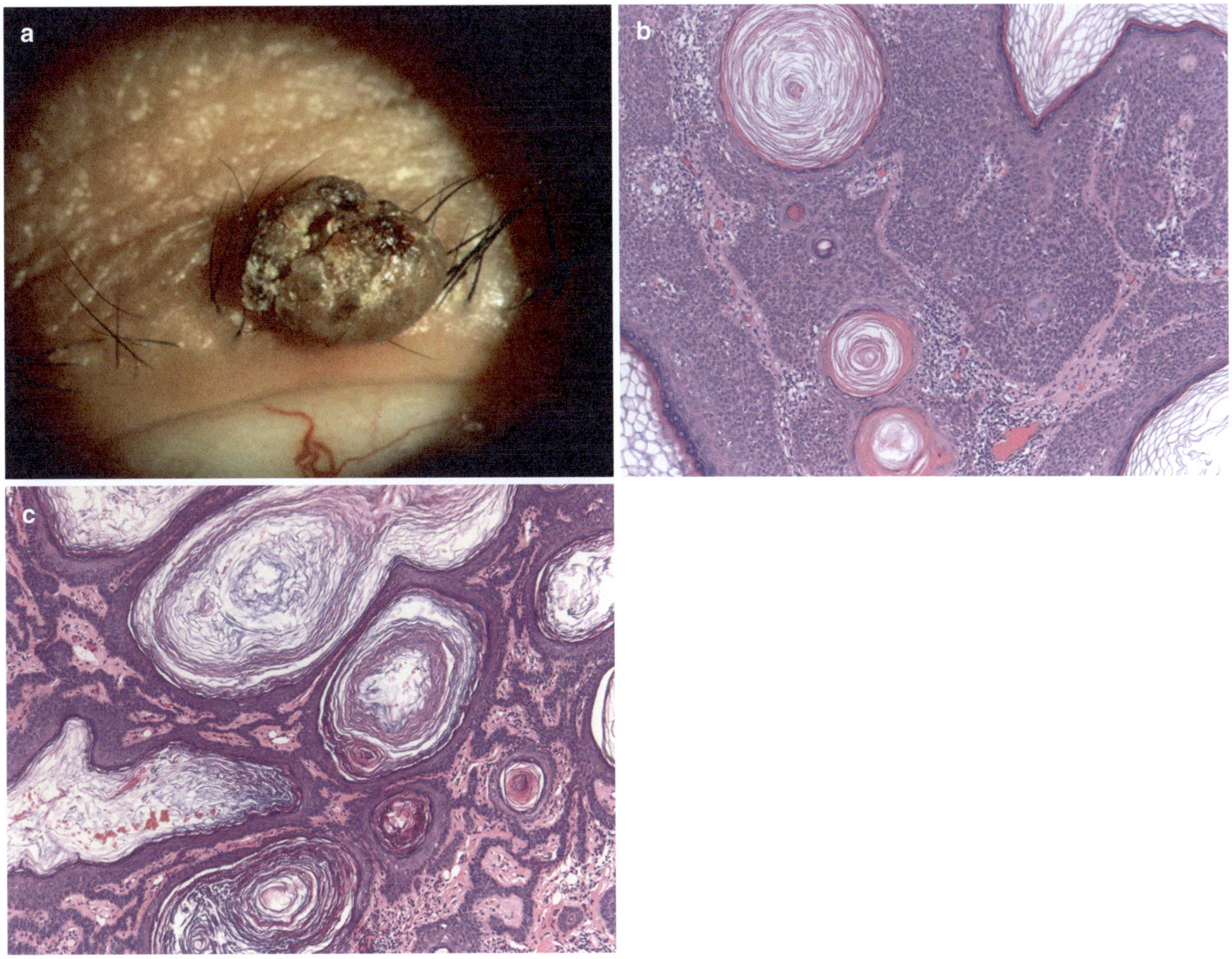

Fig. 3.2 Seborrheic keratosis. Upper eyelid involvement in a 75-year-old man (**a**). Acanthotic SK with proliferation of squamous basaloid cells (**b**); Retiform (network-like) pattern of squamous epithelium surrounding islands of connective tissue with keratin-filled horn pseudocysts (**c**; hematoxylin and eosin; both at magnification 100×)

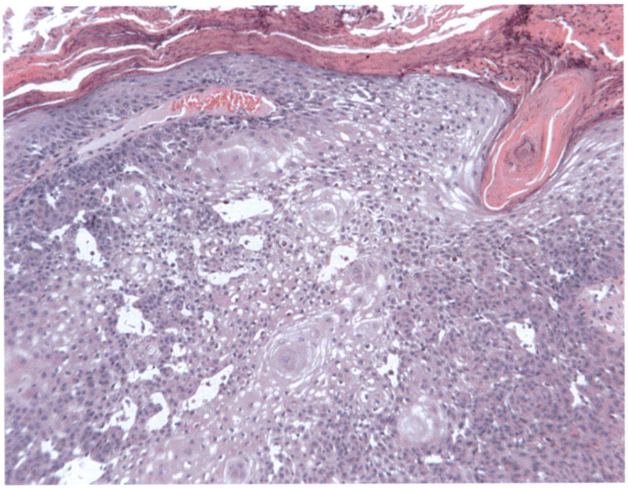

Fig. 3.3 Inverted follicular keratosis. Note endophytic growth pattern with overlying hyperkeratosis and parakeratosis. Flattened concentric epidermal cells within acanthotic areas are called squamous eddies (hematoxylin and eosin; magnification 100×)

which enlarge as they reach the surface and become more basophilic (Fig. 3.4). The central crater consists of disintegrating cells discharging the molluscum bodies and keratin [8]. These lesions usually resolve over months to years in patients with intact immune systems. However, removal of individual lesions can be done surgically or by scraping, decoring, freezing, or electrosurgery. Medications used for warts may also be used, and cantharidin ("beetle juice") is the most common solution used. Tretinoin cream is an alternative.

3.2.5 Verruca Vulgaris

Verruca vulgaris (VV), the common wart, is a hyperkeratotic papilloma caused by infection with human papilloma virus types 2 and 4. Common warts are most often seen on hands of children, but they may be located on any cutaneous surface [9]. On the face and eyelid, verruca may appear filiform

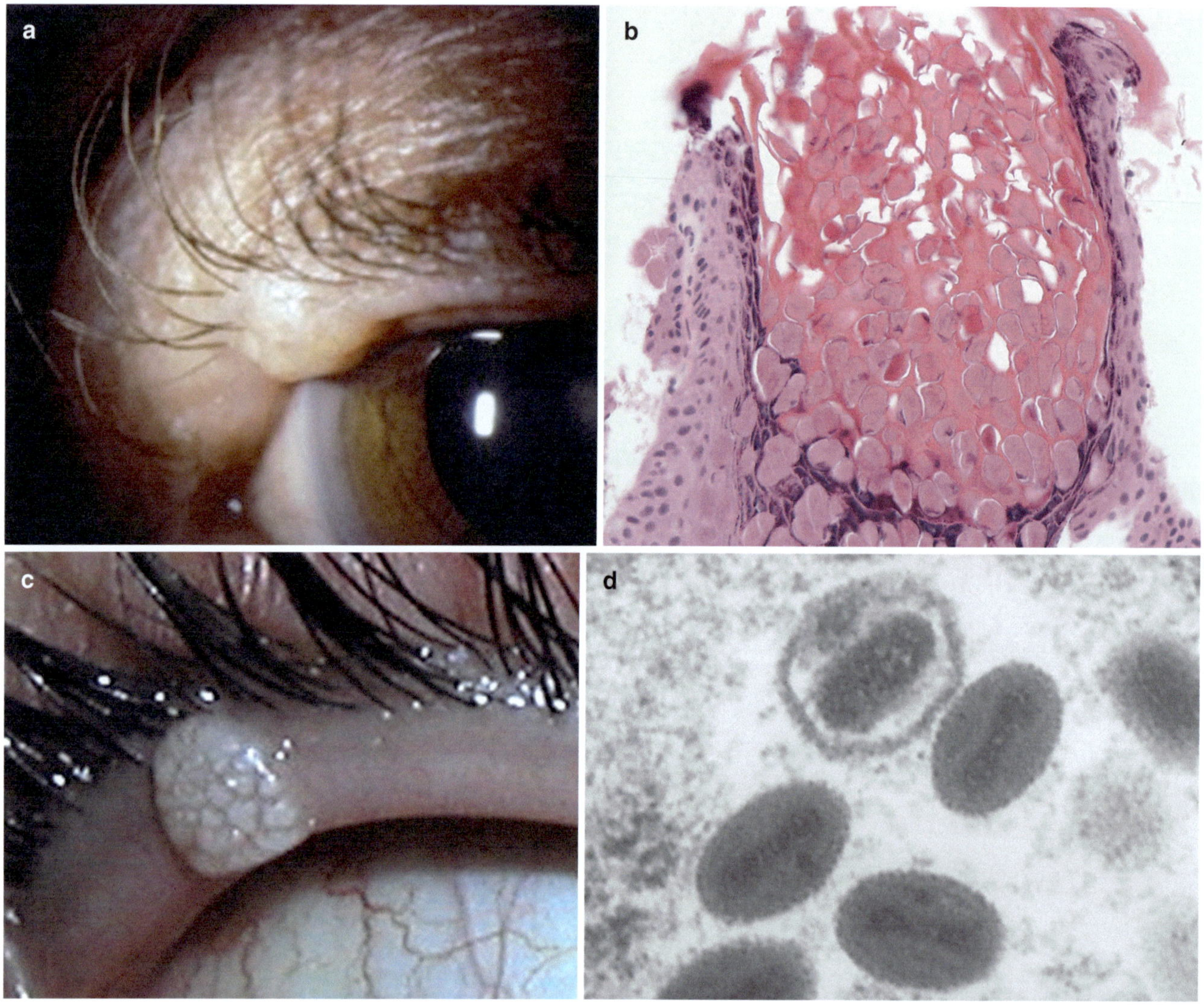

Fig. 3.4 Molluscum contagiosum. Clinical appearance (**a**). Epidermal crater filled with keratinocytes containing molluscum bodies (intracytoplasmic inclusions) (**b**. hematoxylin and eosin; 400× magnification). (**c**) The clinical presentation of a conglomerated lesion which is well-demarcated, white, sessile lesion located on the grey line. (**d**) A molluscum contagiosum virus under electron microscopy. (**c**, **d**) [Reprinted from Rosner M, Zloto O. Periocular molluscum contagiosum: six different clinical presentations. Acta Ophthalmol 2018;96(5):e600-e605. With permission from John Wiley & Sons]

and less firm than on the hands [10]. When present in adults, verruca vulgaris must be distinguished from squamous cell carcinoma. Histopathologically, VV shows hyperkeratosis with parakeratosis (Fig 3.5a) and papillomatosis with dilated capillaries (Fig 3.5b). The granular cell layer has enlarged clumps of basophilic keratohyalin and vacuolated cells (koilocytes; Fig 3.5c); however, these are not as prominent as in genital warts. Regression of VV may be spontaneous. Surgical excision may be performed, but recurrence (especially in immunocompromised patients) may be difficult to treat. In refractory cases, combined treatment with the CO2 laser and perilesionally injected interferon alfa-2b, and treatment with mitomycin C alone, have been successful [11].

3.2.6 Keratoacanthoma

Keratoacanthoma has a complicated history and has been classified as benign or malignant (self-healing squamous cell carcinoma or squamous cell carcinoma (keratoacanthoma-type) (Chap. 6). The latter is favored in many countries. However, in some literature, it has been noted to sometimes spontaneously regress and thus considered to be a benign lesion [12–15]. Typically a keratoacanthoma is a solitary, pink or flesh colored, dome shaped nodule with a central keratin crater, arising on sun-exposed skin of an elderly individual. There may be rapid growth to 1 or 2 cm over the course of 2–10 weeks. This is followed by a stationary period

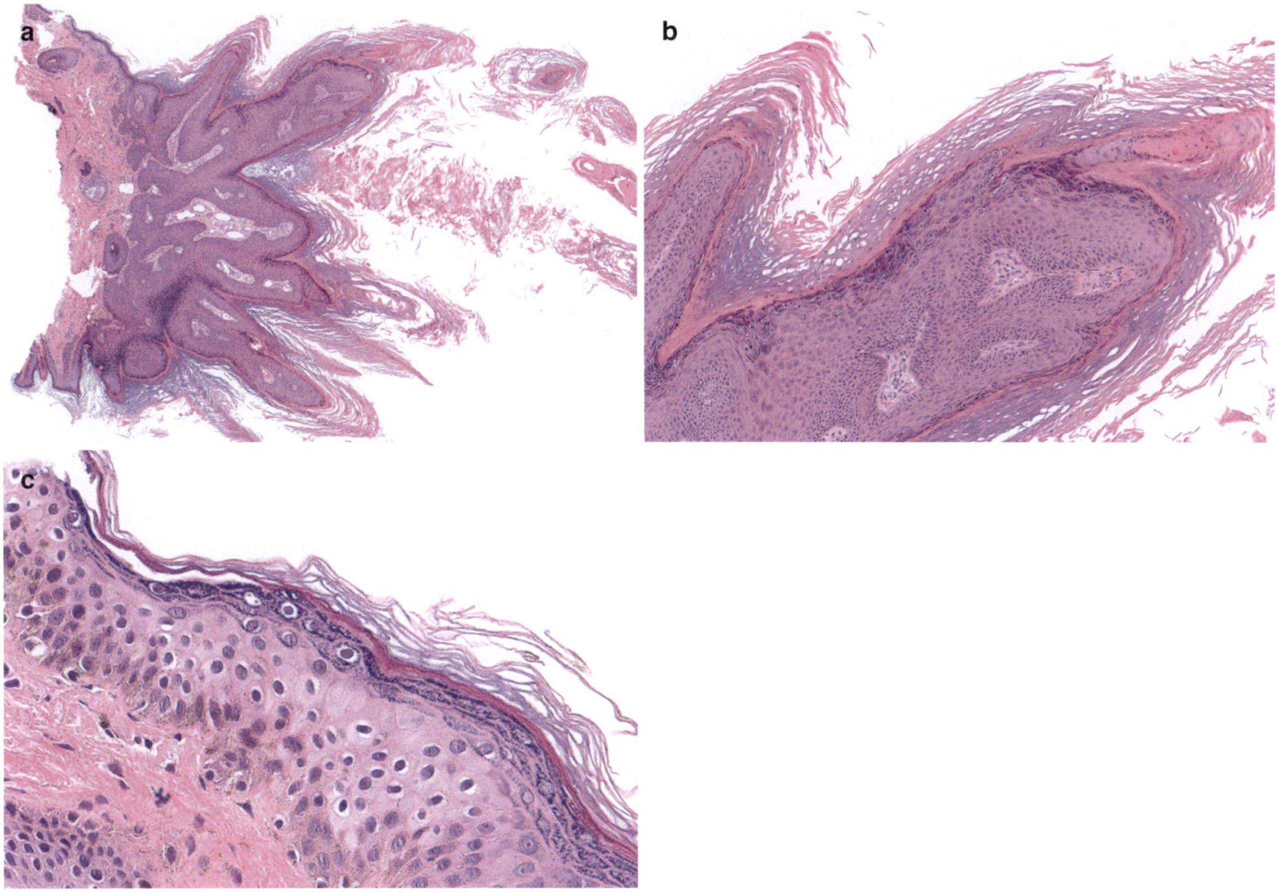

Fig. 3.5 Verruca vulgaris. Papillary lesion with hyperkeratosis, parakeratosis and dilated capillaries high in the epidermis (**a**, **b**; hematoxylin and eosin low power and high power respectively). The granular cell layer has enlarged clumps of basophilic keratohyalin and vacuolated koilocytes (**c**; hematoxylin and eosin magnification 400×)

of similar duration and then involution over the course of 8–50 weeks or more.

The histologic features needed for a confident diagnosis require assessment of the entire lesion, so as not to miss an infiltrating squamous cell carcinoma at the base. The tumor is cup or crater-shaped and consists of centrally proliferating well differentiated squamous cells with strongly eosinophilic cytoplasm that enlarge in the center of the tumor nests. Often there is a central keratin plug, and there may be neutrophilic abscesses in the epithelium. At the periphery, the epithelium forms symmetrical "lips" or "buttresses" which overhang the crater. The underlying dermis is usually inflamed but without desmoplasia unless the lesion is involuting. Deeper sections are recommended in order to rule out the possibility of typical infiltrating squamous cell carcinoma, which may be focal in an otherwise classic picture of keratoacanthoma (thus the term "keratoacanthoma-like squamous cell carcinoma) [15]. Complete excision should be performed.

3.2.7 Reactive Hyperplasia (Pseudoepitheliomatous Hyperplasia)

Squamous epithelial hyperplasia occurs as a reaction to trauma, surgical wound, cryotherapy, burn, radiation, ulcers, or fungal infection [16]. It is not a tumor but rather a reactive process that may clinically be seen as a tumor.

Histopathology can be challenging as well. An elevated nodular or ulcerative lesion resembling basal or squamous cell carcinoma. There may be an ulcer.

There is squamous hyperplasia with elongated, irregular, and sometimes anastomosing rete pegs (rete ridges) which may resemble invasive tongues or nest of squamous carcinoma. Cellular nests may contain neutrophilic microabscesses, especially when associated with infection (Fig. 3.6) [17]. The epithelium shows normal maturation without true dysplasia; however, there may be cytologic atypia and even mitotic activity, further complicating the distinction from carcinoma. Complete excision is recommended when clinically suspicious.

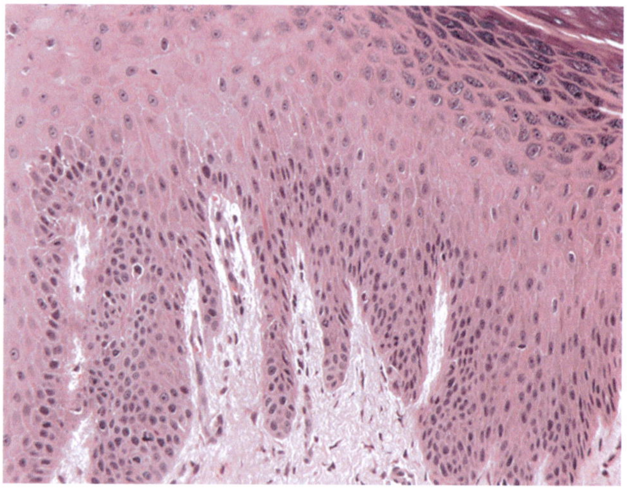

Fig. 3.6 Reactive hyperplasia (pseudoepitheliomatous hyperplasia). Epidermal (squamous) hyperplasia with elongated and sometimes anastomosing rete ridges, normal maturation of epithelium, and variable hyperkeratosis. Note the absence of atypia in this case (hematoxylin and eosin; magnification 200×)

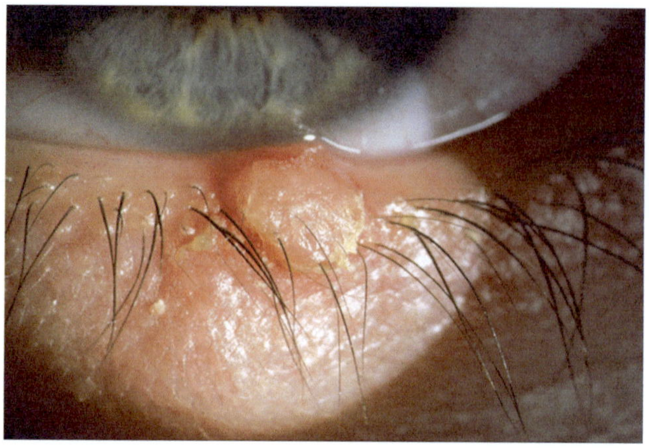

Fig. 3.7 Cutaneous horn is a clinically descriptive, nondiagnostic term for a nonspecific keratosis

3.2.8 Cutaneous Horn or Nonspecific Keratosis

These are nondiagnostic descriptive terms for any hyperkeratotic lesion (benign or malignant) and thus do not imply by themselves predilection for malignant behavior. A protruding keratotic lesion is the presentation (Fig. 3.7). This lesion is associated with a variety of benign or malignant lesions. In a study of 48 cases involving the eyelids, 77% were found to be benign on histopathology, 15% were premalignant, and 8% were malignant skin tumors. The most common associated lesions were seborrheic keratosis, actinic keratosis, basal cell carcinoma, and squamous cell carcinoma [18, 19].

There are no specific histopathologic features other than hyperkeratosis, with or without parakeratosis. The keratosis (or horn) by itself is not diagnostic, but rather the features of the squamous epithelium giving rise to the keratosis is the defining factor as to the biologic behavior of the lesion [18]. Treatment should be determined by the histopathology if possible. If the lesion is clinically suspicious for malignancy, excision is recommended.

3.2.9 Sebaceous Nevus (of Jadassohn)

Sebaceous nevus syndrome (of Jadassohn), an uncommon congenital lesion, is part of the epidermal nevus syndrome and characterized by cutaneous sebaceous nevi and extracutaneous manifestations. It is a benign hamartoma composed of large sebaceous glands, heterotopic apocrine glands, defective hair follicles, acanthosis, and papillomatosis. These lesions evolve with time. They are most commonly found on the head and neck region and appear as irregular linear lesions with alopecia (Fig. 3.8). In spite of their being benign, there is an increased risk in adulthood for the development of secondary benign (such as syringocystadenoma papilliferum) or malignant skin tumors (most commonly basal cell carcinoma) within the area of these nevi [20–22].

3.2.10 Actinic (Solar) Keratosis

Actinic or solar keratosis is most frequently a result of chronic and cumulative exposure of the epidermal cells of the skin to ultraviolet radiation (UV-B) in the form of sunlight, causing mutations to the p53 gene [23]. Fair-skinned older patients and those with a history of excessive sun exposure are typically affected. However there is also an increased incidence in renal transplant patients and thus immunosuppression is a risk factor [24]. There are a variety of clinical presentations, usually characterized by multiple, erythematous, scaly lesions with either discrete or diffuse borders [24]. They feel like sandpaper and may be plaque-like on palpation. Actinic keratosis has historically been considered a precursor to squamous cell carcinoma, and most now consider it to represent squamous cell carcinoma in situ or keratinocyte intraepithelial neoplasia. In a study wherein histopathologic evaluation of 165 cases of resected squamous cell carcinoma was undertaken, 82% of cases had concomitant actinic keratosis close to the carcinoma [25]. However, it is not clear what the rate of conversion of an actinic keratosis to squamous cell carcinoma is; and studies have given a wide range of estimates [26].

Histopathology generally shows hyperkeratosis and parakeratosis with varying degrees of squamous dysplasia, characterized by loss of epithelial cell polarity, cytologic atypia, and dysmaturation. The parakeratosis is usually focal and

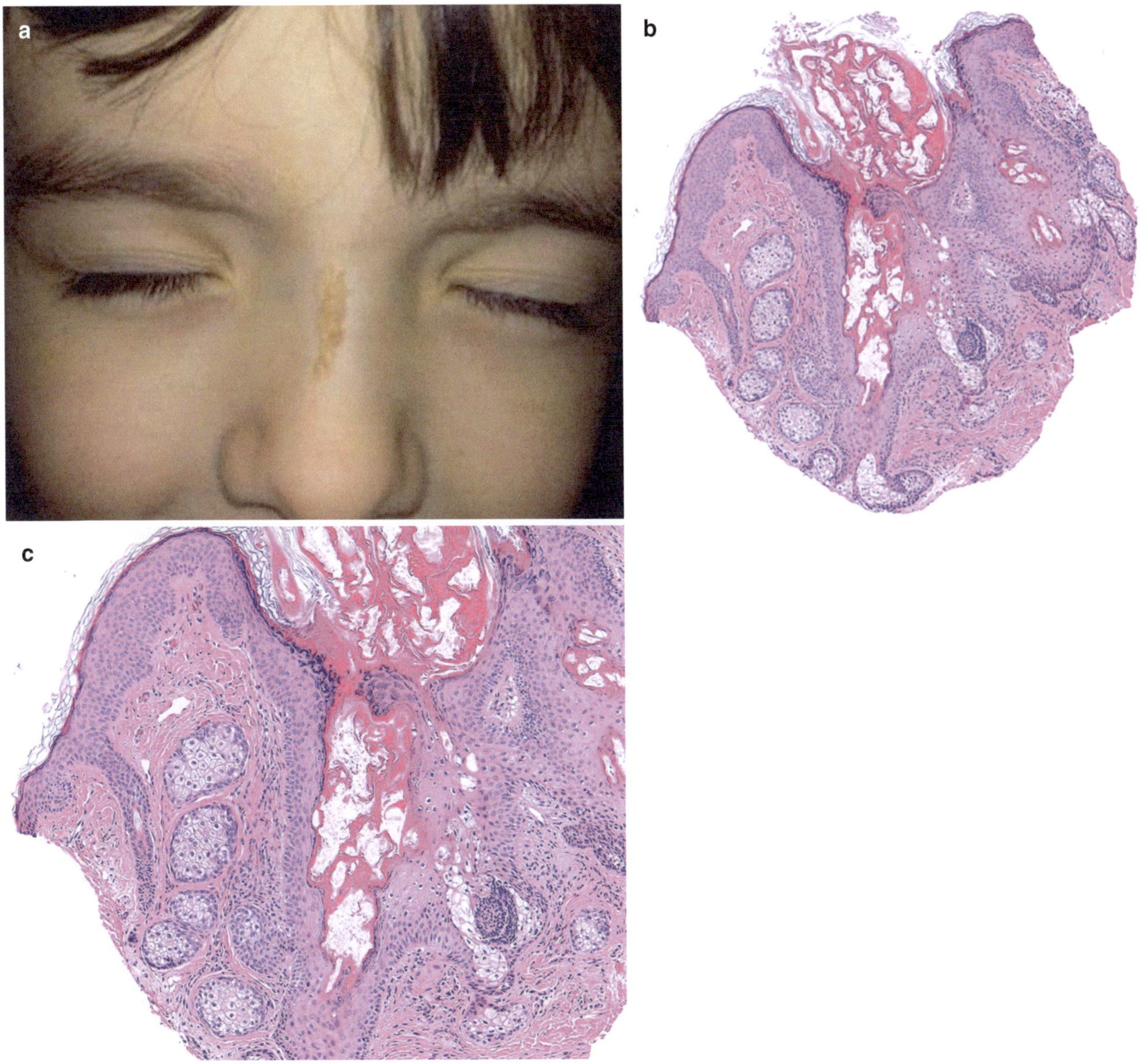

Fig. 3.8 Sebaceous nevus (of Jadassohn). External photo showing tan-colored linear nasal lesion (**a**); Low magnification (**b**, 40×) and higher magnification (**c**, 100×) histopathology of a benign epidermal lesion with presence of acanthosis and hyperkeratosis in association with enlarged gland lobules consistent with nevus sebaceous. [Reprinted from Echegaray JJ, Chen R, Bellerive C, Singh AD [21]. Linear nevus sebaceous syndrome presenting as circumscribed choroidal hemangioma. Ophthalmic Genet 2018;39(2):278–81. With permission from Taylor & Francis]

overlies areas of underlying loss of the granular layer of the epidermis. Solar elastosis of varying degrees is present in the dermis, along with a mild chronic inflammatory infiltrate (Fig. 3.9). Subtypes include hypertrophic (characterized by acanthotic epithelium with irregular psoriasiform hyperplasia), proliferative (characterized by finger-like projections into the dermis), atrophic (thin epithelium), acantholytic (characterized by prominent dyscohesion of the basal cells), and lichenoid (when there is a dense band-like mononuclear cell infiltrate in the upper dermis). The hyperkeratotic or parakeratotic crust may be so thickened as to form a keratotic horn. With severe full thickness dysplasia, the differential includes Bowen's disease (Fig. 3.10). Management is close observation and excision of more suspicious lesions. Multiple lesions can be treated with topical chemotherapeutic agents or cryotherapy. A meta-analysis of published studies indicates that 3% diclofenac in 2.5% hyaluronan gel is effective in treatment of actinic kertatosis [27]. Topical gel must not be applied to the eyelids as it is not approved for ophthalmic use [28].

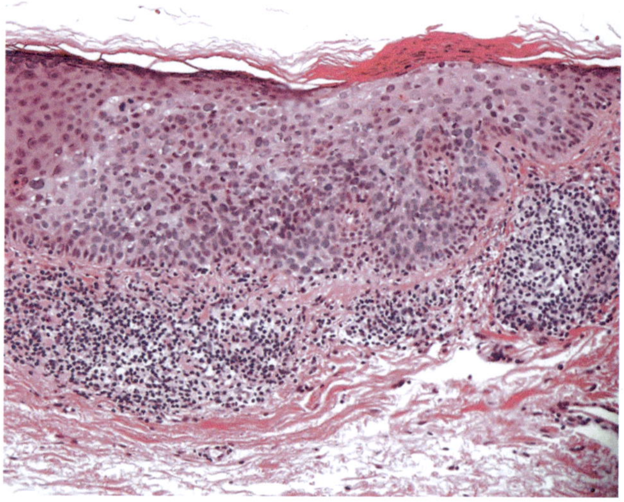

Fig. 3.9 Actinic (solar) keratosis. Note dysmaturation of the squamous epithelium, mitotic figures, loss of granular layer, and parakeratotic crust (hematoxylin and eosin; original magnification 20×)

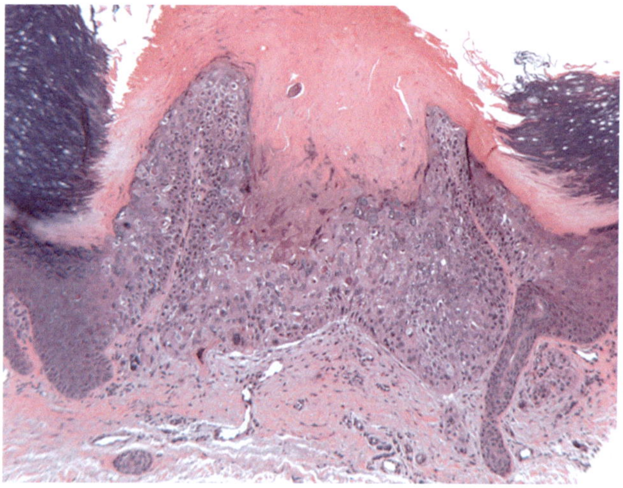

Fig. 3.10 Squamous intraepithelial neoplasia. Marked squamous dysplasia (Bowen's disease, also considered a type of squamous carcinoma in situ); also note suggestion of early or superficial invasion (hematoxylin and eosin; magnification 100×)

3.3 Summary

Benign epidermal tumors of the eyelid are similar to those observed in the other sun-exposed areas of the skin. Some benign eyelid lesions may represent manifestations of systemic disease. They may or may not be pigmented, and with histopathologic examination, they are classified as being melanocytic or non-melanocytic in origin. Once malignancy has been ruled out, they might still have features of a dysplastic or premalignant lesion, warranting closer follow-up or excision.

References

1. Font RL. Eyelids and lacrimal drainage system. In: Spencer WH, editor. Ophthalmic pathology an atlas and textbook, vol. v. 4th ed. Philadelphia: WB Saunders; 1996. p. 4.
2. Sardon C, Dempsey T. The Leser-Trelat sign. Cleve Clin J Med. 2017;84(12):918.
3. Kowalzick L, Truhm B, Eickenscheidt L. Sign and pseudo-sign of Leser-Trelat. J Drugs Dermatol. 2014;13(1):14.
4. Schweitzer JG, Yanoff M. Inverted follicular keratosis. A report of two recurrent cases. Ophthalmology. 1987;94(11):1465–8.
5. Scheie HG, Yanoff M, Sassani JW. Inverted follicular keratosis clinically mimicking malignant melanoma. Ann Ophthalmol. 1977;9(8):949–52.
6. Sim-Davis D, Marks R, Wilson-Jones E. The inverted follicular keratosis. A surprising variant of seborrheic wart. Acta Derm Venereol. 1976;56(5):337–44.
7. Boniuk M, Zimmerman LE. Eyelid tumors with reference to lesions confused with squamous cell carcinoma. II. Inverted follicular keratosis. Arch Ophthalmol. 1963;69:698–707.
8. Rosner M, Zloto O. Periocular molluscum contagiosum: six different clinical presentations. Acta Ophthalmol. 2018;96:e600.
9. Petersen CS, Nurnberg BM. Carbon dioxide laser vaporization combined with perilesionally injected interferon alfa-2b in the treatment of a hyperkeratotic verruca vulgaris on the upper eyelid. Arch Dermatol. 1994;130(11):1369–70.
10. Melton JL, Rasmussen JE. Clinical manifestations of human papillomavirus infection in nongenital sites. Dermatol Clin. 1991;9(2):219–33.
11. Ma'luf RN. Treatment of recurrent eyelid margin verruca vulgaris with mitomycin C. Ophthalmic Plast Reconstr Surg. 2010;26(3):214–5.
12. Grossniklaus HE, Wojno TH, Yanoff M, Font RL. Invasive keratoacanthoma of the eyelid and ocular adnexa. Ophthalmology. 1996;103(6):937–41.
13. Leibovitch I, Huilgol SC, James CL, et al. Periocular keratoacanthoma: can we always rely on the clinical diagnosis? Br J Ophthalmol. 2005;89(9):1201–4.
14. Donaldson MJ, Sullivan TJ, Whitehead KJ, Williamson RM. Periocular keratoacanthoma: clinical features, pathology, and management. Ophthalmology. 2003;110(7):1403–7.
15. Takai T. Advances in histopathological diagnosis of keratoacanthoma. J Dermatol. 2017;44(3):304–14.
16. Wingfield DL, Fraunfelder FT. Possible complications secondary to cryotherapy. Ophthalmic Surg. 1979;10(8):47–55.
17. Zayour M, Lazova R. Pseudoepitheliomatous hyperplasia: a review. Am J Dermatopathol. 2011;33(2):112–22. quiz 23-6
18. Pointdujour-Lim R, Marous MR, Satija CE, et al. Cutaneous horn of the eyelid in 13 cases. Ophthalmic Plast Reconstr Surg. 2017;33(4):233–6.
19. Mencia-Gutierrez E, Gutierrez-Diaz E, Redondo-Marcos I, et al. Cutaneous horns of the eyelid: a clinicopathological study of 48 cases. J Cutan Pathol. 2004;31(8):539–43.
20. Vujevich JJ, Mancini AJ. The epidermal nevus syndromes: multisystem disorders. J Am Acad Dermatol. 2004;50(6):957–61.
21. Echegaray JJ, Chen R, Bellerive C, Singh AD. Linear nevus sebaceous syndrome presenting as circumscribed choroidal hemangioma. Ophthalmic Genet. 2018;39(2):278–81.
22. Miller CJ, Ioffreda MD, Billingsley EM. Sebaceous carcinoma, basal cell carcinoma, trichoadenoma, trichoblastoma, and syringocystadenoma papilliferum arising within a nevus sebaceus. Dermatologic Surg. 2004;30(12 Pt 2):1546–9.
23. Fu W, Cockerell CJ. The actinic (solar) keratosis: a 21st-century perspective. Arch Dermatol. 2003;139(1):66–70.

24. Siegel JA, Korgavkar K, Weinstock MA. Current perspective on actinic keratosis: a review. Br J Dermatol. 2017;177(2):350–8.
25. Mittelbronn MA, Mullins DL, Ramos-Caro FA, Flowers FP. Frequency of pre-existing actinic keratosis in cutaneous squamous cell carcinoma. Int J Dermatol. 1998;37(9):677–81.
26. Werner RN, Sammain A, Erdmann R, et al. The natural history of actinic keratosis: a systematic review. Br J Dermatol. 2013;169(3):502–18.
27. Pirard D, Vereecken P, Melot C, Heenen M. Three percent diclofenac in 2.5% hyaluronan gel in the treatment of actinic keratoses: a meta-analysis of the recent studies. Arch Dermatol Res. 2005;297(5):185–9.
28. Werner RN, Stockfleth E, Connolly SM, et al. Evidence- and consensus-based (S3) guidelines for the treatment of actinic keratosis—International League of Dermatological Societies in cooperation with the European dermatology forum—short version. J Eur Acad Dermatol Venereol. 2015;29(11):2069–79.

Eyelid Tumors: Benign Melanocytic Tumors

4

Tatyana Millman and Arun D. Singh

4.1 Introduction

The eyelid consists of six layers with the epidermis externally and palpebral conjunctiva internally. Between these two (from outer to inner) are dermis, loose subcutaneous layer, orbicularis muscle, and tarsal plate. The epidermis consists of squamous cells and melanocytes primarily with smaller numbers of Langerhans cells and Merkel cells. The presence of Langerhans cells is important to recognize as they, like melanocytes, are positive for the immunohistochemical stain S100. Benign tumors of the eyelid include a variety of nonpigmented and pigmented epidermal tumors, which arise from squamous and melanocytic cells respectively, adnexal tumors (Chap. 9), stromal tumors, and benign lymphoid proliferations. Important to note is that not all clinically pigmented lesions are melanocytic, since squamous cell proliferations (Chap. 3) can include scattered melanocytes or melanin pigment, thus giving a pigmented appearance to a lesion. A classification of melanocytic eyelid tumors is presented in Table 4.1. Only the description of the most common and frequently observed benign melanocytic tumors, along with their corresponding premalignant lesions and tumor-like non-neoplastic lesions, is included in this chapter.

T. Millman (✉)
Ophthalmology and Pathology, Wills Eye Hospital and Jefferson University Hospital, Philadelphia, PA, USA

A. D. Singh
Cole Eye Institute, Cleveland Clinic, Cleveland, OH, USA
e-mail: Singha@ccf.org

Table 4.1 Classification of melanocytic tumors of the eyelid

Benign epithelial pigmentation or hypermelanosis	Ephelis or freckles
	Lentigo simplex
	Solar lentigo
Benign	Junctional nevus
	Intradermal nevus
	Compound nevus
	Spitz nevus
	Balloon cell nevus
	Blue nevus and cellular blue nevus
	Oculodermal nevus of Ota
Potentially premalignant	Congenital dysplastic nevus
	Lentigo maligna (melanotic freckle of Hutchinson)
Malignant	Melanoma arising from nevi
	Melanoma arising in lentigo maligna
	Melanoma arising de novo

4.2 Melanocytic Benign Epidermal Tumors

4.2.1 Freckles or Ephelides

Freckles are flat brown skin macules measuring 1–2 mm that appear in childhood. Freckles characteristically occur in fair-skinned individuals and darken with sunlight exposure and fade in winters in the absence of sunlight exposure. In contrast, solar lentigines do not fade with cessation of sunlight exposure [1]. The epidermal structure in not altered. There is increased melanin pigment in the basal layers without an increase in melanocytes. The delineation of the lesion with the surrounding skin is distinct.

4.2.2 Lentigo Simplex

The lesion of lentigo simplex is a flat, brown to black, sharply circumscribed macule measuring 1–2 mm in diameter.

B. C. K. Patel et al. (eds.), *Clinical Ophthalmic Oncology*, https://doi.org/10.1007/978-3-031-72328-5_4

Pigmentation is usually uniform. They are the precursors of junctional nevi and are clinically indistinguishable from them. Similar appearing multiple lesions of the perioral skin, buccal mucosa, and sometimes eyelid may be associated with the autosomal dominant Peutz-Jeghers syndrome of mucocutaneous pigmentation and intestinal polyposis (Chap 15), Carney syndrome, LEOPARD syndrome, and xeroderma pigmentosum [2].

Histology shows hyperpigmentation of the basal layer with increased number of melanocytes, often with regular elongation of the rete ridges. The papillary dermis may contain a lymphohistiocytic infiltrate and melanophages. If the melanocytic hyperplasia evolves to form early junctional nests (with or without an intradermal component), the lesion is referred to as a lentiginous nevus.

4.2.3 Solar (Actinic) Lentigo

The lesions of solar lentigo are light to dark brown, slowly expanding macules that develop in chronically sun-exposed areas of the skin, including the eyelids. They occur in middle-aged to elderly adults and are considered a hallmark of aged skin. Presenting as small macules 3–5 mm in diameter, the lesions may gradually grow to several centimeters in diameter. They sometimes evolve into the reticulated (adenoid) form of seborrheic keratosis and thus develop a thickened and warty surface. Differentiation from lentigo maligna and lentigo maligna melanoma may be necessary, requiring histopathologic examination. Histology shows hyperpigmentation of the basal layer without appreciably increased number of melanocytes, often with regular elongation of the rete ridges. Actinic elastosis is present in the dermis. Solar lentigo lesions respond to treatment with topical 0.1% tretinoin, 2% hydroquinone, laser therapy, and cryotherapy.

4.2.4 Melanocytic Nevus

A melanocytic nevus is considered as a hamartoma or a benign tumor of neural crest-derived melanocytes [3]. An eyelid nevus, as in other areas of the skin, can be acquired (usually) or congenital.

4.2.4.1 Congenital Melanocytic Nevus

Congenital melanocytic nevi are present in about 1% of newborns (Fig. 4.1) [4, 5]. Congenital nevi may be single or multiple with sharp borders and are usually larger than acquired nevi. They may be light in color in neonates and relatively hairless, and they tend to become darker with papular or nodular change which may be verrucous or cerebriform with age. With age, darkly pigmented hairs may develop. Congenital nevi have been reported to be associated with

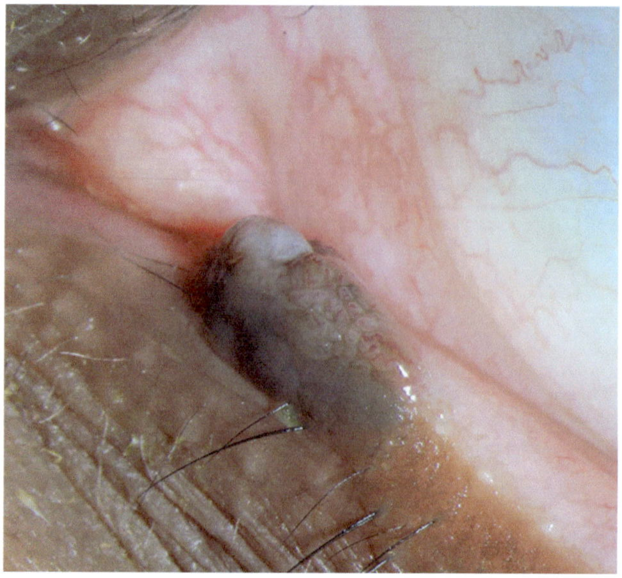

Fig. 4.1 Congenital nevus of the eyelid surrounding the puncta

several developmental abnormalities, including scoliosis, spina bifida, clubfoot, elephantiasis, and cranial bone hypertrophy, as well as syndromes such as neurocutaneous melanocytosis and neurofibromatosis type I [5].

In adults, congenital melanocytic nevi are classified by their largest diameter as small (<1.5 cm), medium (1.5–20 cm), and large or giant congenital melanocytic nevi (>20 cm). However other classifications are based on ease of removal, location and relationship to other anatomic structures, comparison to the size of the patient's palm, and surface area of the body involved. Assessment of proportionate expansion over time is also important in classification [5]. The risk of malignant transformation varies significantly with the size of the lesion. The lifetime risk of developing melanoma in congenital nevi of all sizes is approximately 1–2%. Lifetime risk of developing melanoma in patients with giant congenital nevi has been reported to range from about 2–31%, mostly in the 5–6% range [5]. Despite evidence supporting origin of melanoma in small congenital nevi, it is rare in children [5].

Congenital nevi may be junctional, compound, or intradermal, and they show different patterns depending on the age of the individual. In neonates they are usually junctional and show prominent melanocytic hyperplasia in the epidermis and adnexal epithelium. If biopsied during the first year of life, the histologic picture is that of larger nevus cells in the epidermis and just below it with an intervening uninvolved dermal space and small nevus cells in the reticular dermis. Congenital nevi after the post-natal period have a tendency to involve the lower dermis and subcutaneous tissue with single-file permeation of dermal collagen bundles and perineural, perifollicular, and perivascular distribution of nevus cells. There are differences of opinion as to whether or not these features are pathognomonic and sufficient to distinguish from acquired nevi. The majority (approximately 90%) of large congenital nevi harbor *NRAS* mutations and less frequently *BRAF* pV600E mutations [6, 7]. Surgical excision is recommended for giant congenital nevi because they are disfiguring and potentially malignant.

4.2.4.2 Congenital Nevus Syndrome (Neurocutaneous Melanosis)

Congenital nevus syndrome, formerly termed neurocutaneous melanosis (NCM), is a rare association of multiple and large congenital cutaneous nevi with satellite nevi, various congenital CNS abnormalities including meningeal melanosis or melanoma, and other abnormalities, including facial dysmorphism, metabolic bone disease, and endocrine dysfunction [8, 9].

4.2.4.3 Split Nevus (Kissing Nevus, Divided Nevus)

A variant of congenital compound nevus involving both upper and lower eyelids is the kissing nevus, which can be associated with significant cosmetic and functional defects of the eyelids (Fig. 4.2). Such a contiguous involvement suggests that the nevus develops between ninth and 20th week of gestation when the eyelids are fused. There have been reports citing potential for malignant transformation, but a review of 23 articles (149 cases) revealed no documented cases of this occurring. Most were of medium size. Surgical repair involves excision, and numerous methods of reconstruction have been utilized [10, 11].

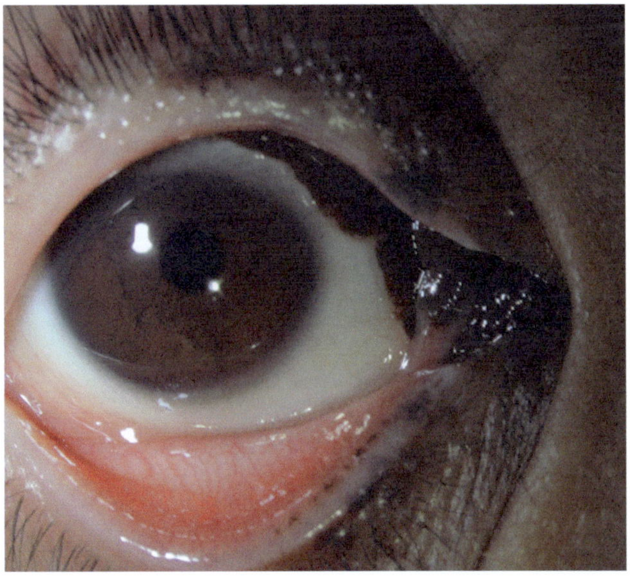

Fig. 4.2 Split nevus. A sharply demarcated, brown discoloration, involving the upper and lower eyelids in a 16-year-old Asian female. Nevomelanocytes migrate from the neural crest to the skin after the tenth week in utero but before 24 weeks when splitting of eyelids occurs. Concomitant conjunctival nevus is also present

4.2.4.4 Blue Nevus

The blue nevus arises from primitive Schwann cell and melanocyte precursors that have been arrested in the dermis before reaching the epidermis (Fig. 4.3) [12]. Within the spectrum of types of blue nevi, different clinicopathologic variants are identified: common blue nevus and cellular blue nevus (localized variants) and oculodermal melanocytosis (diffuse variant) [13, 14].

The blue nevus appears as a typically small dark lesion, the blue color due to the deep location of the melanocytes with absorption of larger wavelengths of light as it passes through the dermis (Tyndall phenomenon). Such eyelid changes can extend to involve adjacent conjunctiva, orbit, and intracranial cavity.

The relationship between blue nevus, blue nevus that has undergone malignant transformation, and melanoma is fraught with classification controversies [15]. Difficulties arise because some metastatic melanomas can resemble blue nevi, spindled sclerotic lesions may be challenging with a differential including scar, dermatofibroma, neurofibroma, and desmoplastic melanoma, and intermediate or hard to classify lesions are often given terms such as atypical or metastasizing nevi, terms which by definition should be avoided [16]. Surgical excision is recommended for cosmesis or to establish a definitive diagnosis.

Histologically, the common blue nevus is composed of dendritic (elongated and finely branching) melanocytes confined to the mid and upper dermis associated with sclerotic stromal collagen. Melanophages are also present. The cellular blue nevus consists of both dendritic melanocytes and a second population of islands of epithelioid and plump spindle-shaped melanocytes. Blue nevi and oculodermal melanocytosis (nevus of Ota) frequently harbor activating mutations in *GNAQ* and *GNA11* genes, similar to the founding mutations in uveal melanoma, and lack *BRAF* and *NRAS* mutations that are enriched in conventional melanocytic nevi [17–20].

4.2.4.5 Nevus of Ota

The nevus of Ota (oculodermal melanocytosis) occurs as a diffuse or speckled bluish or brown discoloration of the eyelids and periorbital skin and episclera due to a proliferation of dermal melanocytes (Fig. 4.4). The temple, forehead, malar region, sclera, and mucosa of the nose and mouth may also be involved. These regions correspond to the ophthalmic and maxillary divisions of the trigeminal nerve. Associated melanocytosis of structures such as uvea, orbit, and ipsilateral meninges may be present but not readily apparent. Nevus of Ota may appear at birth or may develop during the first year of life or during adolescence. It tends to follow the

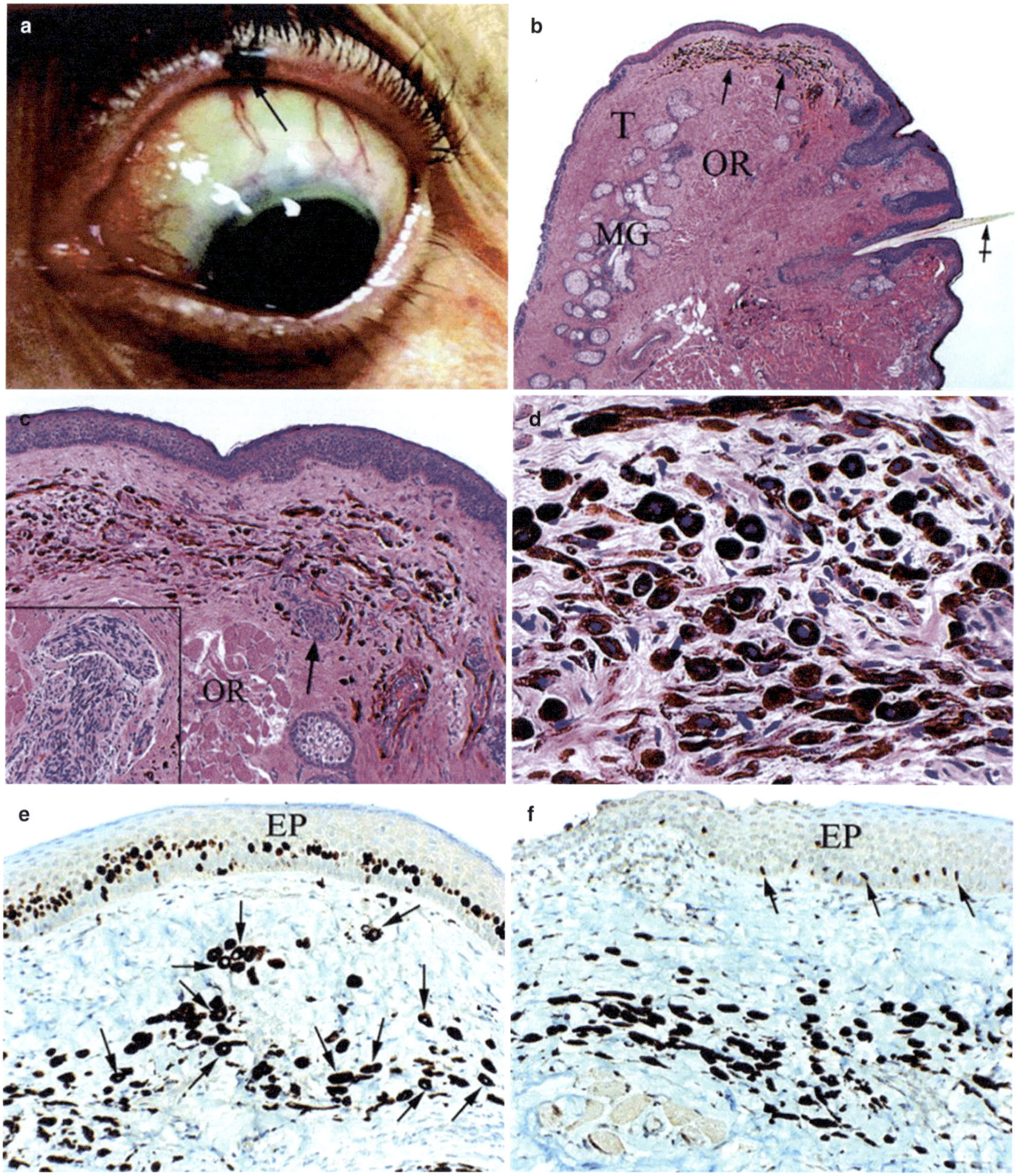
a
b
T
OR
MG
c
OR
d
e
EP
f
EP

distribution of the first and second divisions of the trigeminal nerve. Nevus of Ota may rarely be bilateral.

Histopathologically, nevus of Ota is characterized by proliferation of scattered dendritic and spindle-shaped pigmented melanocytes in the dermis, soft tissues (including the orbit), ocular tissues (episclera, sclera, and uvea), and intracranial structures in the distribution of the ophthalmic and maxillary divisions of the trigeminal nerve.

Frequent follow-up with dilated fundus examination is required because of a small risk of development of a uveal melanoma [21]. Possibility of malignant transformation of the cutaneous component is even more remote [22, 23].

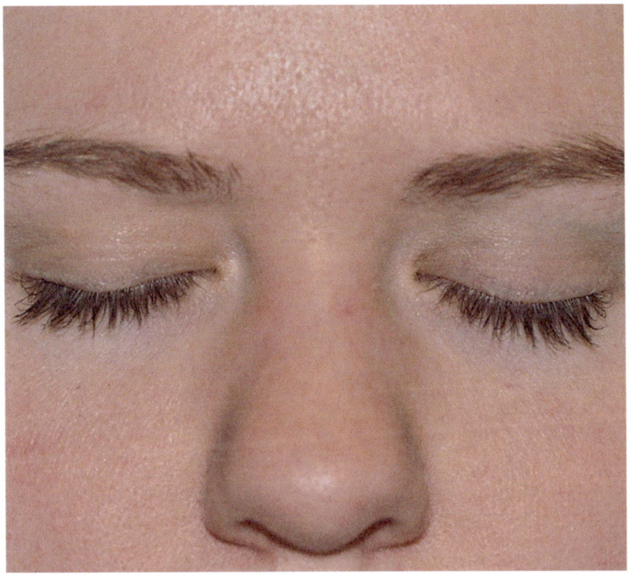

Fig. 4.4 Nevus of Ota. Brown discoloration of the eyelids and periorbital skin along the distribution of the ophthalmic and maxillary divisions of the trigeminal nerve

4.2.4.6 Acquired Nevus

Common acquired nevi (conventional nevi) develop during childhood and adolescence. Mild to moderate sun exposure in early life and genetic susceptibility induce the development of nevi [23, 24]. The acquired nevus appears as a small, flat, or minimally elevated lesion that is light brown in color (Fig. 4.5). Acquired nevi have a limited growth phase, often during adolescence after which they stabilize. Acquired nevi may be located anywhere on the eyelids and frequently involve the eyelid margin and conjunctiva. Surgical excision of large eyelid nevi may necessitate significant tissue loss, so frequent observation rather than routine excision may be warranted in many cases.

The nevus cells (nevoid melanocytes) are found in discrete nests and consist of oval to cuboidal cells with clear cytoplasm and variable melanin pigment. Typically, the cells become smaller and contain less pigment in the deeper dermal component of the lesion if present, a phenomenon known as "maturation." Junctional, compound, and dermal nevi are differentiated by the location of these nests of nevus cells. There is an evolution of acquired nevi in which the nevus cells are initially located only at the dermoepidermal junction (junctional nevus) (Fig. 4.5), followed later with nests at the dermoepidermal junction and dermis (compound nevus) (Fig. 4.6) and finally in the dermis only (dermal nevus) (Fig. 4.7). This progression is referred to as the process of nevogenesis [3]. Thus, junctional nevi are most frequent in the first decade, compound nevus in the second decade, and the proportion of dermal nevi increases with age [23]. Although many melanomas have been shown to be associated with precursor nevi, the risk of malignant transformation for individual nevus is very low [25, 26].

4.2.4.7 Spitz Nevus

A distinctive type of nevus is the Spitz nevus [27], which predominates in childhood and adolescence. Spitz nevi are

Fig. 4.3 (**a**) Eyelid margin blue nevus. A 93-year-old Caucasian woman had an irregular, flat, black lesion (arrow) measuring 3 × 4 mm at the left upper eyelid mucocutaneous junction. (**b**) A full-thickness perpendicular section of the eyelid contains a loose population of pigmented cells mostly located in the dermis (arrows) that has failed to produce any appreciable eyelid thickening. There are no intraepithelial junctional nests. The tarsus (T), Meibomian glands (MG), and orbicularis striated muscle fibers (OR) are overall noninvolved by the tumor cells. The crossed arrow indicates a cilium (hematoxylin-eosin, ×25). (**c**) The cells in the dermis are a mixture of elongated and polygonal melanocytes. The arrow highlights a small fascicle of nonpigmented cells, depicted to greater advantage with gentle waves in the inset. This feature was regarded as a terminal nerve twig with mild Schwann cell hyperplasia. OR, orbicularis muscle fibers devoid of infiltrating cells (hematoxylin-eosin, ×200). (**d**) Spindled and rounded pigmented cells are intermixed. Despite the density of the cytoplasmic pigmentation, a central round nucleus is discernible as a clear zone in the center of most of the cells. Note the absence of both inflammatory cells and a prominent vascularity in the background stroma (hematoxylin-eosin, ×400). (**e**) Ki-67 immunostaining for cells in the S-phase signifying active DNA replication demonstrate positive nuclear staining among the basal germinal cells of the epithelium (EP). The arrows point out central clear zones corresponding to nonstaining melanocytic nuclei in the connective tissue (immunoperoxidase reaction, diaminobenzidine chromogen, ×200). (**f**) Microphthalmia-associated transcription factor immunostains the nuclei of scattered dendritic melanocytes (arrows) within the epithelium (EP) with trail-off on the left within the conjunctiva. There are no visible nuclei among the dendritic dermal melanocytes constituting the tumor, because the immunoproduct of the positively staining nuclei merges imperceptibly with the melanin within the surrounding cytoplasm (immunoperoxidase reaction, diaminobenzidine chromogen, ×200). [Reprinted from Kirzhner M, Jakobiec FA, Kim N. Focal blue nevus of the eyelid margin (mucocutaneous junction): a report of a unique case with a review of the literature. Ophthalmic Plast Reconstr Surg 2011;27(5):338–42. With permission from Wolters Kluwer Health, Inc.]

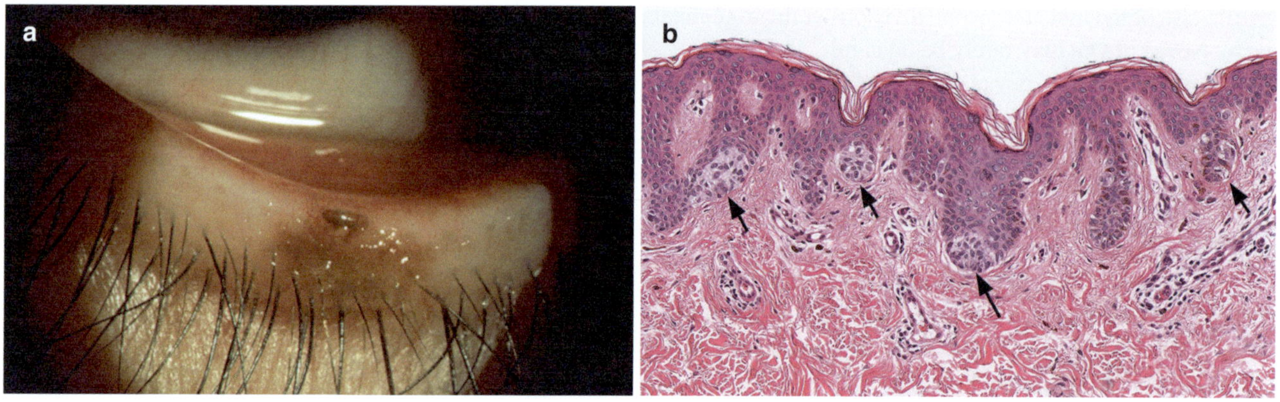

Fig. 4.5 Junctional eyelid nevus. (**a**) Flat pigmented melanocytic nevus on the margin of the upper eyelid (**a**). (**b**) Junctional nevus consisting of melanocyte nests (arrows) without cytologic atypia confined to the dermoepidermal junction (**b**: hematoxylin and eosin; ×200)

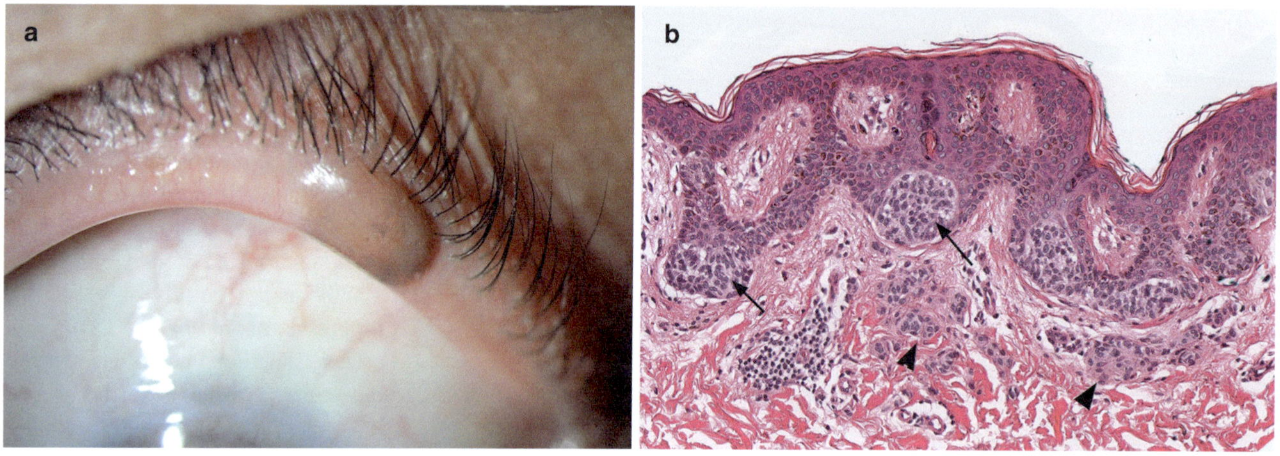

Fig. 4.6 Compound eyelid nevus. (**a**) Dome-shaped pigmented nodule at the eyelid margin. (**b**) Nests of nevus cells at the dermopepidermal junction and in the dermis (hematoxylin and eosin; ×200)

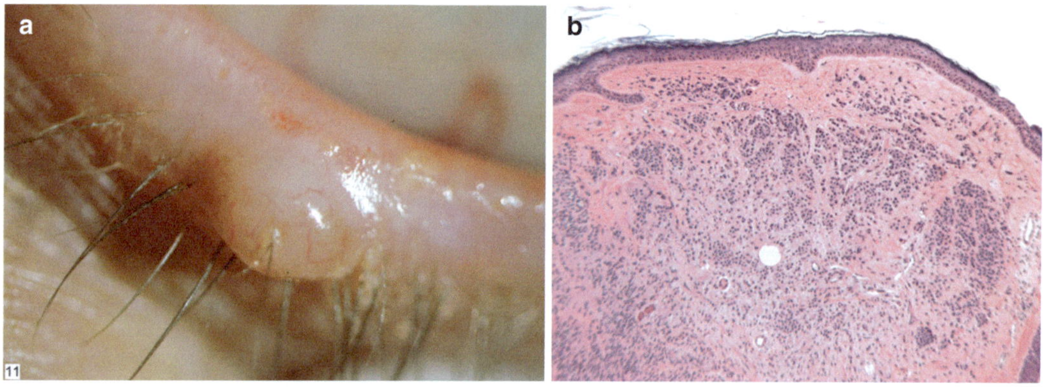

Fig. 4.7 Dermal eyelid nevus. (**a**) Nonpigmented dermal nevus of the eyelid margin. Note that surface epithelium and lashes are intact. (**b**) Dermal nevus composed of nevus cells confined to the dermis and arranged in nests, cords, and singly with maturation (nuclei becoming smaller) in the deeper dermis (hematoxylin and eosin; ×100)

found on the face, trunk, or extremities and they can rarely involve the eyelid (Fig. 4.8) [28, 29]. These lesions are rapidly growing, sharply circumscribed, red- or tan-colored lesions that should be differentiated from pyogenic granuloma or hemangioma and, more importantly, from melanoma which is extremely uncommon in children. Spitz nevus has been referred to in the past as a spindle and epithelioid cell nevus and benign juvenile melanoma, the terms that are cur-

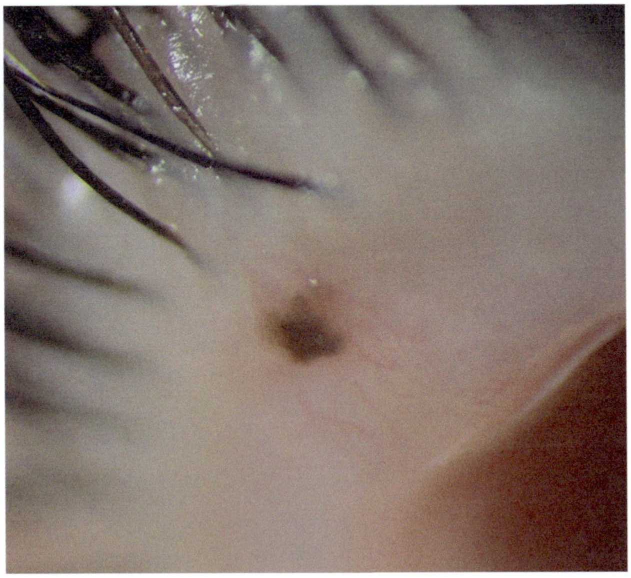

Fig. 4.8 Spitz nevus: recurrent eyelid margin Spitz nevus in a 6-year-old girl

rently not recommended. Formerly a biologically controversial tumor, Spitz nevus is currently regarded as a benign neoplasm with a low risk of malignant transformation. The unusual cases of regional and distant metastases attributed to Spitz nevi are likely due to the fact that morphologic distinction between some Spitz nevi, Spitz melanocytoma (atypical Spitz tumor), and melanoma (Spitzoid melanoma) can be difficult.

Histologically, Spitz nevi are sharply circumscribed, usually less than 5–6 mm in diameter, and typically compound nevi. They are composed of either spindle or epithelioid melanocytes, or both, spindle melanocytes being more common. Superficially located mitotic figures tend to be few in number, and they reflect rapid clinical growth but not an indication of malignancy. Atypical mitoses should not be present, nor should mitoses occur deep in the lesion [30]. These nevi are symmetrical, with no lateral extension of junctional activity beyond the intradermal component. There may be aggregates of nevus cells within the epidermis (but not single cells) in what is referred to as transepidermal elimination. Kamino bodies may be present at the dermoepidermal junction. These are eosinophilic globules which stain with PAS and trichrome histochemical stains, and they are a useful diagnostic feature [29]. Maturation of the nevus cells toward the base is also seen in most cases, a finding that helps distinguish Spitz nevus from melanoma. Minor diagnostic criteria include junctional cleavage (separation of the epidermis from the nevus nests in the junctional zone), pseudoepitheliomatous hyperplasia, absence of pleomorphism, dermal edema and telangiectasia, and giant nevus cells [29].

Immunohistochemical and molecular genetic studies may be useful in morphologically challenging cases. Spitz nevi retain p16 expression, lack PRAME expression, and have a low Ki-67 proliferative index (<5–10%) unlike their morphologic mimics Spitzoid melanocytoma and melanoma. Genomic profiling of Spitz nevi shows frequent *HRAS* mutations and receptor kinase fusions, while Spitz melanocytoma and Spitzoid melanoma may harbor *CDKN2A* deletions and *TERT* promoter mutations [31–33]. Because the clinical features of rapid onset are alarming, excision to exclude the possibility of melanoma should be performed.

4.2.4.8 Dysplastic Nevus

Dysplastic nevi (formerly known as atypical or Clark's nevi) are present in 2–18% of the population, and they may be associated with an increased risk for malignant melanoma. In addition to educating such patients about dangers of sun exposure, periodic total-skin examinations starting at puberty should be recommended. Dysplastic nevi tend to be larger (≥5 mm), with ill-defined borders, and have variegated colors (tan, brown, and pink). The lesions by definition have a flat (macular) component representing junctional melanocytic proliferation and there is frequently a raised portion corresponding to the dermal component (Fig. 4.9). Dysplastic nevi may be multiple.

The characteristic features of dysplastic nevi are architectural disorder and cytologic atypia, which manifest as shouldering or peripheral extension of the junctional component relative to the intradermal component, lentiginous melanocyte hyperplasia, random cytologic melanocyte atypia, and stromal response (lamellar fibroplasia of the papillary dermis) (Fig. 4.9).

Management of dysplastic nevi has been controversial. Options are re-excision of incompletely excised histologically dysplastic nevi vs. observation [34]. Observation may be considered for nevi with mild and low-grade dysplasia [35]. It is recommended that incompletely excised high-grade (severe) dysplastic nevi should be re-excised because of the challenges in unequivocally distinguishing these lesions from melanoma and also because of some concern for progression (Fig. 4.9) [36]. It is also important to note that dysplastic nevi are markers of predisposition to melanoma, along with other risk factors, such as sun exposure, skin pigmentation, and hereditary/genetic alterations [37].

4.2.4.9 Familial Melanoma (Atypical Mole and Melanoma Syndrome, Dysplastic Nevus Syndrome)

Familial melanoma (FAM-M), formerly known as atypical mole or dysplastic nevus syndrome, denotes a specific clinicopathologic entity that is associated with an increased risk for the development of cutaneous melanoma [38]. This syndrome of autosomal dominant predisposition to cutaneous melanoma was originally described by Clark as BK mole syndrome [39]. FAM-M syndrome has been linked to

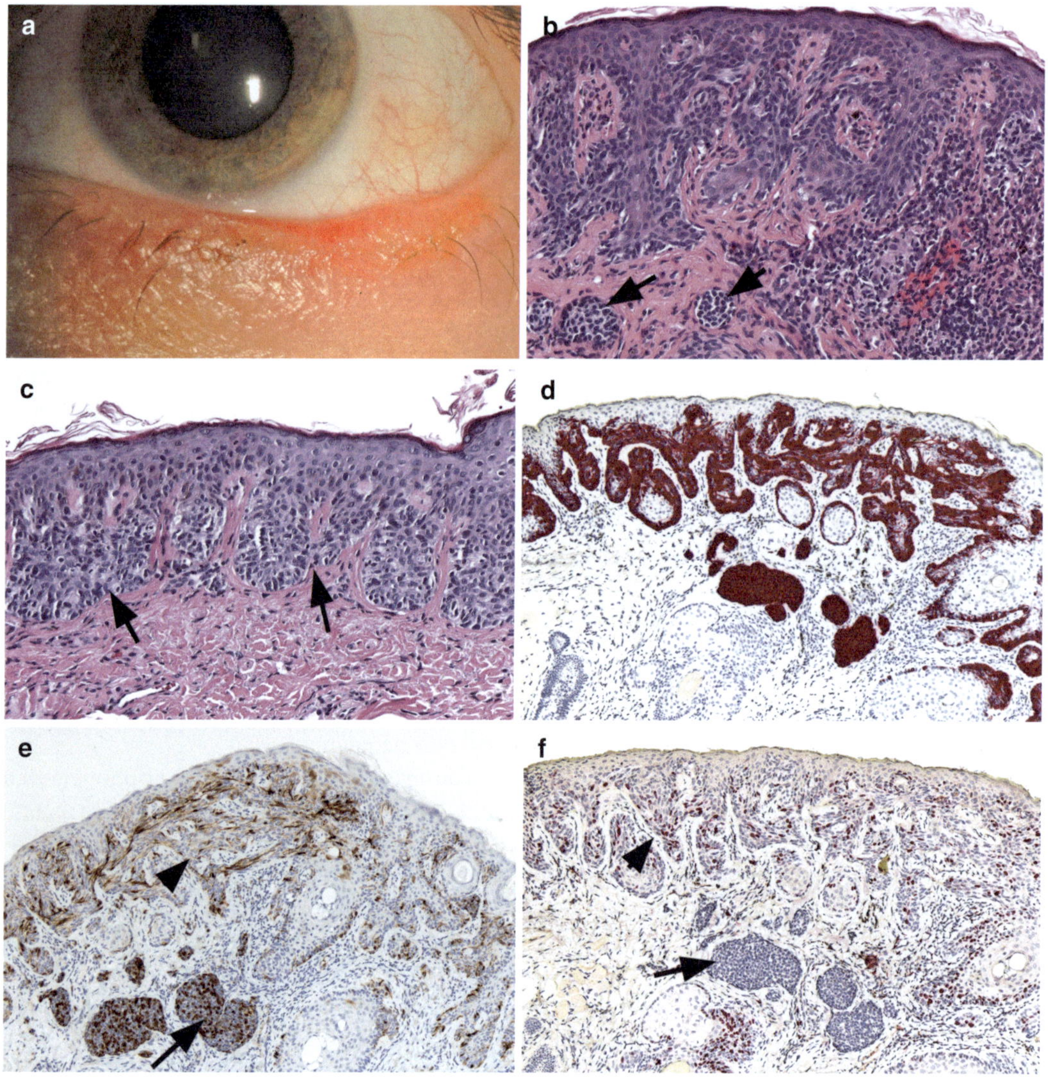

Fig. 4.9 Evolving or early established melanoma in situ arising in a compound nevus with severe dysplasia in a 45 year-old male. (**a**) Variably pigmented, poorly circumscribed, focally mildly elevated lesion involving anterior lamella of the eyelid margin, associated with madarosis. (**b**) Nests of nevoid melanocytes in the dermis (arrows) and proliferation of atypical melanocytes in the overlying epidermis, bridging rete ridges. The dermis is sclerotic with a patchy inflammatory infiltrate. (**c**) Peripheral component of the lesion shows confluent nests of atypical melanocyets bridging rete ridges (arrows). (**d**) Melan-A immunohistochemical stain highlights the dermal nevus nests and the markedly architecturally atypical overlying junctional component that extends peripheral to the dermal component of the lesion. (**e**) P16 immunohistochemical stain shows a typical mosaic pattern of staining in the dermal nevoid component of the lesion (arrow), while this pattern is focally lost in the junctional component (arrowhead), suggestive of evolution to melanoma in situ. (**f**) Ki-67 shows no proliferative activity in the dermal nevoid component of the lesion (arrow) and increased proliferative activity in the overlying junctional component. [hematoxylin-eosin (**b**, **c**), Melan-A (**d**), p16 (**e**), Ki-67 (**f**); ×200 (**b**, **c**); ×100 (**d**–**f**)]

high-penetrance pathogenic variants in *CDKN2A* and *CDK4* genes [40]. Many other high-penetrance and low-penetrance melanoma susceptibility genes have been recently identified, which are beyond the scope of this chapter.

4.2.4.10 Lentigo Maligna (Melanotic Freckle of Hutchinson)

Lentigo maligna refers to an acquired pigmented macule in the sun-exposed skin of middle-aged or elderly individuals [41]. Lentigo maligna was initially described by Hutchinson; hence it is also called melanotic freckle of Hutchinson [12]. Lentigo maligna is now considered the in situ phase (melanoma in situ) of lentigo maligna melanoma (invasive melanoma) (Fig. 4.10).

Lentigo maligna is characterized by a basal lentiginous proliferation (cells occurring mostly singly, contiguously along basal epidermis) of atypical melanocytes with features including pleomorphic and enlarged nuclei, increased and eosinophilic cytoplasm, and mitotic activity (Fig. 4.10). As

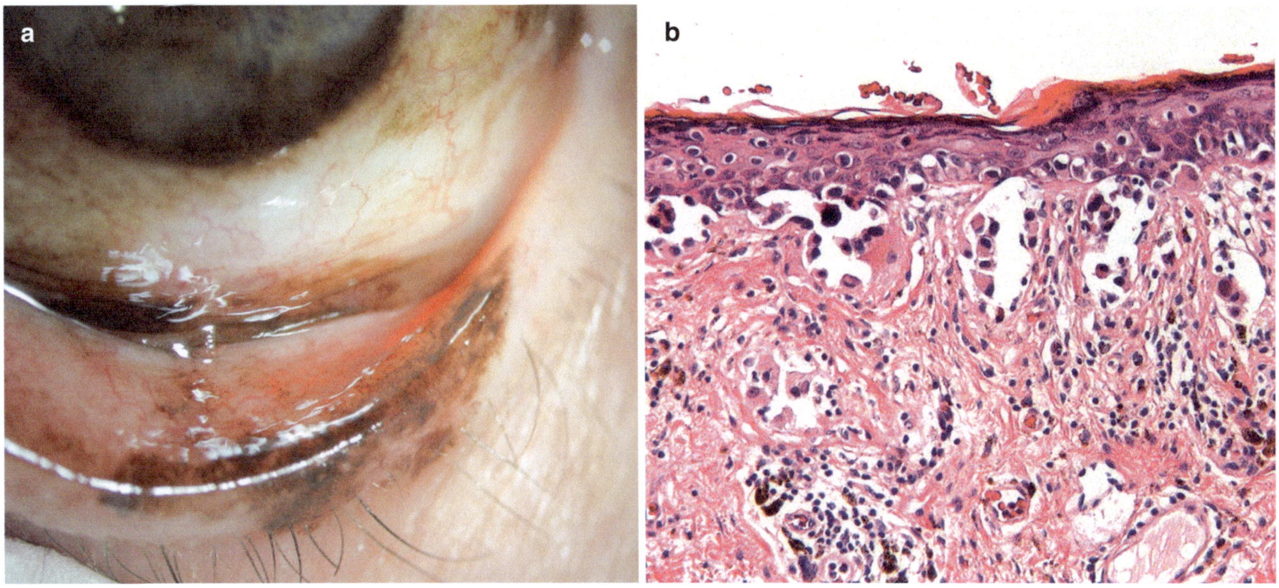

Fig. 4.10 Lentigo maligna melanoma in situ (**a**). Lentiginous proliferation of atypical melanocytes along the basal epidermis (**b**). Focal nesting is also present in a "rain drop"-like pattern. There is no appreciable pagetoid upward scatter. The epidermis is atrophic. The dermis contains chronic inflammatory infiltrate and actinic elastosis (hematoxylin-eosin, ×150)

expected of melanoma of the skin with chronic sun-damage, severe actinic elastosis is present in the dermis.

Lentigo maligna can slowly enlarge horizontally before entering a vertical growth phase and transforming into lentigo maligna melanoma (invasive melanoma). Overall, it is estimated that the lifetime risk of developing invasive melanoma is approximately 5% [42]. Genomically, lentigo maligna is characterized by frequent loss of *NF1* or mutually exclusive activating *NRAS* and *BRAF* mutations [43–45]. *CDKN2A* is frequently lost in vertical growth phase [46]. Frequent *TERT* promoter mutations are also present in both in situ and invasive melanoma [47].

Proposed suitable methods of treatment include surgical excision with mapping, radiotherapy, cryotherapy, topical imiquimod, imiquimod with cryotherapy [48], and a modified Mohs micrographic technique using immunoperoxidase staining with HMB-45 or MART-1 [42]. Management of lentigo maligna melanoma is similar to that of invasive cutaneous melanoma in extraocular location. Advanced tumors are managed in a multidisciplinary approach with oncologic staging, sentinel lymph node biopsy (in appropriate cases), and systemic therapy (in appropriate cases). Current systemic therapy approaches include targeted therapies directed toward tumor genomic profile and immunotherapies.

4.3 Summary

Melanocytic lesions of the eyelid are similar to such lesions elsewhere and range from benign to premalignant to malignant tumors. Some of these lesions are associated genetic predisposition and syndromic manifestations. Therefore, management of such patients should be guided by the general principles of dermatology, dermatopathology, medical oncology, and clinical genetics.

References

1. Praetorius C, Sturm RA, Steingrimsson E. Sun-induced freckling: ephelides and solar lentigines. Pigment Cell Melanoma Res. 2014;27(3):339–50.
2. Korsse SE, van Leerdam ME, Dekker E. Gastrointestinal diseases and their oro-dental manifestations: part 4: Peutz-Jeghers syndrome. Br Dent J. 2017;222(3):214–7.
3. Krengel S. Nevogenesis—new thoughts regarding a classical problem. Am J Dermatopathol. 2005;27(5):456–65.
4. Price HN. Congenital melanocytic nevi: update in genetics and management. Curr Opin Pediatr. 2016;28(4):476–82.
5. Tannous ZS, Mihm MC Jr, Sober AJ, Duncan LM. Congenital melanocytic nevi: clinical and histopathologic features, risk of melanoma, and clinical management. J Am Acad Dermatol. 2005;52(2):197–203.
6. Bauer J, Curtin JA, Pinkel D, Bastian BC. Congenital melanocytic nevi frequently harbor NRAS mutations but no BRAF mutations. J Invest Dermatol. 2007;127(1):179–82.
7. Salgado CM, Basu D, Nikiforova M, et al. BRAF mutations are also associated with neurocutaneous melanocytosis and large/giant congenital melanocytic nevi. Pediatr Dev Pathol. 2015;18(1):1–9.
8. Makkar HS, Frieden IJ. Neurocutaneous melanosis. Semin Cutan Med Surg. 2004;23(2):138–44.
9. Alikhan A, Ibrahimi OA, Eisen DB. Congenital melanocytic nevi: where are we now? Part I. Clinical presentation, epidemiology, pathogenesis, histology, malignant transformation, and neurocutaneous melanosis. J Am Acad Dermatol. 2012;67(4):495. e1-17; quiz 512-4
10. Desai SC, Walen S, Holds JB, Branham G. Divided nevus of the eyelid: review of embryology, pathology and treatment. Am J Otolaryngol. 2013;34(3):223–9.

11. Jacobs SM, Couch SM, Custer PL. Divided eyelid nevus: a lid-sparing, staged surgical approach. Am J Ophthalmol. 2013;156(4):813–8.
12. Hutchinson J. Notes on the cancerous process and on new growths in general. Arch Surg. 1890;2:83–6.
13. Folberg R, Jakobiec FA, Bernardino VB, Iwamoto T. Benign conjunctival melanocytic lesions. Clinicopathologic features. Ophthalmology. 1989;96(4):436–61.
14. Kirzhner M, Jakobiec FA, Kim N. Focal blue nevus of the eyelid margin (mucocutaneous junction): a report of a unique case with a review of the literature. Ophthalmic Plast Reconstr Surg. 2011;27(5):338–42.
15. Mones JM, Ackerman AB. "Atypical" blue nevus, "malignant" blue nevus, and "metastasizing" blue nevus: a critique in historical perspective of three concepts flawed fatally. Am J Dermatopathol. 2004;26(5):407–30.
16. Wang Q, Prieto V, Esmaeli B, et al. Cellular blue nevi of the eyelid: a possible diagnostic pitfall. J Am Acad Dermatol. 2008;58(2):257–60.
17. Van Raamsdonk CD, Bezrookove V, Green G, et al. Frequent somatic mutations of GNAQ in uveal melanoma and blue naevi. Nature. 2009;457(7229):599–602.
18. Roh MR, Eliades P, Gupta S, Tsao H. Genetics of melanocytic nevi. Pigment Cell Melanoma Res. 2015;28(6):661–72.
19. Gerami P, Pouryazdanparast P, Vemula S, Bastian BC. Molecular analysis of a case of nevus of ota showing progressive evolution to melanoma with intermediate stages resembling cellular blue nevus. Am J Dermatopathol. 2010;32(3):301–5.
20. Vivancos A, Caratu G, Matito J, et al. Genetic evolution of nevus of Ota reveals clonal heterogeneity acquiring BAP1 and TP53 mutations. Pigment Cell Melanoma Res. 2016;29(2):247–53.
21. Singh AD, De Potter P, Fijal BA, et al. Lifetime prevalence of uveal melanoma in white patients with oculo(dermal) melanocytosis. Ophthalmology. 1998;105(1):195–8.
22. Patel BC, Egan CA, Lucius RW, et al. Cutaneous malignant melanoma and oculodermal melanocytosis (nevus of Ota): report of a case and review of the literature. J Am Acad Dermatol. 1998;38(5 Pt 2):862–5.
23. Wiecker TS, Luther H, Buettner P, et al. Moderate sun exposure and nevus counts in parents are associated with development of melanocytic nevi in childhood: a risk factor study in 1,812 kindergarten children. Cancer. 2003;97(3):628–38.
24. Newton-Bishop JA, Chang YM, Iles MM, et al. Melanocytic nevi, nevus genes, and melanoma risk in a large case-control study in the United Kingdom. Cancer Epidemiol Biomarkers Prev. 2010;19(8):2043–54.
25. Bevona C, Goggins W, Quinn T, et al. Cutaneous melanomas associated with nevi. Arch Dermatol. 2003;139(12):1620–4. discussion 4
26. Tsao H, Bevona C, Goggins W, Quinn T. The transformation rate of moles (melanocytic nevi) into cutaneous melanoma: a population-based estimate. Arch Dermatol. 2003;139(3):282–8.
27. Spitz S. Melanoma of the childhood. Am J Pathol. 1948;24:591–609.
28. Hiscott P, Seitz B, Naumann GO. Epithelioid cell Spitz nevus of the eyelid. Am J Ophthalmol. 1998;126(5):735–7.
29. Shields PW, Jakobiec FA, Stagner AM, Yoon MK. Spitz nevus arising in the eyelid of a teenager. Surv Ophthalmol. 2016;61(2):228–35.
30. Cheng TW, Ahern MC, Giubellino A. The spectrum of spitz melanocytic lesions: from morphologic diagnosis to molecular classification. Front Oncol. 2022;12:889223.
31. Wiesner T, Kutzner H, Cerroni L, et al. Genomic aberrations in spitzoid melanocytic tumours and their implications for diagnosis, prognosis and therapy. Pathology. 2016;48(2):113–31.
32. Lee S, Barnhill RL, Dummer R, et al. TERT promoter mutations are predictive of aggressive clinical behavior in patients with spitzoid melanocytic neoplasms. Sci Rep. 2015;5:11200.
33. Gerami P, Cooper C, Bajaj S, et al. Outcomes of atypical spitz tumors with chromosomal copy number aberrations and conventional melanomas in children. Am J Surg Pathol. 2013;37(9):1387–94.
34. Vuong KT, Walker J, Powell H, et al. Surgical re-excision versus observation for histologically dysplastic nevi: a systematic review of associated clinical outcomes. Br J Dermatol. 2018;179:590.
35. Kim CC, Berry EG, Marchetti MA, et al. Risk of subsequent cutaneous melanoma in moderately dysplastic nevi excisionally biopsied but with positive histologic margins. JAMA Dermatol. 2018;154(12):1401–8.
36. Fleming NH, Shaub AR, Bailey E, Swetter SM. Outcomes of surgical re-excision versus observation of severely dysplastic nevi: a single-institution, retrospective cohort study. J Am Acad Dermatol. 2020;82(1):238–40.
37. Elder DE. Dysplastic naevi: an update. Histopathology. 2010;56(1):112–20.
38. Salopek TG. The dilemma of the dysplastic nevus. Dermatol Clin. 2002;20(4):617–28. viii
39. Clark WH Jr, Reimer RR, Greene M, et al. Origin of familial malignant melanomas from heritable melanocytic lesions. 'The B-K mole syndrome'. Arch Dermatol. 1978;114(5):732–8.
40. Soura E, Eliades PJ, Shannon K, et al. Hereditary melanoma: update on syndromes and management: genetics of familial atypical multiple mole melanoma syndrome. J Am Acad Dermatol. 2016;74(3):395–407. quiz 8-10
41. Stevenson O, Ahmed I. Lentigo maligna : prognosis and treatment options. Am J Clin Dermatol. 2005;6(3):151–64.
42. Arlette JP, Trotter MJ, Trotter T, Temple CL. Management of lentigo maligna and lentigo maligna melanoma: seminars in surgical oncology. J Surg Oncol. 2004;86(4):179–86.
43. Krauthammer M, Kong Y, Bacchiocchi A, et al. Exome sequencing identifies recurrent mutations in NF1 and RASopathy genes in sun-exposed melanomas. Nat Genet. 2015;47(9):996–1002.
44. Bastian BC. The molecular pathology of melanoma: an integrated taxonomy of melanocytic neoplasia. Annu Rev Pathol. 2014;9:239–71.
45. Viros A, Fridlyand J, Bauer J, et al. Improving melanoma classification by integrating genetic and morphologic features. PLoS Med. 2008;5(6):e120.
46. Shain AH, Garrido M, Botton T, et al. Exome sequencing of desmoplastic melanoma identifies recurrent NFKBIE promoter mutations and diverse activating mutations in the MAPK pathway. Nat Genet. 2015;47(10):1194–9.
47. Shain AH, Yeh I, Kovalyshyn I, et al. The genetic evolution of melanoma from precursor lesions. N Engl J Med. 2015;373(20):1926–36.
48. Read T, Noonan C, David M, et al. A systematic review of non-surgical treatments for lentigo maligna. J Eur Acad Dermatol Venereol. 2016;30(5):748–53.

5 Basal Cell Carcinoma

Ofira Zloto and Mordechai Rosner

5.1 Introduction

Basal cell carcinoma (BCC) is a malignant cutaneous neoplasm capable of extensive tissue destruction. It is often observed on the head and neck, and the eyelids are very common location [1, 2]. BCC was initially described as a distinct entity by Krompecher at the beginning of the twentieth century. Some authorities preferred the term "epithelioma" to carcinoma because of the tumor's limited capacity to metastasize [1, 2]. While the mortality from BCC is low, the morbidity may be considerable.

5.2 Epidemiological Aspects

BCC is the most common human malignancy and accounts for nearly 90% of all nonmelanoma skin cancers. It is also the most common skin cancer of the eyelid, accounting for 86–96% of all cases [3, 4]. It seems that geographical and ethnic differences exist in the occurrence of BCC. In the USA, the incidence of BCC is more than 500 per 100,000, and in parts of Australia, it reaches 2400 per 100,000 [1, 3, 5, 6]. While increasing in frequency was reported during the last century, a possible decreasing trend in the incidence rates was shown in the last decade [7–9].

5.3 Etiology

The risk factors for periocular BCC include ultraviolet (UV) irradiation, local and systemic immune dysfunction, previous ionizing radiation, and focal trauma. It is believed that exposure to UV light causes defects in immune function and that this has a role in the pathogenesis of BCC. Short-wavelength UVB radiation (290–320 nm, sunburn rays) plays a more important role in BCC formation than long-wavelength UVA radiation (320–400 nm, tanning rays) [10–12]. Other risk factors are fair skin color, inability to tan, and exposure to trivalent inorganic arsenic, such as from medications including arsenical compounds [1]. Moreover, larger BCC were associated with a low socioeconomic status [13].

Genetic or congenital diseases predisposing to BCC are Gorlin–Goltz syndrome, xeroderma pigmentosum, albinism, Basex–Dupré syndrome, Muir–Torre syndrome, Rombo syndrome, linear basocellular hamartoma, and sebaceous hamartoma of Jadassohn [9, 14, 15].

5.4 Pathogenesis

The origin of BCC is controversial. It could arise from the basal cell of the epidermis, from the infundibular cells of the hair follicle, or from a pluripotential cell. BCC does not arise from a precursor lesion [1, 5].

5.5 Clinical Features

Approximately 95% of all BCCs occur in people between 40 and 79 years of age, and the average age at diagnosis for BCC of the eyelid is 60. BCC may occur in young adults and in children who have an inherited predisposition to cutaneous neoplasia. However, rarely, a solitary BCC may arise in an adolescent or young adult who has no known risk factors. Men may be more afflicted than women. In most cases, BCC arises as solitary lesion on hair-bearing sun-exposed skin, particularly the face. Most periocular BCCs arise on the lower eyelid (48%) and medial canthus (27%) and least often upper lid (23%). Tumors are usually present for many months prior to diagnosis [1, 2, 6].

O. Zloto · M. Rosner (✉)
Department of Ophthalmology, Goldschleger Eye Institute, Sheba Medical Center, School of Medicine, Tel Aviv University, Tel Aviv, Israel

B. C. K. Patel et al. (eds.), *Clinical Ophthalmic Oncology*, https://doi.org/10.1007/978-3-031-72328-5_5

5.6 Symptoms and Signs

There are several different clinical variants of BCC, including nodular and nodulo-ulcerative, pigmented, cystic, and infiltrating (which is called also morpheaform or sclerotic) BCC. All the clinical variants are usually accompanied by loss of adnexa (hair and lashes); they are firm to palpation and are painless unless secondarily infected. Sometimes, it can present as ulceration and bleeding [1, 2, 6].

5.6.1 Nodular

The nodular BCC begins as a small papule and slowly enlarges to an irregular, dome-shaped tumor (Fig. 5.1). The epithelial surface of the tumor is usually smooth, often described as pearly, with fine telangiectatic vessels beneath it. Ulceration may develop and is filled with a crusty exudate.

5.6.2 Pigmented

The pigmented BCC is usually nodular or nodulo-ulcerative, ranging in color from light tan to deep brown.

5.6.3 Cystic

The cystic BCC may attain significant dimensions (Fig. 5.2).

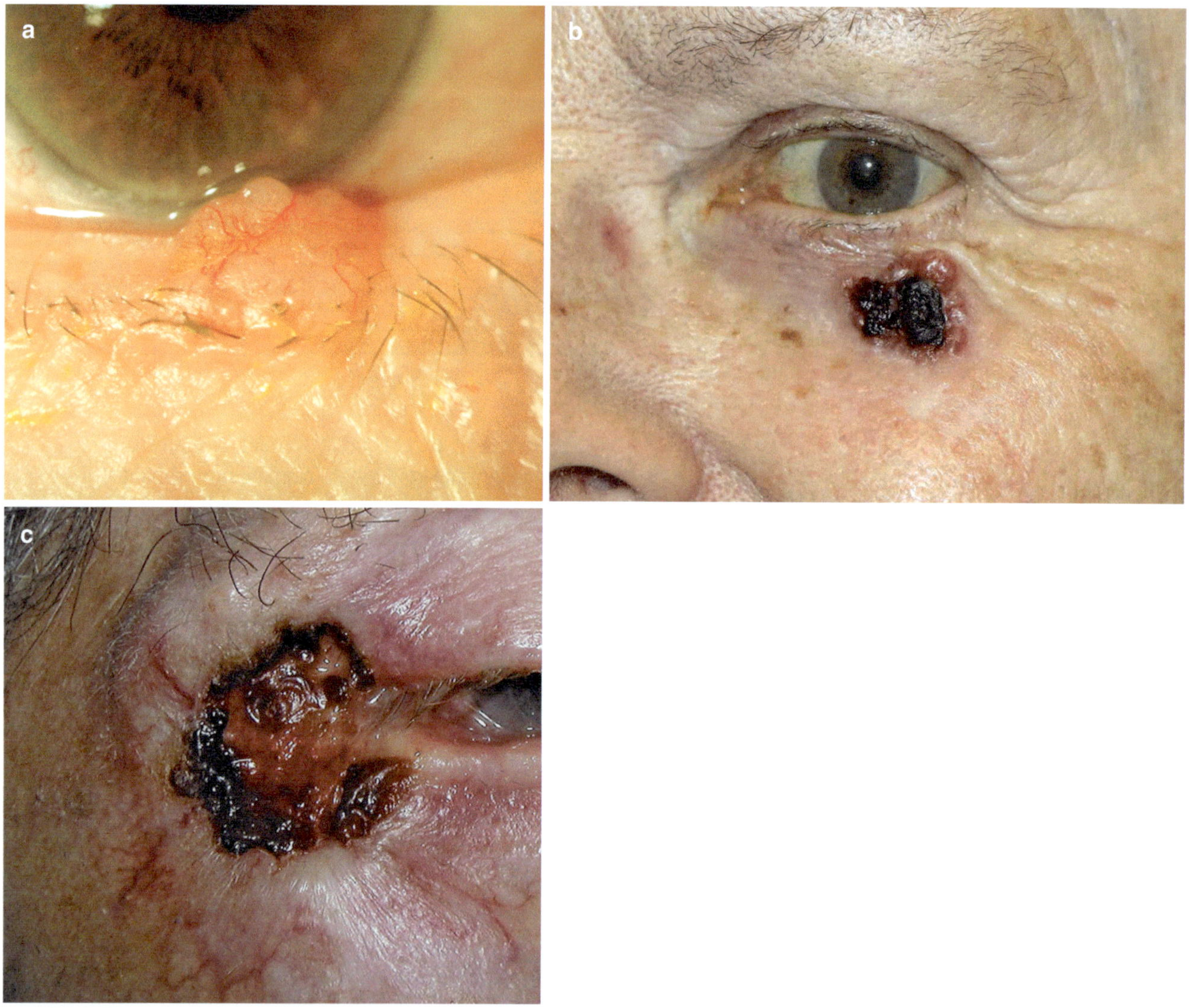

Fig. 5.1 Nodular BCC of the lower lid margin, presenting as an irregular, pearly dome-shaped tumor (**a**). Noduloulcerative basal cell carcinoma of the left lower eyelid and cheek. Note pearly nodular margin (**b**, Courtesy of Bhupender C. Patel, MD Salt Lake City, Utah, USA). Predominantly ulcerative basal cell carcinoma (**c**)

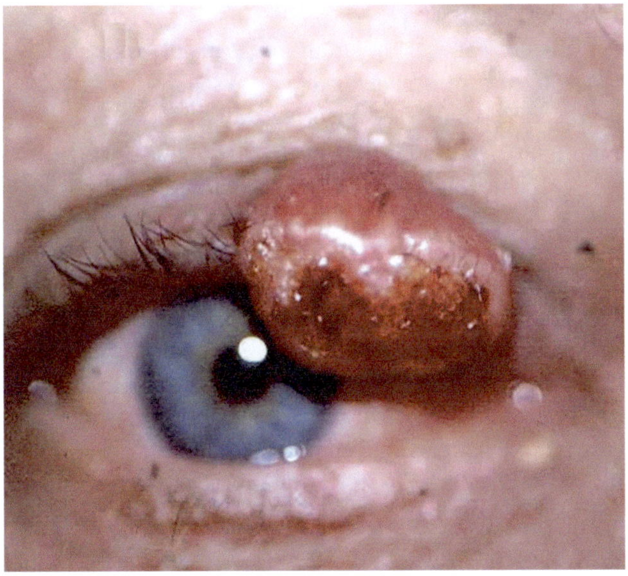

Fig. 5.2 Cystic BCC of the upper lid

5.6.4 Infiltrating

The infiltrating BCC presents as an indurated, yellowish to tan patch or plaque with occasional focal ulceration and poorly defined margins (Fig. 5.3). Patchy crusts, papules, and nodules are scattered throughout some morpheaform tumors. Infiltration within the eyelid can cause deformities and malpositioning of the lid margin.

5.7 Histopathologic Features

BCC is characterized by a proliferation of cells with oval nuclei and scant cytoplasm that form infiltrative nests or strands (Fig. 5.4). The neoplastic cells are relatively uniform in appearance and seldom display significant anaplasia or mitotic figures. At the periphery of the nests, they are usually arranged in a radial pattern called "palisading" (Fig. 5.5):

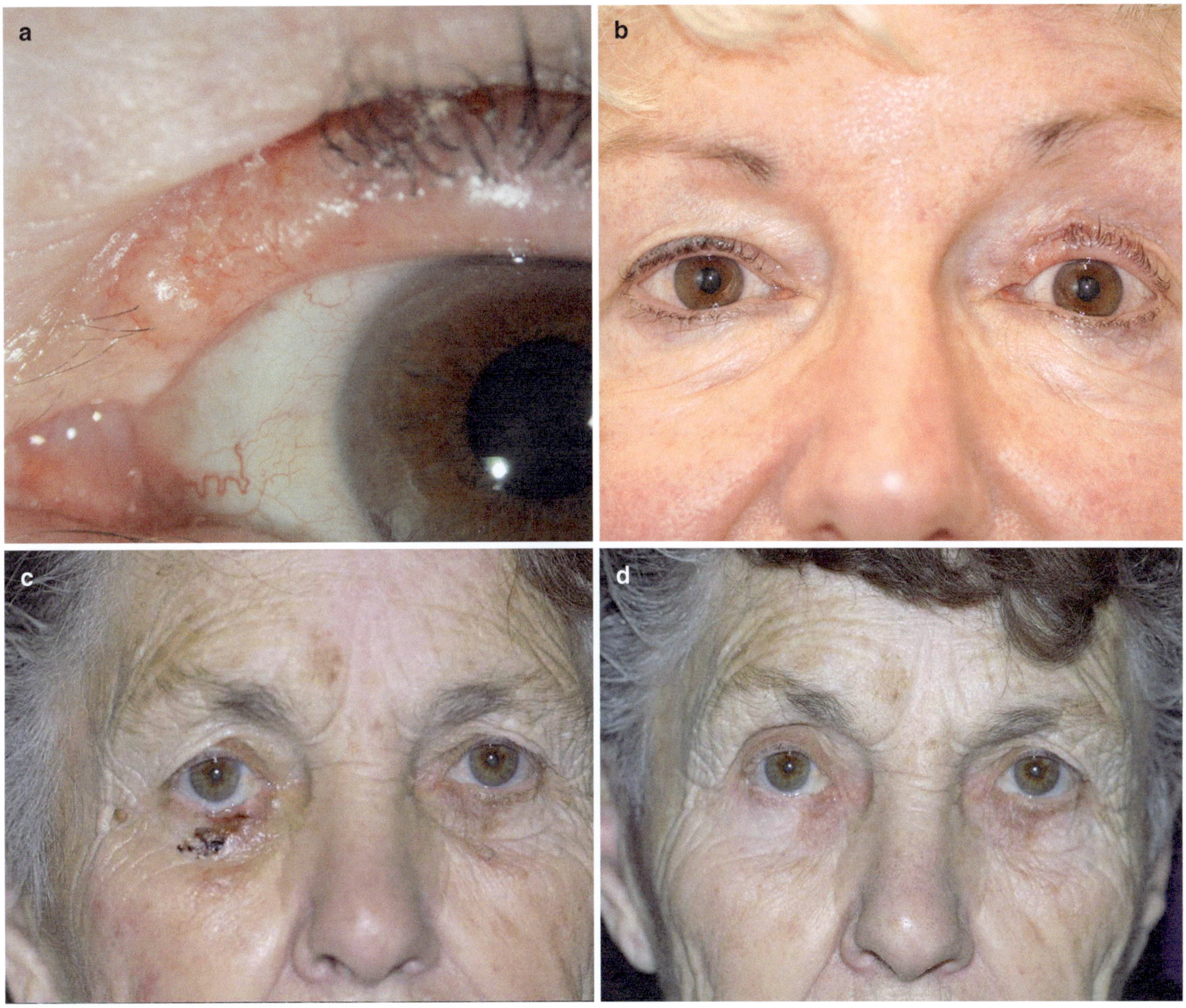

Fig. 5.3 Infiltrating BCC presenting as an indurated, yellowish to tan patch or plaque with focal ulceration and poorly defined margins (**a**, **b**). Infiltrating BCC before and after Mohs resection and repair of right lower eyelid and cheek (**c**, **d**). (Courtesy of Bhupender C. Patel, MD Salt Lake City, Utah, USA)

although this is not diagnostic, in its absence, the diagnosis of BCC should be questioned. The nests of tumor cells characteristically retract from the stroma, creating a gap (Fig. 5.5). Initially thought to be a processing artifact, this gap reflects defects in the production of adhesion-like substances by tumor cells. Necrosis is a common finding in BCC, and the necrotic debris eventually calcifies or is replaced by fibrous scar tissue. BCC also demonstrates an inflammatory infiltrate of variable intensity around the nests of tumor cells that consists predominantly of lymphocytes. The junction between the stroma of the neoplasm and normal connective tissue is ill defined [5, 6].

There is no universally accepted histopathologic subclassification of BCC according to patterns of growth and cellular differentiation. The two most important growth patterns are the circumscribed and the infiltrative. Circumscribed BCC is characterized by nests and sheets of tumor cells and usually corresponds clinically to a nodular tumor. In contrast, an infiltrative BCC is composed mainly of elongated strands of tumor cells that are several cell layers thick, with no peripheral cellular palisading (Fig. 5.6), and usually corresponds to a morphemic variety. However, in many cases different growth patterns occur in the same tumor (Fig. 5.7).

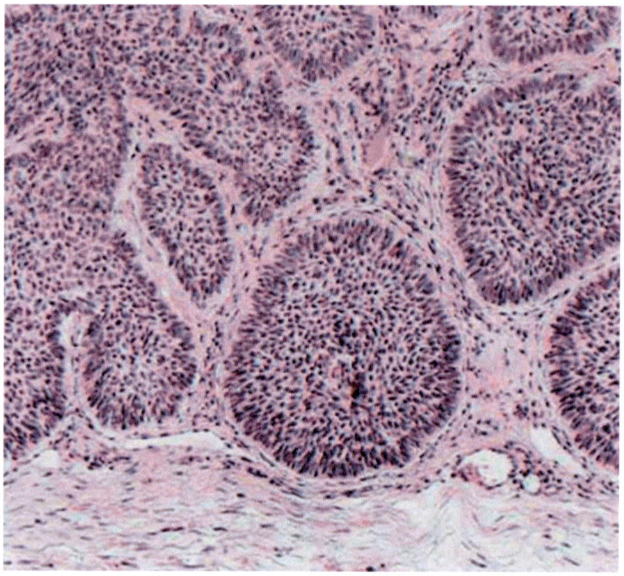

Fig. 5.4 Histopathologically, BCC is characterized by a proliferation of cells with oval nuclei and scant cytoplasm that form infiltrative nests or strands

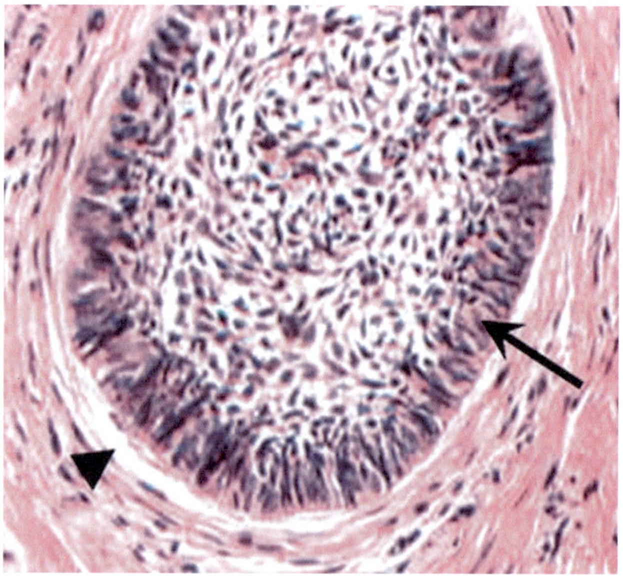

Fig. 5.5 At the periphery of the nests, the tumor cells are usually arranged in a radial pattern called "palisading" (*arrow*), and these are characteristically retracted from the stroma, creating a gap (*arrowhead*)

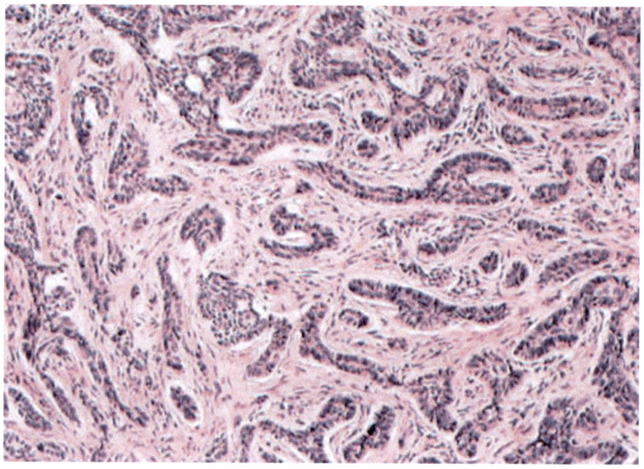

Fig. 5.6 An infiltrative BCC is composed mainly of elongated strands of tumor cells that are several cell layers thick, with no peripheral cellular palisading

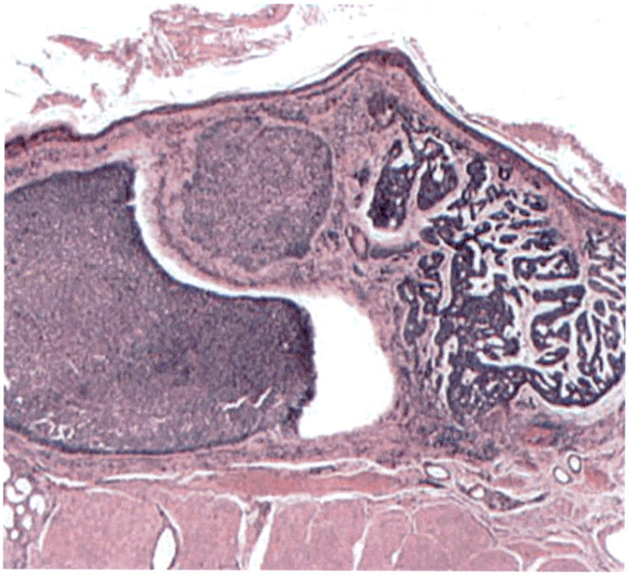

Fig. 5.7 In many cases, different growth patterns of BCC occur in the same tumor

There is a third important histologic pattern, the superficial BCC, which is presumed to be of multicentric origin and with horizontal spread. Superficial BCC is described mainly on the trunk and extremities [5, 6]. More than 20 types of cellular differentiation or histologic patterns have been described in BCC as signs of sebaceous, apocrine, or eccrine gland, as well as pillar differentiation in an otherwise typical BCC [5, 6, 13]. However, only the metatypical (basosquamous) carcinomas have an impact on prognosis. Basosquamous carcinoma displays various degrees of squamous differentiation and has been suggested to occupy a conceptual intermediate ground between squamous cell carcinoma and BCC (Box 5.1) [5, 6].

Box 5.1 Salient Diagnostic Findings

Painless, firm, nodular, or flat skin lesion with smooth, pearly epithelium, and subepithelial telangiectatic vessels, accompanied by loss of adnexa

Microscopic findings of infiltrative nests, sheets, or strands of cells with oval nuclei and scant cytoplasm, which are arranged at the periphery of the nests in a radial "palisading" pattern

Presence of a gap between the nests of tumor cells and the stroma

5.8 Diagnostic Evaluation

5.8.1 Histopathologic Examination of Excisional or Incisional Biopsy

The most important diagnostic evaluation of BCC is histopathologic examination of the excised tissue. Incisional biopsy should be taken only in cases where the clinical diagnosis is highly questionable; otherwise excisional biopsy should be performed.

5.8.2 Exfoliative Cytology

Exfoliative cytology has been shown to have a high diagnostic accuracy for BCC but may be considered only occasionally, when the plan is to treat the tumor nonsurgically [3, 6, 9, 16].

5.8.3 Imaging

When orbital or intraocular invasion is suspected, imaging is used to evaluate it. T1 contrast-enhanced fat-suppressed MRI scans are the modality of choice for demonstrating a soft tissue mass or infiltration. Computed tomographic (CT) bone windows with axial and coronal views of the orbit are best for demonstrating bony destruction—which, however, is uncommon in BCC patients [3, 15, 17].

5.8.4 Other Noninvasive Methods

Pulsed ultrasound at 20 MHz has been used for the noninvasive measurement of BCC thickness in order to plan photodynamic therapy (PDT) and to evaluate the rate of tumor regression after treatment. It was found that such measurements can distinguish between skin, fibrosis, and tumor and can even trace recurrences of BCC prior to clinical findings [4, 18].

Near-infrared reflectance-mode confocal scanning laser microscopy is a novel imaging technique for microscopic analysis of skin lesions that may offer a sensitive and specific tool for the noninvasive diagnosis of BCC in vivo [15, 19, 20].

5.9 Differential Diagnosis

The clinical and histopathologic differential diagnosis is broad. Challenging examples are trichoepithelioma and desmoplastic trichoepithelioma, chalazion, metastatic carcinoma, sebaceous carcinoma, squamous cell carcinoma, Merkel cell carcinoma, and keratoacanthoma. However, as BCC is by far the most common malignant lesion of the periocular skin, most periocular nodular or cystic skin lesions should be treated as suspicious [3, 9, 15].

5.10 Treatment

The main treatment modality for BCC is surgical excision of the lesion with microscopic monitoring of its margins or Mohs' microsurgery [2, 3, 9, 15]. The other surgical and nonsurgical modalities include curettage and electrodessication, cryosurgery, radiotherapy, chemotherapy, photodynamic therapy, and immunotherapy. Selection of the appropriate therapy depends on the patient's age, anticipated life expectancy, and the location, size, and pattern of growth characteristics of the tumor. However, therapies that are not surgical and do not include microscopic monitoring should be avoided for BCCs when they are not very small, when they are located in the medial canthus, or when the margins are clinically ill defined. The importance of preventing sun exposure needs to be stressed to children and young adults in order to reduce the incidence of BCC in the future [1].

5.10.1 Surgical Excision

Only by surgical excision of the tumor with safe margins it is possible to assess the adequacy of extirpation. However, in cases with deep infiltration into the orbit or in proximity to the eyeball tissues, excision with safe margins is not possible and exenteration is inevitable. A variety of ways are used to examine the surgical margins, and good results have been reported when frozen-section control is used. Mohs' micrographic surgery has been considered to be the most reliable method for tumor extirpation or as reliable as excision with frozen-section or permanent-section control, with the lowest recurrence rate and best cure rate [15, 21, 22]. As significant extra difficulty, time, and expense of Mohs' surgery may not be justified in all BCCs of the eyelid, and thus it is usually reserved for deeply infiltrative tumors with a high risk of recurrence [6]. An intermediate technique that incorporates Mohs' surgery using formalin-fixed, paraffin-embedded sections (slow Mohs) may offer a histologically superior and cheaper alternative to standard Mohs' surgery [23].

The carbon dioxide laser has a few advantages over the conventional scalpel in the excision of BCC, including the possibility of bloodless excision of tissue in thin layers for histological examination of the margins and the possibility of obviating electrocautery, which is important for patients taking anticoagulants or who have a cardiac pacemaker [1, 6].

Special reconstructive techniques are used to maintain the functions of the eyelid and to achieve the best cosmetic results after surgical excision of periocular BCC (Chap. 10).

5.10.2 Curettage and Electrodesiccation

Curettage and electrodesiccation and, lately, vaporization of the tumor by CO2 laser are commonly used techniques to treat small BCC in areas remote from the eye. As the adequacy of margins is not determined, there is always the risk that residual tumor will escape destruction, especially near embryonic fusion planes. Also, the amount of secondary scarring and contracture with electrodesiccation may be cosmetically unacceptable in the periocular area [1, 6].

5.10.3 Cryotherapy

Cryotherapy is a tissue-sparing modality with no control of the adequacy of tumor removal. It has been suggested that cryotherapy of eyelid BCC with a well-defined border, including tumors larger than 10 mm and tumors in the medial canthal area, has a high cure rate, is cost-effective, well tolerated, and with good cosmetic and functional outcomes [23–26].

5.10.4 Radiation Therapy

The role of radiation therapy in the management of BCC is controversial. It has been found that there is significant recurrence after radiotherapy for BCC [2, 25], and such recurrences, particularly those in the midface, are exceptionally difficult to treat successfully by any means and are at high risk ultimately to cause death [1, 6, 7]. Radiotherapy can be used as an adjuvant therapy to exenteration in cases with orbital invasion by periocular basal cell carcinoma [17].

5.10.5 Chemotherapy and Other Therapies

Chemotherapy is used for cases of non-resectable BCC, when for some reason surgery cannot be undertaken, or for rare cases of metastatic BCC. Cisplatinum chemotherapy, used alone or in combination with doxorubicin or with paclitaxel, has been beneficial in case reports [3, 6, 27]. The results of preliminary studies using retinoids (etretinate and isotretinoin) in the management of BCC have been varied [1, 2, 9, 15].

5.10.5.1 Interferon

Intralesional injection of human recombinant α-interferon was used to treat BCC, with some success [9, 28]. A class of immune response modifier, represented by topical imiquimod cream, was suggested as a potential topical treatment of BCC, either alone or in combination with retinoids [9, 28, 29].

5.10.5.2 Photodynamic Therapy

Photodynamic therapy (PDT) with aminolevulinic acid was suggested as a promising approach in the therapy of dermal lesions of the eyelids [30].

5.10.5.3 Imiquimod

Topical treatments such as imiquimod cream (IMQ) have the advantage of assisting in the removal of BCC without causing collateral structural damage. IMQ is an immune response modifier that causes eventually production of cytokines such as interferon-a. It was reported to be effective for treatment eyelid nodular BCCs with good cosmesis and good functional results [31].

5.10.5.4 Vismodegib

Vismodegib (Erivedge) is a molecular inhibitor of the Hedgehog signaling pathway. The hedgehog signal transduction pathway plays an important role in cell proliferation, and alterations in hedgehog signaling may transform a conjunctival intraepithelial neoplasia into invasive squamous cell carcinoma [32]. It was approved by the FDA in January 2012 for the oral therapy of metastatic and locally advanced BCC. As oral Vismodegib has been shown to be effective in preventing disease progression in patients with metastatic or locally advanced BCC not amenable to surgical excision or radiotherapy [15, 33]. Vismodegib is also used to treat basal cell nevus syndrome (Gorlin syndrome), which is not amenable to surgery and involves numerous cutaneous lesions of the periocular region and face.

Side effects of vismodegib include muscle spasms, alopecia, dysgeusia, dysosmia, weight loss, fatigue, nausea, decreased appetite, diarrhea and even keratoacanthoma and squamous cell carcinoma. Although some patients give up therapy with vismodegib because of these side effects, vismodegib is generally well tolerated with acceptable side effects [34].

5.10.5.5 Pembrolizumab

The PD-L1 inhibitor pembrolizumab has also been used successfully when hedgehog pathway inhibition has failed, suggesting that targeting PD-1 or PD-L1 may be of utility as a salvage treatment or in conjunction with hedgehog inhibition [35].

Although new nonsurgical procedures were found to be promising approaches in the therapy of BCC of the eyelids, none of them are yet an acceptable alternative to surgical excision and are reserved for research or for selected patients.

5.11 Follow-Up

As two-thirds of recurrences appear within 3 years of treatment and 18% appear between 5 and 10 years, long-term clinical follow-up is necessary [1, 3, 9, 15].

5.12 Prognosis

5.12.1 Prognostic Factors

The prognosis of BCC depends mainly on the size of the tumor, its anatomic location, its pattern of infiltrative growth, and the age of the patient [1–3]. Large tumors and location in the medial canthal region are the most important clinical features predicting recurrence.

A high risk for orbital invasion was found for BCC of the medial and lateral canthus [1, 5, 6, 15]. The morpheaform clinical pattern, the histologic finding of an infiltrative growth pattern, or metatypical (basosquamous carcinoma) differentiation have been correlated with deep invasion and greater recurrence after treatment. More aggressive tumors and a higher frequency of recurrence was found in patients under 35 years of age [1, 5, 6, 15].

5.12.2 Local Spread

The vast majority of BCC grow in a slow but relentless manner. However, localized spontaneous regression has been documented [36]. BCC invades along the paths of least resistance and then destroys adjacent tissues (Fig. 5.8). Destruction of bone, cartilage, and muscle is usually seen only in the very late stages of the disease. Invasion of lymphatics is common, but does not correlate with the rarely occurring regional metastasis. Some BCCs follow peripheral nerves and can thereby gain access to deeper tissues. Spread to the central nervous system may occur via cranial nerves, the orbital fissure, and cranial foramina. Intraocular invasion by BCC is rare and usually occurs in advanced cases with orbital invasion. The globe is entered through a sclera emissary canal or an old surgical wound [2, 4, 5].

5.12.3 Recurrence

The recurrence rate of treated BCC of the eyelid averages 4.2% in the short term and 8.7% for more than 5 years. This varies according to the therapeutic method used. Tumors that recur tend to be more aggressive and difficult to manage [1–5, 9].

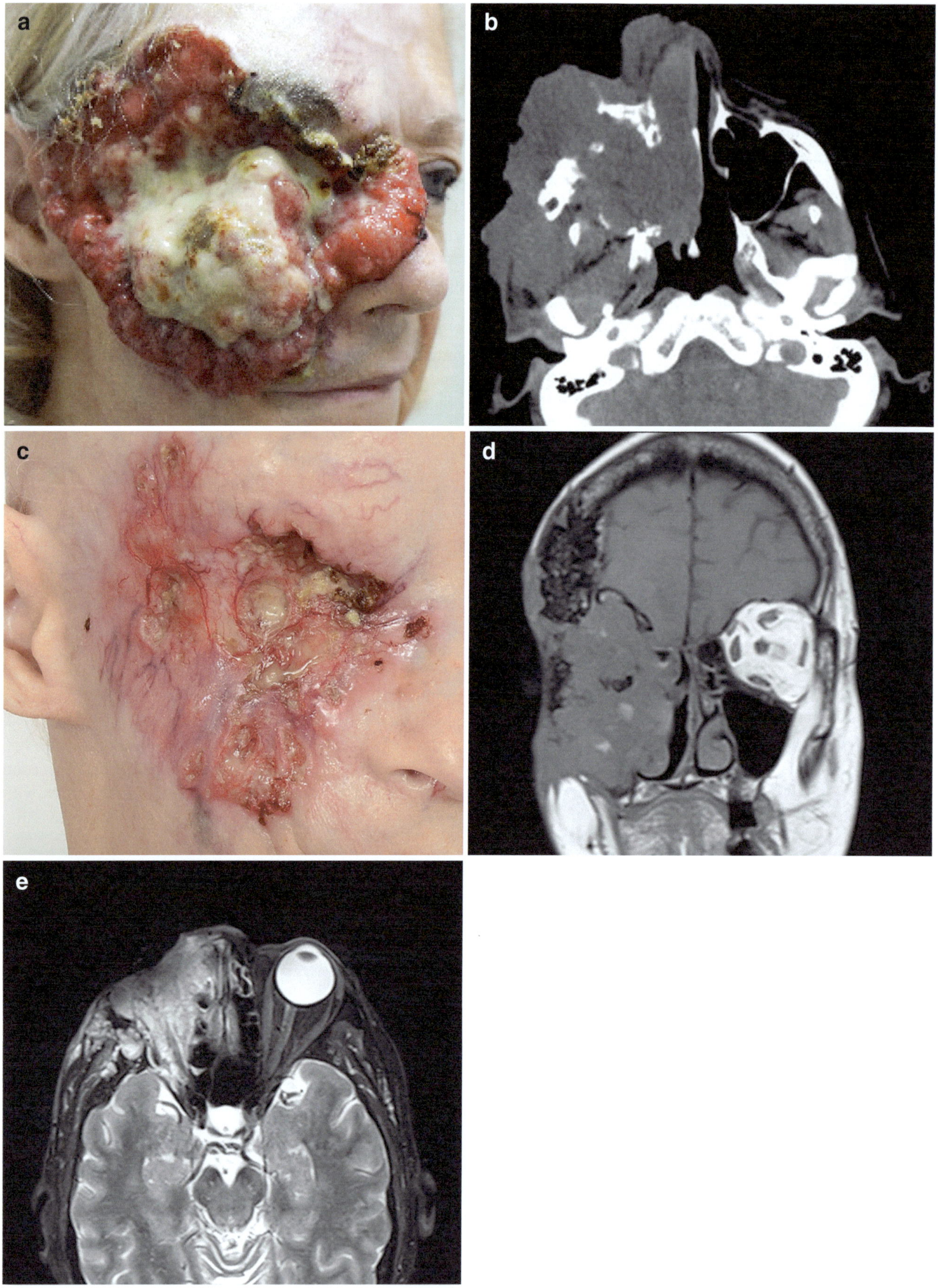

Fig. 5.8 Advanced locally infiltrative infiltrative Basal cell carcinoma (BCC) Advanced locally infiltrative BCC clinically and imaging fidures (**a**–**e**)

5.13 Metastases and Mortality

Metastatic BCC is extremely rare and its rate has been estimated to be between 0.0028 and 0.01%. The most frequent sites of metastasis are the lymph nodes, lungs, bone, liver, and spleen [1–5, 9]. Clinical features suggesting a greater probability of metastasis include multiple recurrences, an aggressive histological appearance, perineural invasion, and a history of previous ionizing radiation. Mortality from eyelid and medial canthal BCC is rare, and all deaths recorded were related to intracranial extension [1–5, 9].

5.14 Staging

According to the applied practical review of the *American Joint Committee on Cancer (AJCC)* seventh edition (Box 5.2) [32, 34, 37], primary BCC 5 mm or less, between 5 and 20 mm in greatest dimension, not invading the tarsal plate or eyelid margin with no involvement of regional lymph nodes and no distant metastasis, were classified as stage I tumors. BCC more than 20 mm in greater dimension or any tumor that invades adjacent ocular or orbital structures were classified as stage II. Stage III was when tumor complete resection requires enucleation, exenteration, or bone resection, when regional lymph node metastasis is evident, or when the tumor is not resectable due to extensive invasion of ocular, orbital, craniofacial structures, or brain. Stage IV is the rare cases with distant metastasis. This classification was found to be a practical tool for staging of carcinoma of the eyelids [3, 9, 15].

Box 5.2 AJCC Cancer Staging of Carcinoma of the Eyelids

Stage I A—primary BCC 5 mm or less in greatest dimension, not invading the tarsal plate or eyelid margin with no involvement of regional lymph nodes and no distant metastasis

Stage I B—primary BCC between 5 and 10 mm in greatest dimension, not invading the tarsal plate or eyelid margin with no involvement of regional lymph nodes and no distant metastasis

Stage I C—primary BCC between 10 and 20 mm in greatest dimension, not invading the tarsal plate or eyelid margin with no involvement of regional lymph nodes and no distant metastasis

Stage II—primary BCC more than 20 mm in greater dimension or any tumor that invades adjacent ocular or orbital structures

Stage III A—when tumor complete resection requires enucleation, exenteration, or bone resection

Stage III B—when regional lymph node metastasis is evident

Stage III C—when the BCC is not resectable due to extensive invasion of ocular, orbital, craniofacial structures, or brain

Stage IV—primary BCC with distant metastasis

References

1. Margo CE, Waltz K. Basal cell carcinoma of the eyelid and periocular skin. Surv Ophthalmol. 1993;38:169–92. https://doi.org/10.1016/0039-6257(93)90100-l.
2. Shi Y, Jia R, Fan X. Ocular basal cell carcinoma: a brief literature review of clinical diagnosis and treatment. Onco Targets Ther. 2017;10:2483–9. https://doi.org/10.2147/OTT.S130371.
3. Yin VT, Merritt HA, Sniegowski M, Esmaeli B. Eyelid and ocular surface carcinoma: diagnosis and management. Clin Dermatol. 2015;33:159–69. https://doi.org/10.1016/j.clindermatol.2014.10.008.
4. Mannor GE, Chern PL, Barnette D. Eyelid and periorbital skin basal cell carcinoma: oculoplastic management and surgery. Int Ophthalmol Clin. 2009;49:1–16. https://doi.org/10.1097/IIO.0b013e3181b7ebe8.
5. Wu A, Sun MT, Huilgol SC, et al. Histological subtypes of periocular basal cell carcinoma. Clin Experiment Ophthalmol. 2014;42:603–7. https://doi.org/10.1111/ceo.12298.
6. Allali J, D'Hermies F, Renard G. Basal cell carcinomas of the eyelids. Ophthalmologica. 2005;219:57–71. https://doi.org/10.1159/000083263.
7. Paavilainen V, Tuominen J, Pukkala E, Saari KM. Basal cell carcinoma of the eyelid in Finland during 1953-97. Acta Ophthalmol Scand. 2005;83:215–20. https://doi.org/10.1111/j.1600-0420.2005.00445.x.
8. Malhotra R, Huilgol SC, Huynh NT, Selva D. The Australian Mohs database, part I: periocular basal cell carcinoma experience over 7 years. Ophthalmology. 2004;111:624–30. https://doi.org/10.1016/j.ophtha.2003.12.003.
9. Gniesmer S, Sonntag SR, Schiemenz C, et al. Diagnosis and treatment of malignant eyelid tumors. Die Ophthalmol. 2024;121:33–9. https://doi.org/10.1007/s00347-023-01945-y.
10. Buljan M, Bulat V, Situm M, et al. Variations in clinical presentation of basal cell carcinoma. Acta Clin Croat. 2008;47:25–30.
11. Rass K, Reichrath J. UV damage and DNA repair in malignant melanoma and nonmelanoma skin cancer. Adv Exp Med Biol. 2008;624:162–78. https://doi.org/10.1007/978-0-387-77574-6_13.
12. Tchernev G, Kordeva S, Lozev I. Giant basal cell carcinoma of the scalp: rotation advancement flap as a successful dermatosurgical approach. Dermatol Reports. 2023;15:9664. https://doi.org/10.4081/dr.2023.9664.
13. Lim LT, Agarwal PK, Young D, et al. The effect of socio-economic status on severity of periocular basal cell carcinoma at presentation. Ophthalmic Plast Reconstr Surg. 2015;31:456–8. https://doi.org/10.1097/IOP.0000000000000386.
14. Yin VT, Pfeiffer ML, Esmaeli B. Targeted therapy for orbital and periocular basal cell carcinoma and squamous cell carcinoma. Ophthalmic Plast Reconstr Surg. 2013;29:87–92. https://doi.org/10.1097/IOP.0b013e3182831bf3.
15. Zgolli H, Choura R, Elzarrug HKH, et al. Management of eyelids' primary malignancies. Libyan J Med. 2023;18:2258668. https://doi.org/10.1080/19932820.2023.2258668.
16. Wade TR, Ackerman AB. The many faces of basal-cell carcinoma. J Dermatol Surg Oncol. 1978;4:23–8. https://doi.org/10.1111/j.1524-4725.1978.tb00375.x.
17. Bakis S, Irwig L, Wood G, Wong D. Exfoliative cytology as a diagnostic test for basal cell carcinoma: a meta-analysis. Br J Dermatol. 2004;150:829–36. https://doi.org/10.1111/j.1365-2133.2004.05716.x.
18. Leibovitch I, McNab A, Sullivan T, et al. Orbital invasion by periocular basal cell carcinoma. Ophthalmology. 2005;112:717–23. https://doi.org/10.1016/j.ophtha.2004.11.036.
19. Nori S, Rius-Díaz F, Cuevas J, et al. Sensitivity and specificity of reflectance-mode confocal microscopy for in vivo diagnosis of basal cell carcinoma: a multicenter study. J Am Acad Dermatol. 2004;51:923–30. https://doi.org/10.1016/j.jaad.2004.06.028.
20. Allan E, Pye DA, Levine EL, Moore JV. Non-invasive pulsed ultrasound quantification of the resolution of basal cell carcinomas after photodynamic therapy. Lasers Med Sci. 2002;17:230–7. https://doi.org/10.1007/s101030200034.
21. Cook BE, Bartley GB (2001) Treatment options and future prospects for the management of eyelid malignancies: an evidence-based update . Ophthalmology 108:2088–2098; quiz 2099–100, 2121. https://doi.org/10.1016/s0161-6420(01)00796-5.
22. Marra DE, Torres A, Schanbacher CF, Gonzalez S. Detection of residual basal cell carcinoma by in vivo confocal microscopy. Dermatologic Surg. 2005;31:538–41. https://doi.org/10.1111/j.1524-4725.2005.31157.
23. Malhotra R, Huilgol SC, Huynh NT, Selva D. The Australian Mohs database, part II: periocular basal cell carcinoma outcome at 5-year follow-up. Ophthalmology. 2004;111:631–6. https://doi.org/10.1016/j.ophtha.2003.11.004.
24. Morris DS, Elzaridi E, Clarke L, et al. Periocular basal cell carcinoma: 5-year outcome following Slow Mohs surgery with formalin-fixed paraffin-embedded sections and delayed closure. Br J Ophthalmol. 2009;93:474–6. https://doi.org/10.1136/bjo.2008.141325.
25. Jaramillo-Ayerbe F. Cryosurgery in difficult to treat basal cell carcinoma. Int J Dermatol. 2000;39:223–9. https://doi.org/10.1046/j.1365-4362.2000.00952.x.
26. Lindgren G, Larkö O. Long-term follow-up of cryosurgery of basal cell carcinoma of the eyelid. J Am Acad Dermatol. 1997;36:742–6. https://doi.org/10.1016/s0190-9622(97)80328-3.
27. Lindgren G, Larkö O. Cryosurgery of eyelid basal cell carcinomas including 781 cases treated over 30 years. Acta Ophthalmol. 2014;92:787–92. https://doi.org/10.1111/aos.12441.
28. Avril MF, Auperin A, Margulis A, et al. Basal cell carcinoma of the face: surgery or radiotherapy? Results of a randomized study. Br J Cancer. 1997;76:100–6. https://doi.org/10.1038/bjc.1997.343.
29. Jefford M, Kiffer JD, Somers G, et al. Metastatic basal cell carcinoma: rapid symptomatic response to cisplatin and paclitaxel. ANZ J Surg. 2004;74:704–5. https://doi.org/10.1111/j.1445-1433.2004.03130.x.
30. Wang I, Bauer B, Andersson-Engels S, et al. Photodynamic therapy utilising topical delta-aminolevulinic acid in non-melanoma skin malignancies of the eyelid and the periocular skin. Acta Ophthalmol Scand. 1999;77. https://doi.org/10.1034/J.1600-0420.1999.770213.X.
31. Ingves C, Jemec GBE. Combined imiquimod and acitretin for non-surgical treatment of basal cell carcinoma. Scand J Plast Reconstr Surg Hand Surg. 2003;37:293–5. https://doi.org/10.1080/02844310310001724.
32. Celebi ARC, Kiratli H, Soylemezoglu F. Evaluation of the "hedgehog" signaling pathways in squamous and basal cell carcinomas of the eyelids and conjunctiva. Oncol Lett. 2016;12:467–72. https://doi.org/10.3892/ol.2016.4625.
33. Rhodes LE, de Rie M, Enström Y, et al. Photodynamic therapy using topical methyl aminolevulinate vs surgery for nodular basal cell carcinoma: results of a multicenter randomized prospective

trial. Arch Dermatol. 2004;140:17–23. https://doi.org/10.1001/archderm.140.1.17.
34. Demirci H, Worden F, Nelson CC, et al. Efficacy of Vismodegib (Erivedge) for basal cell carcinoma involving the orbit and periocular area. Ophthalmic Plast Reconstr Surg. 2015;31:463–6. https://doi.org/10.1097/IOP.0000000000000388.
35. Lipson EJ, Lilo MT, Ogurtsova A, et al. Basal cell carcinoma: PD-L1/PD-1 checkpoint expression and tumor regression after PD-1 blockade. J Immunother Cancer. 2017;5:23. https://doi.org/10.1186/s40425-017-0228-3.
36. Garcia-Martin E, Gil-Arribas LM, Idoipe M, et al. Comparison of imiquimod 5% cream versus radiotherapy as treatment for eyelid basal cell carcinoma. Br J Ophthalmol. 2011;95:1393–6. https://doi.org/10.1136/bjo.2010.193078.
37. Sekulic A, Migden MR, Oro AE, et al. Efficacy and safety of vismodegib in advanced basal-cell carcinoma. N Engl J Med. 2012;366 https://doi.org/10.1056/NEJMOA1113713.

Squamous Cell Carcinoma

6

Ofira Zloto and Mordechai Rosner

6.1 Introduction

Squamous cell carcinoma (SCC) is an invasive epithelial malignancy that arises from the prickle–squamous cell layers of the epidermis and shows keratinocytic differentiation. It is capable of metastasis to regional lymph nodes, orbital and/or intracranial invasion, and distant spread and is potentially lethal. SCC was first distinguished from basal cell carcinoma by Kompecher in 1902 [1, 2]. The terms "squamous cell epithelioma," "epidermoid carcinoma," "epithelioma spinocellular," "prickle cell epithelioma," and "spinalioma" have all been used in the literature, but "squamous cell carcinoma" is the preferred terminology.

6.2 Epidemiological Aspects

The incidence of eyelid SCC varies from 0.9 to 2.42 cases per 100,000, with the highest incidence reported from Australia [2–6]. In most populations, SCC is the second most common malignant neoplasm of the eyelids after basal cell carcinoma (BCC) comprising 5–10% of all eyelid malignancies [1, 4, 5]. However, in India, China, and Japan, the proportion of BCC and sebaceous gland carcinoma (SGC) was found to be almost equal, and even reverse [7], in contrast to most other countries, where the reported incidence of SCC relative to BCC ranges from 1:11 to 1:40 [8–10].

6.3 Etiology

Extrinsic risk factors for SCC include ultraviolet light and actinic damage, exposure to arsenic, hydrocarbons, radiation, or immunosuppressive drugs [2, 11]. Intrinsic risk factors include albinism, preexisting chronic skin lesions, and genetic skin disorders such as xeroderma pigmentosum and epidermodysplasia verruciformis [2, 12].

O. Zloto · M. Rosner (✉)
Department of Ophthalmology, Goldschleger Eye Institute, Sheba Medical Center, School of Medicine, Tel Aviv University, Tel Aviv, Israel

6.4 Clinical Features

SCC occurs most commonly in fair-skinned elderly individuals who have a history of chronic sun exposure [2, 12–14]. The majority of patients with SCC are 60 years of age or older [8, 12, 13]. It has been suggested that the distinct male predominance may represent increased occupational sunlight exposure by males, rather than a genetic predisposition [12].

Periocular SCC occurs most frequently on the lower eyelid, followed by the medial canthus, the upper eyelid, and the lateral canthus, in that order of frequency. The preponderance of lower-lid involvement in SCC is not as pronounced as in BCC. In some series, SCC of the medial canthus has outnumbered those confined to the eyelid. SCC also has a predilection for the eyelid margin [8, 14, 15].

6.5 Symptoms and Signs

Although the clinical presentation of SCC varies, most often it appears as a painless, elevated, nodular, or plaque-like lesion with chronic scaling and fissuring of the skin. Pearly irregular borders and a tendency to develop ulceration with irregular rolled edges are also characteristic features (Box 6.1) [2, 13]. In a well-differentiated tumor, keratin gives the lesion a grayish-white, granular appearance (Fig. 6.1). Additional presenting features include a small erythematous scaly patch, a cyst-like lesion, a papillomatous lesion, a cutaneous horn, and a large ulcerated lesion. The edges of the lesion are well circumscribed in some cases and ill defined in others [1, 12, 13].

Patients with SCC tend to have other tumors of the skin, including intraepidermal carcinoma (Bowen's disease),

B. C. K. Patel et al. (eds.), *Clinical Ophthalmic Oncology*, https://doi.org/10.1007/978-3-031-72328-5_6

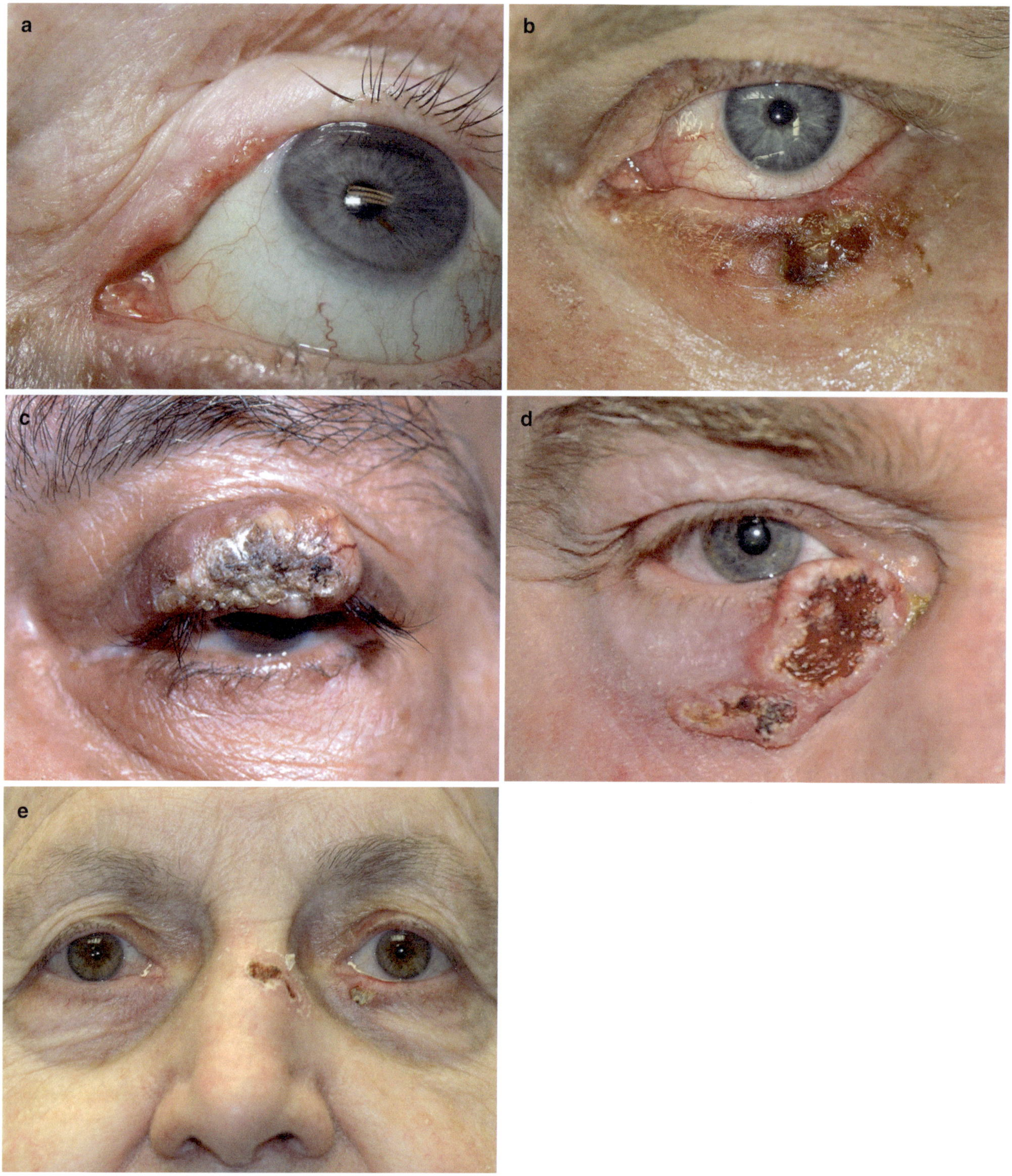

Fig. 6.1 Spectrun of clinical features. Ulcerative squamous cell carcinoma right upper eyelid (**a**, Courtesy of Bhupender **c**. Patel, MD Salt Lake City, Utah, USA). Note the destruction of the eyelid margin with loss of Meibomian gland orifices and loss of lashes. Patient was treated as having blepharitis for more than a year. Left lower eyelid ulcerative squamous cell carcinoma (**b**, Courtesy of Bhupender **c**. Patel, MD Salt Lake City, Utah, USA). Although most squamous cell carcinomas will not have a pearly nodular rim, ulceration can make these lesions look like basal cell carcinomas. Squamous cell carcinoma of the upper lid (**c**) and lower eyelid (**d**) presenting as an irregular, elevated lesion with masses of keratin. Squamous cell carcinoma of the nasal bridge and left lower eyelid. Beware of multiple skin malignancies (**e**, Courtesy of Bhupender C. Patel, MD Salt Lake City, Utah, USA)

senile keratosis, and basal cell carcinoma [1]. Bowen's disease represents full-thickness involvement of the epidermis by neoplastic cells (carcinoma in situ) with a relatively high risk of progression to invasive SCC [10]. Its clinical manifestation is of a persistent and slowly enlarging erythematous, scaly, or crusted lesion with a sharp, irregular outline [1, 2, 12, 13].

6.6 Histopathologic Features

6.6.1 Pathogenesis

SCC arises from the epidermal prickle and squamous cells. Although it may develop de novo, actinic keratosis, Bowen's disease, and radiation dermatoses are all precursors to the development of SCC [2, 9, 12, 16].

6.6.2 Evolution

SCC of the eyelid usually begins with an early epithelial phase referred to as actinic keratosis (senile keratosis, solar keratosis), with subtotal replacement of the epidermis by atypical cells (intraepithelial squamous dysplasia). Intraepithelial squamous cell carcinoma or squamous cell carcinoma in situ is diagnosed when there is complete disorganization of the epidermis, with numerous atypical cells that are rounded, large, and with homogeneous, eosinophilic cytoplasm. Invasion of the dermis is the hallmark for the histopathologic diagnosis of invasive SCC (Fig. 6.2) [2, 16].

6.6.3 Light Microscopic Features

The invading cells show different degrees of differentiation leading to variable histologic features. In well-differentiated tumors, the cells are polygonal, with abundant acidophilic cytoplasm and prominent hyperchromatic nuclei that vary in size and staining properties. Characteristic findings are of abnormal keratinization with dyskeratotic cells and keratin pearls and intercellular bridges. Poorly differentiated lesions show an increased degree of cellular anaplasia, with irregularly shaped and sized cells, enlarged nuclei, abnormal mitoses, little or no evidence of keratinization, and loss of intercellular bridges (Fig. 6.3).

Histological subtypes associated with metastatic risk include adenosquamous and desmoplastic lesions. The adenosquamous subtype, though rare, exhibits a propensity for locoregional recurrence, displaying both squamous and glandular features of differentiation. The latter can be identified through positive staining for anticarcinoembryonic antigen.

Desmoplasia refers to the formation of a dense peritumoral collagenous stroma in response to tumor cell activation. This process involves the degradation of the normal extracellular matrix to facilitate tumor growth [12]. Histologically, desmoplastic SCC is characterized by atypical keratinocytes arranged in an infiltrative pattern of nests and strands, accompanied by prominent stromal changes. Particularly in the periocular region, these aggressive lesions pose a significant risk of orbital invasion.

Another histological subtype inclined toward unfavorable outcomes is spindle cell (sarcomatoid) SCC, especially when

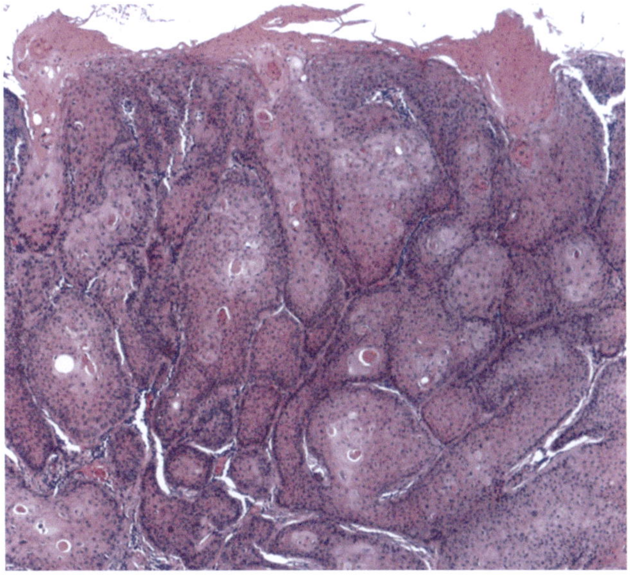

Fig. 6.2 Invasive well-differentiated squamous cell carcinoma showing invasion of the dermis by tumor polygonal cells that vary in size and staining properties

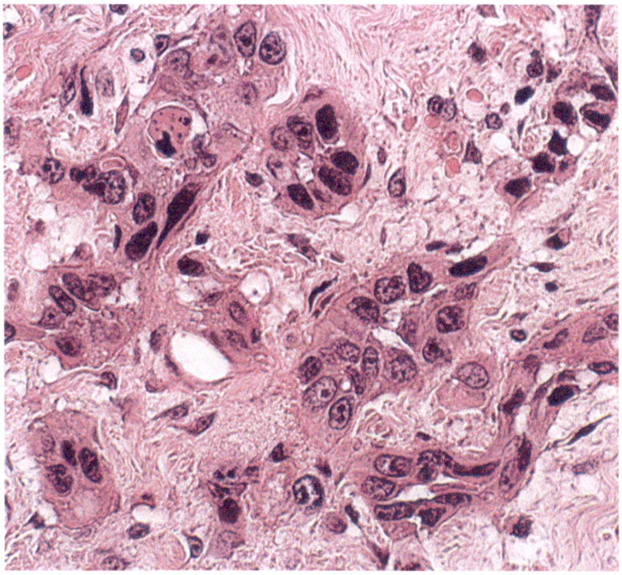

Fig. 6.3 Poorly differentiated squamous cell carcinoma showing cellular anaplasia with irregularly shaped and sized cells, enlarged nuclei, and no evidence of keratinization

originating from previous radiotherapy sites rather than developing as a de novo lesion.

6.7 Diagnostic Evaluation

Because of its variable clinical presentation, biopsy and histological examination are required for an accurate diagnosis [1]. Examination of the face or extremities for other types of premalignant lesions may aid in the diagnosis [1, 13].

In comparison to BCC, SCC exhibits a more aggressive nature characterized by faster and more invasive growth, and it frequently demonstrates orbital invasion. Moreover, lymph node metastases have been reported in up to 25% of cases, with the possibility of distant metastases. Consequently, it is imperative to conduct ultrasound staging of locoregional lymph nodes, potentially supplemented by CT imaging of the neck/chest and lymph node biopsy if there are suspicions of lymph node metastases. In cases where distant metastases are suspected, whole-body CT in the form of fluorodeoxyglucose (FDG) positron-emission tomography (PET)/CT is a suitable diagnostic approach.

6.8 Differential Diagnosis

SCC of the eyelid and periocular region typically has no pathognomonic feature that allows its differentiation from other cutaneous lesions, and it may mimic many other types of skin lesion, both benign and malignant [1, 2, 9, 12].

6.9 Tumor Markers

6.9.1 Programmed Cell Death Ligand 1

Programmed cell death ligand 1 (PD-L1) is a transmembrane glycoprotein with the capability to bind to Tumor-Infiltrating Lymphocytes (TILs), allowing it to elude immune detection and facilitate lymphatic metastasis [2, 8, 9, 14]. The intensity of PD-1 staining is categorized into three grades: grade 1 (5–10% of tumor cells with positive membranous staining), grade 2 (10–25% positive staining), or grade 3 (>25% positive staining). A histological examination involving 40 primary and 5 metastatic cutaneous SCC revealed an association between PD-L1 expression and high-risk pathological features, including tumor thickness, large-caliber Perineural Invasion (PNI), and poor differentiation.

6.9.2 P300

P300 is a transcriptional coactivating protein that plays a role in various cellular processes such as proliferation, differentiation, and apoptosis. It was shown in cutaneous SCC specimens, that elevated p300 expression, defined as positive immunohistochemical staining in more than 55% of tumor cells, was linked to poorer recurrence-free survival and overall survival in multivariate analysis [6, 8, 9].

6.9.3 Epidermal Growth Factor Receptor

Activation of the epidermal growth factor receptor in cutaneous SCC has been proposed to promote the proliferation of tumor cells by evading apoptosis. Nevertheless, the literature on its prognostic significance in predicting metastatic risk from advanced cutaneous SCC remains inconclusive [17–19]. While upregulation of the epidermal growth factor receptor has been linked to nodal metastasis in primary cutaneous SCC, a study involving patients with advanced head and neck SCC found no significant association between epidermal growth factor receptor expression and metastasis (either regional or distant). Furthermore, there was no correlation with clinicopathologic variables.

6.10 Gene Expression Profiling

An innovative approach to enhance the precision of metastasis prediction in cutaneous SCC involves the use of a 40-gene expression profile (40-GEP) test. This introduces the possibility of personalized prognostication, categorizing patients into three risk groups: Class 1 (low risk), Class 2A (high risk), or Class 2B (very high risk) [20]. The Class 2B subgroup, with a risk of ≥50% for metastasis, is recommended to undergo aggressive high-intensity management strategies. Conversely, patients in the Class 1 category would require only low-intensity management, involving 1–2 visits per year, clinical nodal assessment, and thereby eliminating the necessity for systemic therapy or adjuvant radiotherapy [15].

6.11 Treatment

6.11.1 Preventive

Prevention by minimizing sun exposure, especially in childhood and adolescence, remains of prime importance in minimizing the morbidity and mortality associated with SCC [8, 12, 15, 21].

6.11.2 Therapeutic

The main treatment modality used for eyelid SCC is surgical excision, with microscopic monitoring of the margins or Mohs' microsurgery. A variety of other forms of therapy were suggested, such as radiation therapy, cryotherapy, chemotherapy, curettage with carbon dioxide laser, photodynamic therapy, and treatment with retinoids or α-interferon. When used alone, these therapies have high recurrence rates, which are not acceptable for SCC of the eyelid, where recurrent tumors can be more aggressive and invasive. However, they may be appropriate for patients who cannot tolerate or who decline surgery [1, 8, 21, 22].

6.11.2.1 Surgery

Only surgical excision with monitoring of the margins, using either a frozen-section, or a paraffin-section control, or Mohs' micrographic surgery is an acceptable treatment option for periocular SCC [1, 8, 21, 22]. The treatment of choice for secondary orbital invasion of SCC is orbital exenteration [1, 6, 15].

6.11.2.2 Sentinel Lymph Node Biopsy

The presence of regional lymph node metastases is the single most important prognostic factor for most solid neoplasms, and complete lymph node dissection with pathologic examination of a cross section of a lymph node is considered the gold standard in staging patients for adjuvant therapy. However, its therapeutic value is questionable, and it may be associated with considerable morbidity [4]. The sentinel lymph node biopsy has been suggested as a potentially useful technique to stage periocular SCC, especially in patients with recurrent, large, or highly invasive lesions or those with perineural invasion (Chap. 12) [8, 11, 12, 15].

6.11.2.3 Radiation Therapy

Radiation therapy has been used in the treatment of eyelid malignancies since the beginning of the twentieth century. SCC is relatively radioresistant and responds even less than BCC to radiation [2, 6, 13, 15, 21, 22]. However, postoperative radiotherapy has been recommended in all patients with microscopic perineural invasion, as the role of surgery in the treatment of perineural spread seems to be only palliative [1, 23].

Three-dimensional conformal planning or intensity-modulated radiation therapy is needed to minimize damage to adjacent structures, and synchronous chemotherapy should be considered to potentiate the effectiveness of radiation. It was suggested that primary radiotherapy for SCC of the eyelid provides high control rates with good function and cosmesis and should be considered an alternative to surgery in selected patients [23].

6.11.2.4 Chemotherapy

Chemotherapy may be used for patients with systemic disease and for those who cannot tolerate surgical excision or who decline surgery [6, 13, 15, 24]. It is usually used as an adjuvant to surgery and radiotherapy in aggressive infiltrating SCC.

6.11.2.5 Topical Therapy

Topical treatments such as with fluorouracil (5-FU) cream and imiquimod cream (IMQ) were found to be effective treatments for SCC of the eyelids in only very small series of patients. Topical 5% 5-FU cream was found to be useful in the treatment of squamous cell carcinoma in situ involving the eyelid, including the eyelid margin [1, 6, 25]. Topical 5% IQ treatment was reported as successful in cases with intraepidermal as well as invasive SCC of the eyelids.

6.11.2.6 Photodynamic Therapy

Photodynamic therapy (PDT) was suggested as treatment for patients with multiple or large SCC or in whom surgery is not appropriate [4, 15, 26, 27].

6.11.2.7 Checkpoint Inhibitors

PD-1 inhibitors (Cemiplimab) have been FDA approved SCC. Additionally, EGFR inhibitors, including Cetuximab, were suggested in certain cases [28].

6.12 Prognosis

6.12.1 Prognostic Factors

High-risk eyelid SCC lesions are those larger than 2 cm, with poor histological differentiation, deep invasion, and the presence of perineural invasion [12, 15, 16, 29]. Recurrent tumors and tumors developing in scars or in immunocompromised patients also imply a poor prognosis [30, 31]. The histologic variant of adenoid SCC is associated with a better prognosis [8, 9, 12].

6.12.2 Staging

According to the applied practical review of the American Joint Committee on Cancer (AJCC) seventh edition [9, 12, 30], primary SCC is classified into stages I, II, III, and IV stages according to size, adjacent invasion, complete resection that requires enucleation, exenteration or bone resection, involvement of regional lymph nodes, extensive invasion making the tumor not resectable, and evidence of distant metastasis. This classification was found to be a practical tool for staging of carcinoma of the eyelids [32].

Box 6.1 Salient Diagnostic Features of Squamous Cell Carcinoma

- Painless nodular, plaque-like, or ulcerated lesions with scaling and fissuring of the skin and irregular, rolled, pearly borders
- Microscopic findings of infiltrative neoplasm arising from the epidermis and composed of polygonal cells with abundant acidophilic cytoplasm and prominent, hyperchromatic, pleomorphic nuclei
- The presence of dyskeratotic cells with the formation of keratin pearls and intercellular bridges

6.12.3 Local Spread

Eyelid SCC is potentially fatal and responsible for considerable morbidity [15]. Aggressive or neglected cases of eyelid SCC may spread into the lacrimal passages, the orbit, and the intracranial cavity. SCC is by far the most frequent of the secondary epithelial neoplasms in the orbit [33]. However, orbital invasion is a rare complication that has been reported to occur in 2.5% of all eyelid BCC and SCC [1]. Orbital invasion of eyelid SCC may take years to occur, often preceded by several surgical interventions, irradiations, and recurrences of the tumor. If left unattended, the entire orbital region and a major portion of the face are destroyed in an ulcerating fungating crater [1]. Orbital spread is usually associated with complete ptosis, ophthalmoplegia, and proptosis. Eventually, involvement of the orbital nerves and bones causes severe and constant pain [1, 12, 33].

6.12.4 Perineural Spread

Perineural spread of SCC occurs in up to 14% of facial lesions [34, 35]. The perineural infiltration of SCC of the eyelids along branches of the trigeminal nerve, the extraocular motor nerves, and the facial nerve facilitates its spread into the orbit, periorbital structures, and intracranial cavity (Fig. 6.4) [34, 35]. Once clinical signs or symptoms of perineural spread have developed, the prognosis is poor, with around 50% recurrence after simple excision [34, 35].

6.12.5 Local Recurrence

The 5-year local recurrence rate for SCC is about 23%. The 5-year metastatic rates vary between 5% and 45% [36]. The recurrence rate of periocular squamous intraepithelial carcinoma is 5% and 12% for primary and recurrent lesions, respectively [2, 15].

6.12.6 Metastasis

Unlike BCC, SCC has a tendency to metastasize to regional lymph nodes and distant sites through hematogenous and lymphatic pathways. The incidence of lymph node metastasis from eyelid SCC has ranged from 0% to as high as 21%, and of distant metastasis varies from 1% to 21% [6, 14, 15, 33]. The incidence of metastasis of SCC arising from actinic keratoses is lower than for SCC arising de novo.

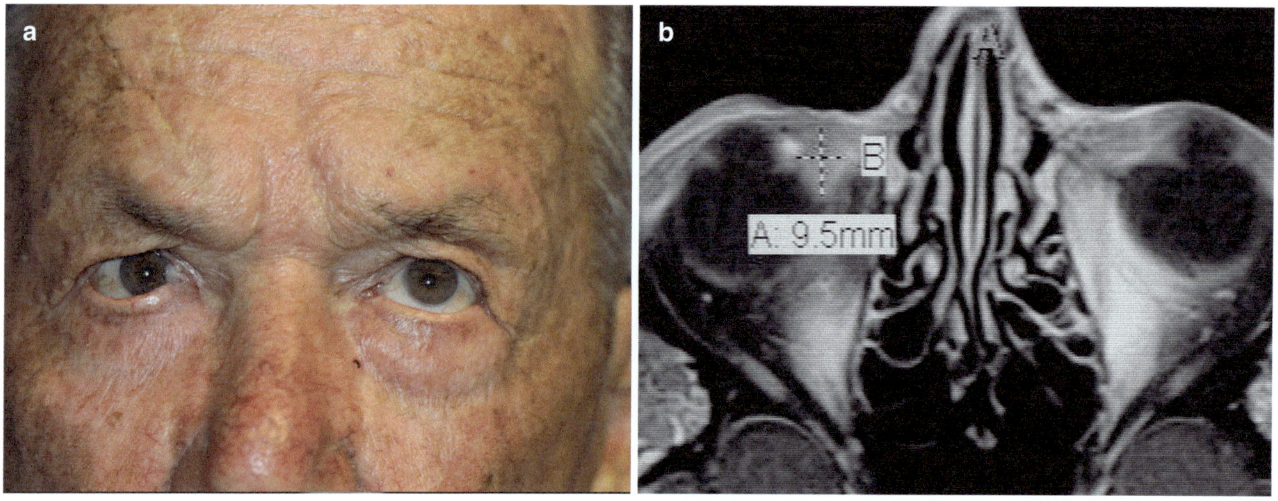

Fig. 6.4 Invasive right medial canthal squamous cell carcinoma with limitation of movement of the right eye (**a**) with deep orbital extension (**b**). Courtesy of Bhupender C. Patel, MD Salt Lake City, Utah, USA

6.12.7 Mortality

The tumor-related mortality rates have been reported to be as high as 40%, and an increased rate is associated with lesions of the upper lid and medial canthus [6, 8, 9]. However, if detected early and treated adequately, the prognosis of SCC is generally excellent and the risk of death and disability can be minimized [1, 2, 6, 33].

6.13 Variants of SCC Including Keratoacanthoma

Less common histologic variants of SCC include the spindle cell and adenoid (adenoacanthoma or pseudoglandular) squamous cell carcinoma. The adenoid SCC variant is characterized by extensive acantholysis and tubular and pseudoglandular patterns [1, 2, 6]. Keratoacanthoma is indistinguishable from squamous cell carcinoma clinically as well as histopathologically (keratocarcinoma or keratoacanthoma-like squamous cell carcinoma) [36]. However, because keratoacanthoma may regress, it is considered to be a variant of squamous cell carcinoma.

6.13.1 Keratoacanthoma

Keratoacanthoma was first described by Sir Jonathan Hutchinson in 1889 as a crateriform ulcer of the face and was classified for many years as a benign skin lesion [37]. Although there are many variants of the disease, it usually presents as a solitary rapidly growing lesion. The suggested etiology is diverse, ranging from ultraviolet exposure, viral infection by human papilloma virus, immunosuppression, and genetic susceptibility [38].

6.13.1.1 Epidemiology

The annual incidence of cutaneous keratoacanthoma varies according to geographical location and is estimated to be 100–150 cases per 100,000 in sun-exposed areas (e.g., northern parts of Australia). It is considered more prevalent in males and affects patients in their fifth to seventh decades [37].

6.13.1.2 Clinical Features

The lesion begins as a small flesh-colored papule that develops rapidly over 4–8 weeks to a lesion typically 5–25 mm in diameter with a central, keratin-filled crater (Fig. 6.5), followed by a stationary phase of similar duration, and a resolution phase may develop in up to 6 months duration (Fig. 6.6). The keratoacanthoma has smooth borders that merge with the surrounding skin, and some present with erythema surrounding the base of the lesion and with telangiectases running over the surface of the tumor. The macroscopic sequelae are rare, generally only a mildly depressed scar. The tumor is most commonly seen on sun-exposed hair-bearing areas, mainly on the face, forearms, and hands. In the eyelids, it is considered not common [39, 40].

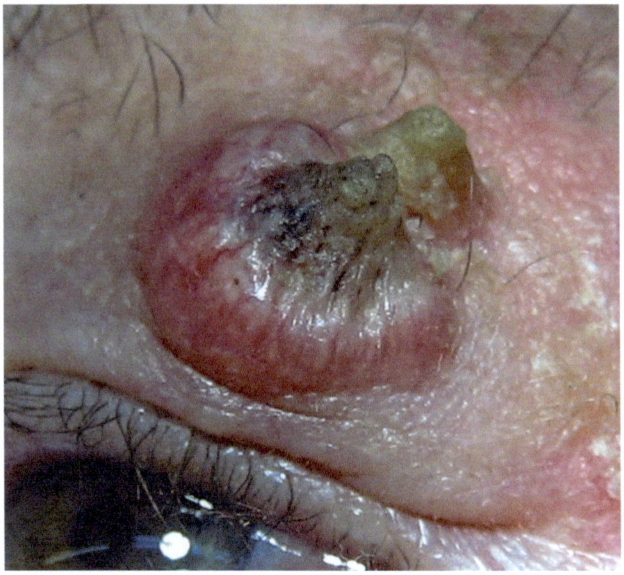

Fig. 6.5 Keratoacanthoma is a nodular lesion with a central keratin-filled crater

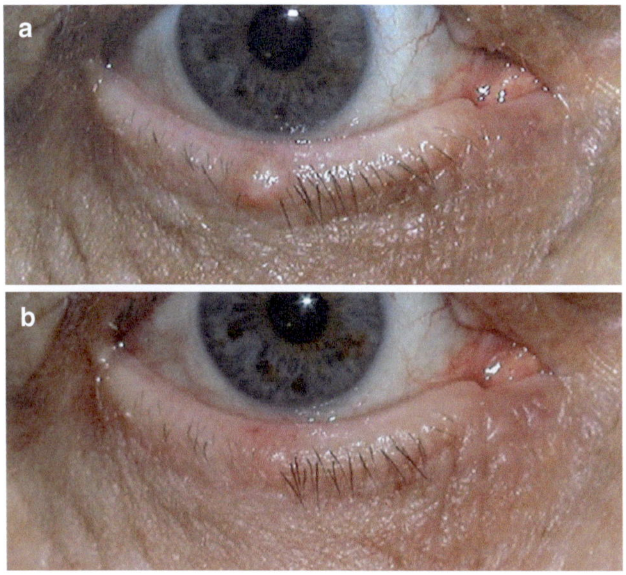

Fig. 6.6 Keratoacanthoma (**a**) with spontaneous resolution 2 weeks later (**b**)

There are several rare variants of keratoacanthoma, which include the giant keratoacanthoma (>3 cm in diameter), keratoacanthoma centrifugum marginatum, subungual keratoacanthoma (keratoacanthoma of the nail), and mucosal keratoacanthoma. Keratoacanthomas are usually solitary lesions. However, there are a number of syndromes that feature multiple keratoacanthomas, including the Muir–Torre syndrome, a generalized eruptive variant of Grzybowski, and the Ferguson-Smith syndrome.

6.13.1.3 Histopathologic Features

Keratoacanthoma typically has a dome-shaped elevation and thickening of the epidermis, surrounding a central mass of keratin (Fig. 6.7). Microabscesses may be present within islands of squamous epithelium that may show atypia. The dermis shows a polymorphous inflammatory infiltrate [39, 40].

6.13.1.4 Treatment

Some advocate a wait-and-watch strategy for keratoacanthoma, since the tumor can regress spontaneously. However, since tumor excision provides tissue for accurate histological diagnosis, hastens cure, and prevents growth of possible squamous cell carcinoma, surgical excision with margin control using frozen sections or Mohs' surgery should be considered for such lesions in the periocular area [6, 8, 13, 33]. Alternative treatment modalities described include radiotherapy, cryotherapy, topical or intralesional 5-fluorouracil, and topical application of 5% imiquimod cream.

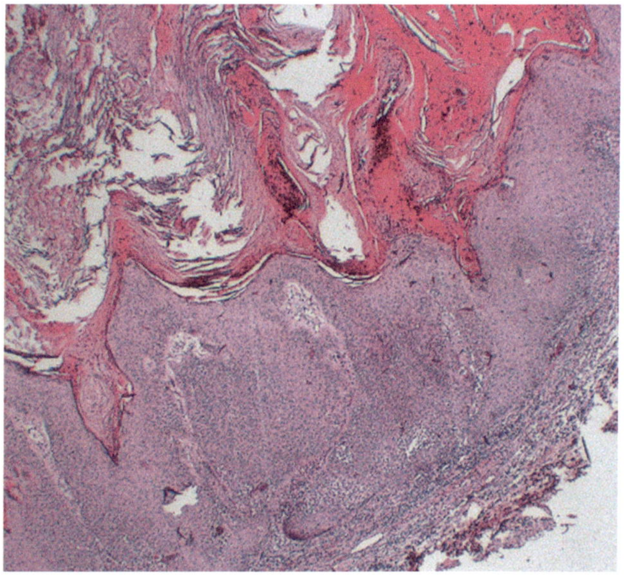

Fig. 6.7 Histologically, variable squamous atypia may be seen at the base of the lesion, and inflammatory infiltrate is present in the dermis

References

1. Reifler DM, Hornblass A. Squamous cell carcinoma of the eyelid. Surv Ophthalmol. 1986;30:349–65. https://doi.org/10.1016/0039-6257(86)90089-5.
2. Thosani MK, Schneck G, Jones EC. Periocular squamous cell carcinoma. Dermatologic Surg. 2008;34:585–99. https://doi.org/10.1111/j.1524-4725.2007.34115.x.
3. Scotto J, Kopf AW, Urbach F. Non-melanoma skin cancer among Caucasians in four areas of the United States. Cancer. 1974;34:1333–8. https://doi.org/10.1002/1097-0142(197410)34:4<1333::aid-cncr2820340447>3.0.co;2-a.
4. Cook BE, Bartley GB. Epidemiologic characteristics and clinical course of patients with malignant eyelid tumors in an incidence cohort in Olmsted County, Minnesota. Ophthalmology. 1999;106:746–50. https://doi.org/10.1016/S0161-6420(99)90161-6.
5. Malhotra R, Huilgol SC, Huynh NT, Selva D. The Australian Mohs database: periocular squamous cell carcinoma. Ophthalmology. 2004;111:617–23. https://doi.org/10.1016/j.ophtha.2003.07.020.
6. Limawararut V, Leibovitch I, Sullivan T, Selva D. Periocular squamous cell carcinoma. Clin Experiment Ophthalmol. 2007;35:174–85. https://doi.org/10.1111/j.1442-9071.2006.01411.x.
7. Lim VSY, Amrith S. Declining incidence of eyelid cancers in Singapore over 13 years: population-based data from 1996 to 2008. Br J Ophthalmol. 2012;96:1462–5. https://doi.org/10.1136/bjophthalmol-2012-302032.
8. Silverman N, Shinder R. What's new in eyelid tumors. Asia Pac J Ophthalmol (Philadelphia, Pa). 2017;6:143–52. https://doi.org/10.22608/APO.201701.
9. Maheshwari A, Finger PT. Cancers of the eye. Cancer Metastasis Rev. 2018;37:677–90. https://doi.org/10.1007/s10555-018-9762-9.
10. Kwitko ML, Boniuk M, Zimmerman LE. Eyelid tumors with reference to lesions confused with squamous cell carcinoma. I. Incidence and errors in diagnosis. Arch Ophthalmol (Chicago, Ill 1960). 1963;69:693–7. https://doi.org/10.1001/archopht.1963.00960040699003.
11. Maclean H, Dhillon B, Ironside J. Squamous cell carcinoma of the eyelid and the acquired immunodeficiency syndrome. Am J Ophthalmol. 1996;121:219–21. https://doi.org/10.1016/s0002-9394(14)70593-8.
12. Donaldson MJ, Sullivan TJ, Whitehead KJ, Williamson RM. Squamous cell carcinoma of the eyelids. Br J Ophthalmol. 2002;86:1161–5. https://doi.org/10.1136/bjo.86.10.1161.
13. Cook BE, Bartley GB. Treatment options and future prospects for the management of eyelid malignancies: an evidence-based update. Ophthalmology. 2001;108:2088–98.; quiz 2099–100, 2121. https://doi.org/10.1016/s0161-6420(01)00796-5.
14. Watson AH, Akbani S, Homer N, et al. Adnexal squamous cell carcinoma: incidence of eyelid margin involvement. Orbit. 2023;42:269–72. https://doi.org/10.1080/01676830.2022.2092156.
15. Tong JY, Huilgol SC, James C, Selva D. Recommendations for risk stratification of periocular squamous cell carcinoma. Surv Ophthalmol. 2023;68:964–76. https://doi.org/10.1016/j.survophthal.2023.05.001.
16. Yin VT, Merritt HA, Sniegowski M, Esmaeli B. Eyelid and ocular surface carcinoma: diagnosis and management. Clin Dermatol. 2015;33:159–69. https://doi.org/10.1016/j.clindermatol.2014.10.008.

17. Szabó B, Nelhubel GA, Kárpáti A, et al. Clinical significance of genetic alterations and expression of epidermal growth factor receptor (EGFR) in head and neck squamous cell carcinomas. Oral Oncol. 2011;47:487–96. https://doi.org/10.1016/j.oraloncology.2011.03.020.
18. Smilek P, Neuwirthova J, Jarkovsky J, et al. Epidermal growth factor receptor (EGFR) expression and mutations in the EGFR signaling pathway in correlation with anti-EGFR therapy in head and neck squamous cell carcinomas. Neoplasma. 2012;59:508–15. https://doi.org/10.4149/neo_2012_065.
19. Alter M, Satzger I, Mattern A, et al. Treatment of advanced cutaneous squamous cell carcinomas with epidermal growth factor receptor inhibitors. Dermatology. 2013;227:289–94. https://doi.org/10.1159/000355181.
20. Borman S, Wilkinson J, Meldi-Sholl L, et al. Analytical validity of DecisionDx-SCC, a gene expression profile test to identify risk of metastasis in cutaneous squamous cell carcinoma (SCC) patients. Diagn Pathol. 2022;17:1–9. https://doi.org/10.1186/s13000-022-01211-w.
21. Clark TJE, Harris GJ. Management of periocular cutaneous squamous cell carcinoma with perineural invasion: a case series and literature review. Orbit. 2022;41:34–43. https://doi.org/10.1080/01676830.2021.1893342.
22. Franco E, Salgari N, Dugo M, et al. Management of bilateral conjunctival squamous carcinoma following ocular cicatricial pemphigoid: a case report and review of literature. Eur J Ophthalmol. 2023;33:NP112–7. https://doi.org/10.1177/11206721221090698.
23. Petsuksiri J, Frank SJ, Garden AS, et al. Outcomes after radiotherapy for squamous cell carcinoma of the eyelid. Cancer. 2008;112:111–8. https://doi.org/10.1002/cncr.23143.
24. Luxenberg MN, Guthrie TH. Chemotherapy of basal cell and squamous cell carcinoma of the eyelids and periorbital tissues. Ophthalmology. 1986;93:504–10. https://doi.org/10.1016/s0161-6420(86)33708-4.
25. Couch SM, Custer PL. Topical 5-fluorouracil for the treatment of periocular actinic keratosis and low-grade squamous malignancy. Ophthalmic Plast Reconstr Surg. 2012;28:181–3. https://doi.org/10.1097/IOP.0b013e3182467c68.
26. Rossi R, Puccioni M, Mavilia L, Campolmi P, Mori M, Cappuccini A, Reali EF, Cappugi P. Squamous cell carcinoma of the eyelid treated with photodynamic therapy. J Chemother. 2004;16 https://doi.org/10.1179/JOC.2004.16.3.306.
27. Marmur ES, Schmults CD, Goldberg DJ. A review of laser and photodynamic therapy for the treatment of nonmelanoma skin cancer. Dermatologic Surg. 2004;30:264–71. https://doi.org/10.1111/j.1524-4725.2004.30083.x.
28. Esmaeli B. Immune checkpoint inhibitor therapy for orbital and ocular adnexal squamous cell carcinomas: International Society of Ocular Oncology President's Lecture, 2022. Invest Ophthalmol Vis Sci. 2023;64:29. https://doi.org/10.1167/iovs.64.7.29.
29. Faustina M, Diba R, Ahmadi MA, Esmaeli B. Patterns of regional and distant metastasis in patients with eyelid and periocular squamous cell carcinoma. Ophthalmology. 2004;111:1930–2. https://doi.org/10.1016/j.ophtha.2004.02.009.
30. Alam M, Armstrong A, Baum C, et al. Guidelines of care for the management of cutaneous squamous cell carcinoma. J Am Acad Dermatol. 2018;78(3):560–78. https://doi.org/10.1016/j.jaad.2017.10.007. PMCID: PMC6652228 NIHMSID: NIHMS1038477 PMID: 29331386
31. Rowe DE, Carroll RJ, Day CL. Prognostic factors for local recurrence, metastasis, and survival rates in squamous cell carcinoma of the skin, ear, and lip. Implications for treatment modality selection. J Am Acad Dermatol. 1992;26:976–90. https://doi.org/10.1016/0190-9622(92)70144-5.
32. Crawford C, Fernelius C, Young P, et al. Application of the AJCC 7th edition carcinoma of the eyelid staging system: a medical center pathology based, 15-year review. Clin Ophthalmol. 2011;5:1645–8. https://doi.org/10.2147/OPTH.S26418.
33. Burton KA, Ashack KA, Khachemoune A. Cutaneous squamous cell carcinoma: a review of high-risk and metastatic disease. Am J Clin Dermatol. 2016;17:491–508. https://doi.org/10.1007/s40257-016-0207-3.
34. Cottel WI. Perineural invasion by squamous-cell carcinoma. J Dermatol Surg Oncol. 1982;8:589–600. https://doi.org/10.1111/j.1524-4725.1982.tb00317.x.
35. Goepfert H, Dichtel WJ, Medina JE, et al. Perineural invasion in squamous cell skin carcinoma of the head and neck. Am J Surg. 1984;148:542–7. https://doi.org/10.1016/0002-9610(84)90385-4.
36. Petter G, Haustein UF. Histologic subtyping and malignancy assessment of cutaneous squamous cell carcinoma. Dermatologic Surg. 2000;26:521–30. https://doi.org/10.1046/j.1524-4725.2000.99181.x.
37. Cribier B, Asch P, Grosshans E. Differentiating squamous cell carcinoma from keratoacanthoma using histopathological criteria. Is it possible? A study of 296 cases. Dermatology. 1999;199:208–12. https://doi.org/10.1159/000018276.
38. Schwartz RA. Keratoacanthoma: a clinico-pathologic enigma. Dermatologic Surg. 2004;30:326–33.; discussion 333. https://doi.org/10.1111/j.1524-4725.2004.30080.x.
39. Donaldson MJ, Sullivan TJ, Whitehead KJ, Williamson RM. Periocular keratoacanthoma: clinical features, pathology, and management. Ophthalmology. 2003;110:1403–7. https://doi.org/10.1016/S0161-6420(03)00402-0.
40. Grossniklaus HE, Wojno TH, Yanoff M, Font RL. Invasive keratoacanthoma of the eyelid and ocular adnexa. Ophthalmology. 1996;103:937–41. https://doi.org/10.1016/s0161-6420(96)30583-6.

7 Sebaceous Gland Carcinoma

Ofira Zloto and Mordechai Rosner

7.1 Introduction

Sebaceous gland carcinoma (SGC), called also sebaceous cell carcinoma, sebaceous carcinoma, Meibomian gland carcinoma, is a malignant neoplasm capable of aggressive local behavior and metastasis to regional lymph nodes and distant organs. It originates from cells of the sebaceous glands and occurs most often in the periorbital area, usually in the eyelid [1]. This lesion is considered among the most lethal of all ocular adnexal tumors [2].

Thiersch may have reported the first case of periorbital SGC in 1865, and Baldauf reported another case in 1870. However, Allaire is credited with the first well-documented case of adenocarcinoma of the meibomian gland in 1891, and most of the modern understanding of eyelid SGC was initiated by the review of Straatsma in 1956 [2]. Progressive education about this disease and early diagnosis reduced the mortality rate from 50% to around 2–10%.

7.2 Epidemiological Aspects

SGC represents a small percentage (1–3%) of all malignant tumors and constitutes 0.6–10.2% of eyelid tumors. Its prevalence varies across ethnic groups, notably being higher in countries like China and India, where it may equal or surpass periocular basal cell carcinoma (BCC) and squamous cell carcinoma (SCC) in frequency [3, 4].

In the United States, the yearly incidence of eyelid SGC in the White population aged over 20 is approximately 0.5 per million, with a potential upward trend. In contrast, in India, SGC has emerged as the predominant malignant ocular lesion, accounting for 37% of cases, surpassing SCC at 21%. The global incidence of SGC has shown a significant increase, reaching 3.2 (male) and 1.6 (female) per 1 million person/years in 2012, compared to an estimated 1–2 cases per 1 million individuals/year in 2009. This places SGC as the third most prevalent eyelid malignancy, following BCC and SCC [5].

7.3 Etiology

There are no systemic conditions that convincingly predispose to SGC. Ocular or facial irradiation for the treatment of hereditary retinoblastoma, acne, cutaneous hemangioma, and eczema are important risk factors [1]. The relationship between the use of diuretic medications and the development of SGC is not firmly proven [1, 6]. Occasional reports have suggested an association between SGC at a relatively young age and immune dysfunction. A possible relationship between SGC and human papillomavirus (HPV) has also been observed, [1] as well as Muir–Torre syndrome (MTS), immunosuppression, and human immunodeficiency virus. Gender predilection is an object of debate. Reports regarding gender have varied, and while some studies have suggested that men are 1.35–1.4 times as likely as women to have SGC, other studies have found a higher incidence in women.

7.4 Clinical Features

SGC is generally a disease of older individuals, with a reported mean age at diagnosis of 57–73 years [2, 7, 8]. However, it may develop in older children and young adults, particularly after irradiation for retinoblastoma [1]. SGC has a marked tendency to arise in the ocular region, but it is estimated that approximately 25% occur in regions other than the head and neck [9]. According to the Surveillance, Epidemiology, and End Results (SEER) study from 2002 to 2012, SGC can be classified into two groups: ocular type and extraocular type. The majority of SGC arise from the meibo-

O. Zloto (✉) · M. Rosner
Department of Ophthalmology, Goldschleger Eye Institute, Sheba Medical Center, Sackler School of Medicine, Tel Aviv University, Tel Aviv, Israel

B. C. K. Patel et al. (eds.), *Clinical Ophthalmic Oncology*, https://doi.org/10.1007/978-3-031-72328-5_7

mian glands within the tarsus. About 65% occur in the upper eyelid, 25% in the lower eyelid, 5% involve both eyelids [2, 8], and 5% arise in the caruncle [1, 10]. Occasional cases of primary SGC of the conjunctiva and even of the lacrimal gland are reported [1]. Sebaceous carcinoma of the eyelid also has the tendency to exhibit multicentric origins [5] and pagetoid spread, which makes local recurrence a potential problem (Box 7.1). When patients present with a history of multiple SGCs the possibility of Muir–Torre syndrome, should be considered [11].

Box 7.1 Salient Diagnostic Features of Sebaceous Gland Carcinoma

- A unilateral, solitary, sessile subcutaneous round nodule that is firm, painless, and yellow, masquerading as chalazion
- Unilateral diffuse thickening of the eyelid and/or the conjunctiva masquerading as blepharoconjunctivitis
- Microscopic findings of an infiltrating mass composed of cells with lipid vacuoles in the cytoplasm, pronounced nuclear pleomorphism, and mitotic activity
- Flat superficial involvement of the epithelium—"pagetoid growth pattern"
- Positive oil red-O stain for lipid
- Immunohistologic expression of HMFG1, EMA, and BRST-1, but not of cytokeratins

7.5 Symptoms and Signs

7.5.1 Solitary Nodule of the Eyelid

The most common clinical variant of SGC is a solitary, firm, painless, sessile subcutaneous round nodule fixed to the tarsus (Fig. 7.1). With enlargement, the tumor may assume a yellow color owing to the lipids it contains [12]. However, SGC that arises from the glands of Zeis is located at the eyelid margin and has no firm attachment to the tarsus. The tumor eventually causes loss of cilia, as observed with other eyelid malignant tumors (Fig. 7.2) [1]. Rarely, SGC may become ulcerated.

7.5.2 Diffuse Thickening of the Eyelid

Unilateral diffuse thickening of the eyelid is the second most frequent presentation of SGC. The diffuse tumor may extend into the epithelium of the forniceal or bulbar conjunctiva, and even the cornea (Fig. 7.2) [11]. Rarely, SGC arising from the glands of Zeis can become pedunculated, keratinized, and even appear as a cutaneous horn. When SGC develops in the caruncle, it appears as an irregular yellow mass that usually is not fixed to adjacent structures (Fig. 7.3) [1, 13].

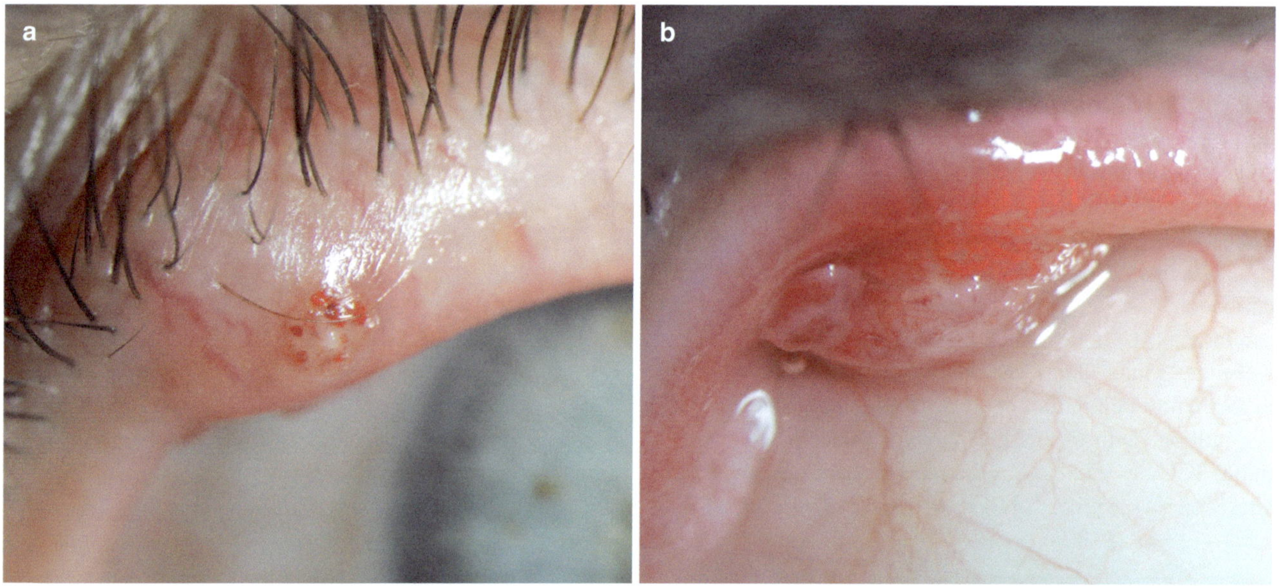

Fig. 7.1 Sebaceous gland carcinoma arising in left upper eyelid—a firm, sessile subcutaneous round nodule fixed to the tarsus (**a**, **b**). (Courtesy of Dr. Santosh Honavar)

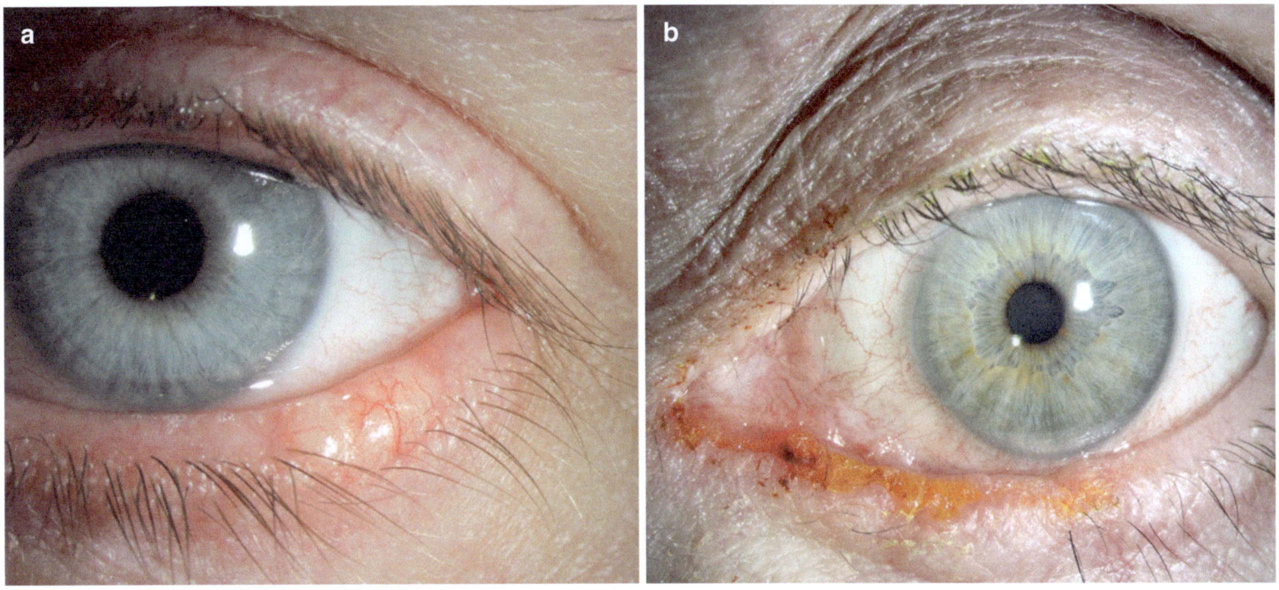

Fig. 7.2 Diffuse involvement of the eyelids by sebaceous gland carcinoma causing loss of cilia (a, **b**), and extending into the fornical or bulbar conjunctiva (**b**). Courtesy of Dr. Santosh Honavar

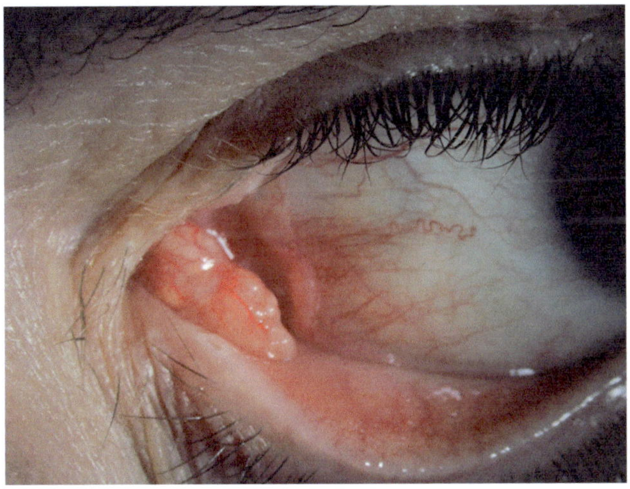

Fig. 7.3 Sebaceous gland carcinoma of the caruncle in a 56-year-old man, growing gradually during 2 months. The lesion was multilobulated and was yellowish red in color with fine intrinsic vessels

7.6 Histopathologic Features

7.6.1 Pathogenesis

Periocular SGC arises from the sebaceous glands in the ocular region, including meibomian glands in the tarsus, glands of Zeis of the cilia, pilosebaceous glands of the caruncle, and from the conjunctival epithelium [1, 12]. It may exhibit multicentric origins. Most SGC appear to arise de novo and not from a preexisting sebaceous adenoma, sebaceous hyperplasia, or sebaceous (organoid) nevus [1, 14, 15].

7.6.2 Light Microscopic Features

Histopathologically, SGC is an unencapsulated infiltrating mass composed of cells with finely vacuolated, frothy cytoplasm, pronounced nuclear pleomorphism, and usually high mitotic activity (Fig. 7.4a, b) [1, 12, 16]. The presence of lipid can be demonstrated with the oil red-O stain (Fig. 7.4c). This lipid can incite a foreign body giant cell reaction. SGC is associated with a chronic inflammatory response that is less intense than in BCC [1, 13].

7.6.3 Pagetoid Spread

SGC exhibits peculiar intraepithelial spread into the eyelid epidermis and the conjunctival epithelium in 44–80% of cases [1, 6, 8]. This flat superficial involvement of the epithelium is usually referred to as "pagetoid spread" (Fig. 7.5).

7.6.4 Immunohistochemistry

The histopathologic diagnosis of SGC can usually be made readily on routine light microscopy. However, immunohistochemistry replaces the need for fat stains on frozen sections and may help to differentiate SGC from basal and squamous cell carcinoma. The central foamy cells of SGC express human milk fat globulin-1 (HMFG1) and epithelial membrane antigen (EMA), but not cytokeratins, whereas the small peripheral basal and duct cells generally express cytokeratin but not HMFG1 or EMA (Fig. 7.6). SGC also

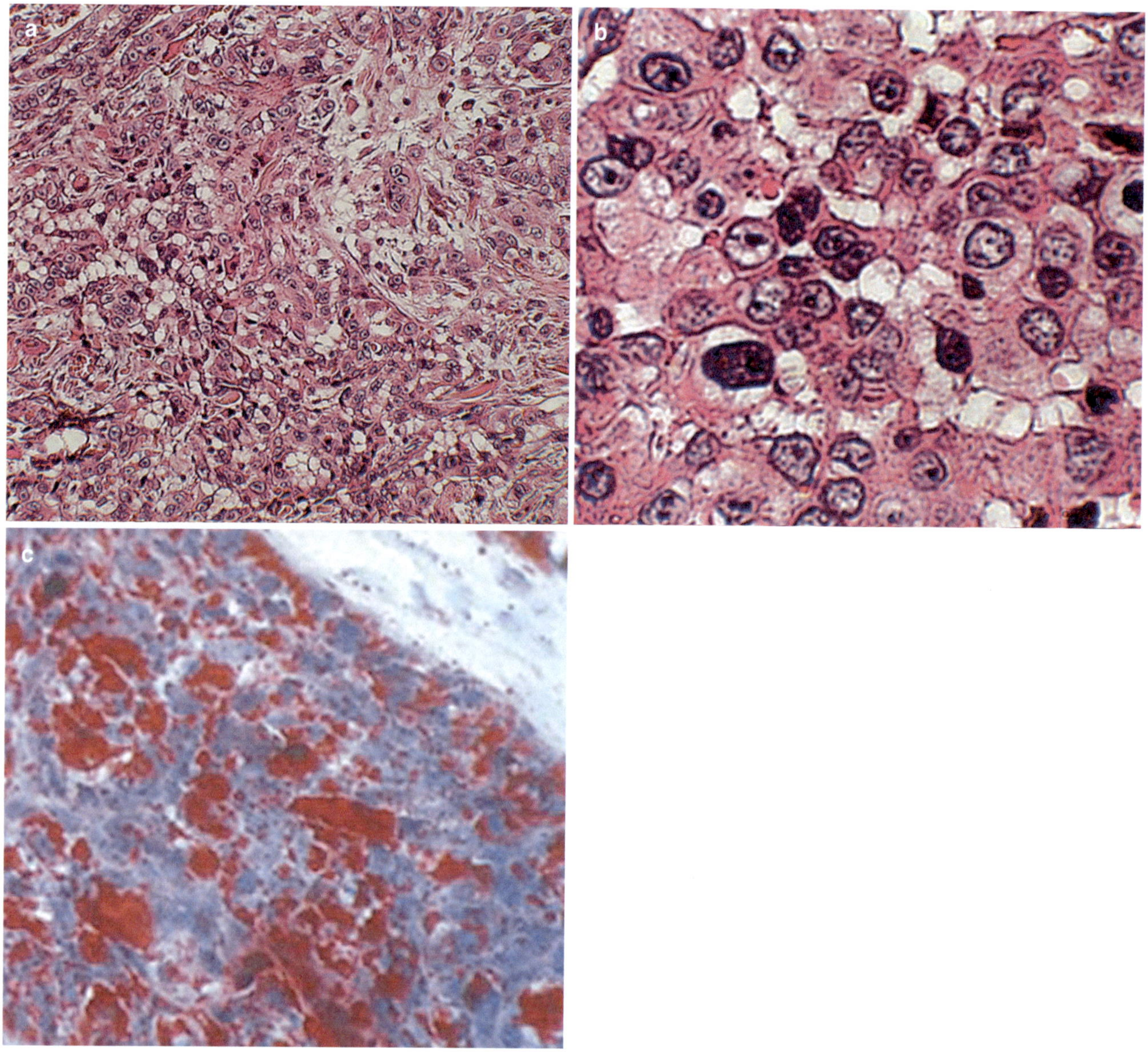

Fig. 7.4 Histopathologically, sebaceous gland carcinoma is an unencapsulated infiltrating mass (**a**, hematoxylin–eosin ×100). The tumor is composed of cells with finely vacuolated, frothy cytoplasm and pronounced nuclear pleomorphism (**b**, hematoxylin & eosin ×400). Accentuation of the lipid using oil red-O stain. The lipid globules have a red color (**c**, Frozen section, oil red-O ×250)

expresses Cam 5.2 and BRST-1, whereas BCC expresses neither EMA nor BRST-1, and SCC expresses EMA but not Cam 5.2 (Table 7.1) [1, 12, 14, 17]. Androgen receptor reactivity (AR) was also found as a sensitive marker for SEB, especially in less differentiated tumors. Along with other markers and morphologic features, AR can be helpful in the diagnosis of SEB and its differentiation from SCC and BCC [18].

7.6.5 Histopathological Classification

In addition to being well, moderately, or poorly differentiated [2, 12], SGC can be readily classified into one of four patterns: lobular, comedocarcinoma, papillary, and mixed [1, 12].

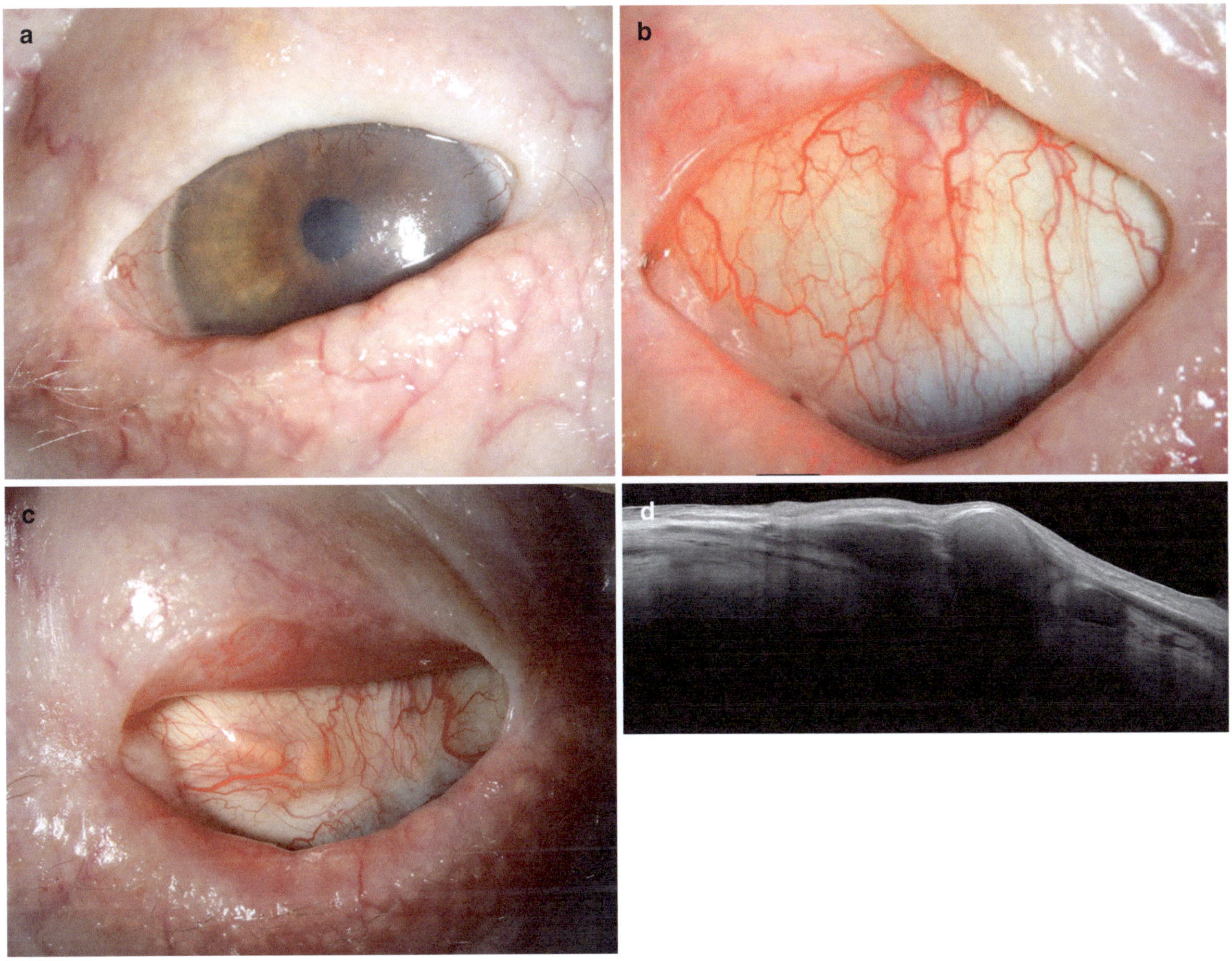

Fig. 7.5 A 90-year-old man with sebaceous cell carcinoma of left upper eyelid, s/p Mohs excision and repair (Cutler Beard procedure) 18 months prior. In addition to invasive sebaceous gland carcinoma (2.1 mm deep), there was pagetoid spread that was treated with 3 cycles of topical mitomycin eye drops (0.04% QID, 1 week on 3 weeks off) as he could not tolerate 4th cycle due to surface toxicity (**a**). 6 months after topical mitomycin a small area of superior bulbar conjunctival recurrence was excised (with extensive cryotherapy applied to bulbar conjunctiva) which showed sebaceous cell carcinoma in situ without invasive component (**b**). Subsequent diffuse conjunctival recurrence (**c**) appeared as subepithelial nodules by OCT (**d**) that eventually led to exenteration

7.6.5.1 Lobular Pattern

Lobular pattern is the most common and has architecture similar to that of a normal sebaceous gland, with fewer differentiated cells peripherally and more differentiated lipid-producing cells located centrally.

7.6.5.2 Comedocarcinoma Pattern

A large necrotic central core surrounded by viable cells characterizes the comedocarcinoma pattern.

7.6.5.3 Papillary Pattern

Papillary pattern which occurs frequently in small conjunctival lesions is distinguished by papillary projections and areas of sebaceous differentiation.

7.6.5.4 Mixed Pattern

Mixed pattern exhibits any combination of these three patterns.

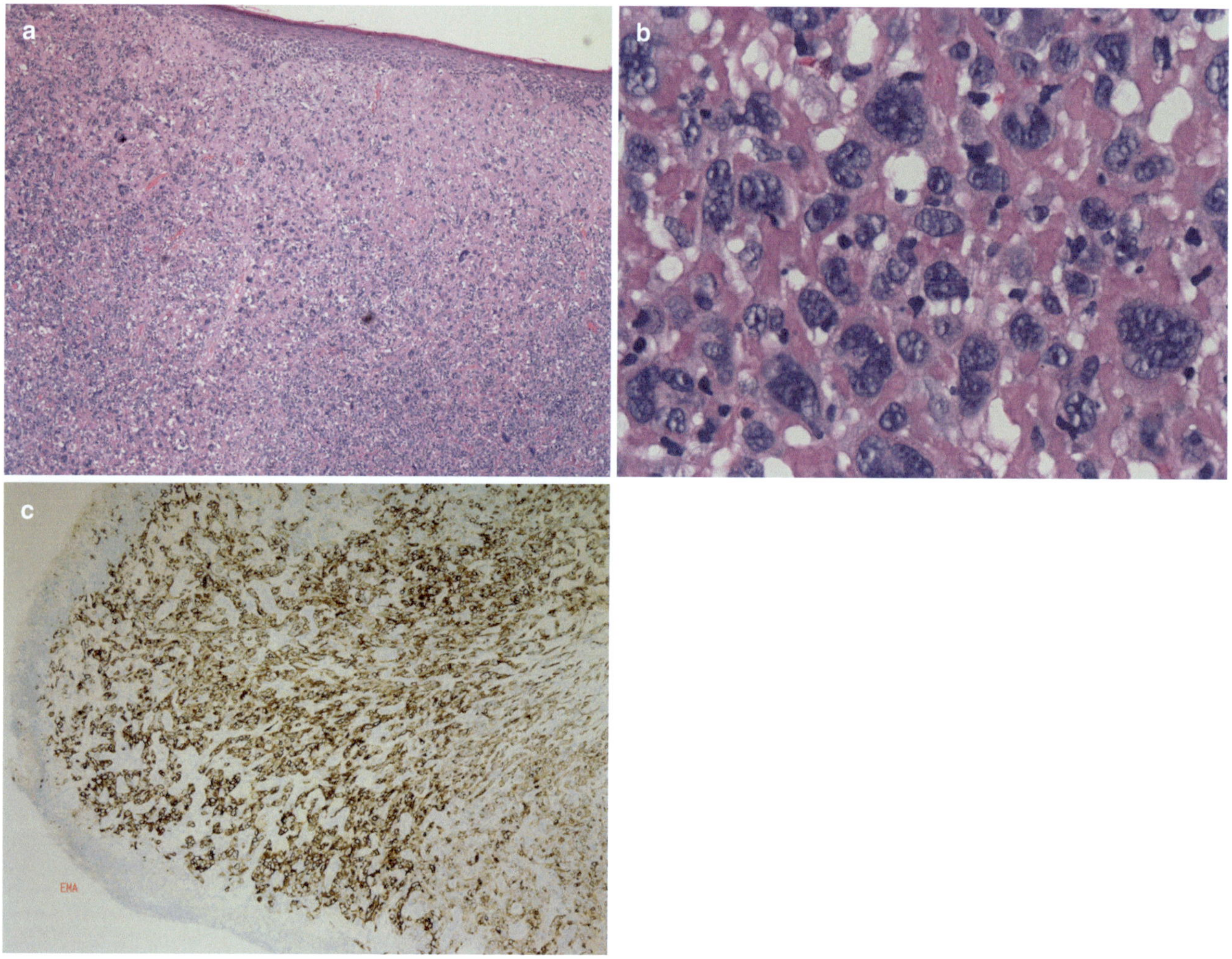

Fig. 7.6 Poorly differentiated tumor cells infiltrate the dermis with inflammatory response (**a**, H&E 10×). Higher power shows pleomorphic nuclei and cytoplasmic vacuolation (**b**, H&E 60×). Immunohistochemistry for epithelial membrane antigen is positive in cords of tumor cells (**c**, EMA 20×)

Table 7.1 Immunohistochemistry profile of common malignant eyelid tumors

	Tumor type (% positive cases)		
Tumor antibody	Sebaceous gland carcinoma	Basal cell carcinoma	Squamous cell carcinoma
EMA and BRST-1	64	0	36
EMA and Cam 5.2	73	6	0
EMA and Cam 5.2	55	0	0

Modified from Sinard [14]

EMA anti-epithelial membrane antigen, *BRST-1* anti-BCA 225, *Cam 5.2* anti-low molecular weight keratin

7.6.6 Genetic Immunomarkers and Prognostic Implications

Around 67% of SGC tumors exhibit missense or nonsense mutations in the gene p53, with immunoreactivity reported in 50–100% of SGC cases [14]. P53 overexpression is suggested as a diagnostic indicator in differentiating SGC from benign sebaceous proliferation (11%), basal cell carcinoma (BCC) (20%), and squamous cell carcinoma (SCC) (50–60%) [14, 15, 17–21]. A similar diagnostic role has been attributed to p16 [14].

The Ki-67 proliferation index (PI), representing the fraction of Ki-67-positive tumor cells in SGC, is estimated to be 38–72%, slightly higher than in other solid malignancies (25–50%) [14, 17, 20, 21]. Elevated Ki-67 PI is associated with an unfavorable clinical outcome concerning tumor recurrence and regional lymph node metastasis [14, 17, 21].

Significantly increased levels of the Bcl-2-associated athanogene 3 (BAG3) and ZEB2/SIP1 have been observed in SGC cases [22, 23]. ZEB2, a transcription factor linked to the epithelial-to-mesenchymal transition phenomenon, represses the expression of the E-cadherin gene [14, 17, 21]. Immunohistochemical overexpression of ZEB2, along with loss of E-cadherin and CDH1 promoter methylation, has been correlated with a higher risk of lymph node metastasis, orbital invasion, large tumor size, advanced stage, and poorer survival. Multivariate analysis has identified ZEB2 as the most significant poor prognostic indicator for eyelid SGC. Similarly, BAG3 overexpression has been associated with cancer development, invasiveness, metastasis, angiogenesis, tumor adhesion, migration, and resistance to chemotherapy [22, 23]. Yunoki et al. found that BAG3 is overexpressed in SGC of the eyelid [23].

7.6.7 Hormonal Immunophenotype

The hormonal panel analysis of SGC has unveiled immunostaining results for estrogen, progesterone, and androgen receptors (AR) in 43%, 26%, and 81% of cases, respectively [20, 21, 24]. The immunoreactivity observed for these proteins holds promise for potential therapeutic avenues in the future treatment of SGC. Positive AR staining has been detected in a variable nuclear or cytoplasmic pattern within SGC cells, particularly in tumors with a pagetoid spread [20, 21]. This marker proves valuable in distinguishing SGC from SCC (predominantly negative, 90–100%) and BCC (occasionally positive, 50–86%). Findings indicate that a high AR score is associated with an increased risk of cancer recurrence following excision [17, 21, 25].

Similarly, the C-erbB-2 oncoprotein, a significant oncogene in breast carcinoma, has been demonstrated to be overexpressed in 85% of SGC cases, often linked with ERBB2 amplification detected through fluorescence in situ hybridization [26].

7.6.8 Immunophenotype in Syndromic SGC

Utilizing immunohistochemical screening for aberrations in mismatch repair proteins (MMRP) offers a straightforward and convenient method for diagnosing Microsatellite Instability Syndrome (MST) [14, 17, 21]. This syndrome stems from an autosomal dominant inherited defect in one of the genes responsible for encoding MMRP, resulting in genomic microsatellite instability. Carcinogenesis is inevitably triggered by a second-hit somatic mutation or methylation suppression of the remaining functioning allele [14, 17, 21]. The deficient immunohistochemical expression of MLH1, MSH2, MSH6, and PMS2 strongly indicates the need for prompt counseling regarding hereditary neoplasia.

7.7 Tumor Staging

The staging is assessed by the TNM (tumor node metastasis) definitions of the American Joint Committee on Cancer (AJCC). The recent staging of SGC based on the eighth edition of AJCC classification is listed in Table 7.1.

7.8 Diagnostic Evaluation

Full-thickness excisional or incisional biopsy of the eyelid is the preferred method of confirming the suspected clinical diagnosis of SGC. When diffuse involvement of eyelid and conjunctiva is suspected, multiple conjunctival map biopsies should be performed to determine the extent of the disease [1, 7]. Fine-needle aspiration biopsy and impression cytology have been used in the early diagnosis of SGC [27, 28] and to detect conjunctival spread, but these methods are generally not advisable because of the limited amount of tissue obtained. However, fine-needle biopsy may be acceptable for the diagnosis of regional lymph node metastases [1, 12]. Only in cases with suspected diffuse involvement of the eyelid and conjunctiva is orbital imaging indicated, either before or after the initial biopsy, to rule out posterior extension [1, 12].

7.9 Differential Diagnosis

SGC is notorious for its variable clinical presentation and its ability to masquerade, both clinically and histopathologically, as common benign or less invasive conditions, resulting in delayed diagnosis and treatment [1, 2, 7].

7.9.1 Chalazion

In the early stages, SGC of the eyelids can be very similar to chalazion. However, in contrast to SGC, chalazion generally occurs in younger individuals, is more circumscribed and painful, and is usually not associated with loss of cilia. However, recurrent chalazia, as well as chalazia in older patients, should undergo a biopsy to rule out SGC.

7.9.2 Inflammatory Conditions

Virtually any inflammatory condition of the eyelid and the conjunctiva must be included in the differential diagnosis of SGC. These include unilateral blepharitis, conjunctivitis, meibomitis, superior limbic keratoconjunctivitis, papillary conjunctivitis, cicatricial pemphigoid, conjunctival granuloma, and sarcoidosis. Thus, SGC should be suspected in every middle-aged or older patient with a diagnosis of unilateral blepharitis or other inflammatory conditions that do not respond to usual therapy [1, 12, 16].

7.9.3 Benign and Malignant Tumors

Several benign and malignant tumors can have a clinical appearance similar to that of SGC. These include BCC, SCC, melanoma, Merkel cell carcinoma, lymphoma, sweat gland neoplasm, junctional squamous papilloma, hereditary benign intraepithelial dyskeratosis, metastatic carcinoma, and other rare tumors [1, 12, 16].

7.9.3.1 Basal Cell Carcinoma

The nodular BCC is more common on the lower lid and is white rather than yellow. BCC is also more likely to become ulcerated than SGC. Although diffuse sclerosing BCC may closely simulate SGC, it very rarely exhibits diffuse invasion of the conjunctiva. Histologically, BCC typically shows peripheral palisading of nuclei and retraction artifact that are not seen in SGC.

7.9.3.2 Squamous Cell Carcinoma

SCC is more superficial and lacks a yellow color. Conjunctival intraepithelial neoplasia can be very similar to diffuse epithelial invasion by SGC, except for eyelid involvement, which is less likely to be present in SGC. Histopathologically, SCC is the lesion most often confused with SGC [29]. Unlike SGC, SCC cells have more abundant eosinophilic cytoplasm, lack lipid vacuoles, and demonstrate eddy formation and keratin cysts.

7.9.3.3 Melanoma

Nodular or diffuse cutaneous melanoma in the eyelid or conjunctiva can usually be distinguished from SGC by its black or brown pigmentation, but amelanotic melanoma can resemble SGC.

7.9.3.4 Other Tumors

Merkel cell carcinoma of the eyelid is distinguished by its red or red-blue color. Lymphoma of the eyelid arises from deeper layers than does SGC, and in the conjunctiva it has a characteristic "salmon patch" color. Moreover, inflammatory signs that are commonly associated with SGC are lacking in lymphoma.

7.10 Treatment

7.10.1 Surgery

The most acceptable management of periocular SGC is complete surgical removal [30]. Excisional biopsy of a small lesion is recommended even before histopathologic verification of the diagnosis [12, 16, 30]. Either frozen section control or Mohs' microsurgery is usually used at the time of tumor excision, to evaluate the margins, and the resection is continued until the margins are histopathologically clear.

However, there is controversy as to which is preferable and whether either technique is better than waiting for permanent sections, because of the difficulty in diagnosing SGC in frozen sections [30]. It has been suggested that wide margins, of at least 5 mm, should be taken in order to prevent recurrence. Orbital exenteration is currently performed less often but is still indicated for advanced and diffuse SGC with orbital invasion in the absence of metastasis [1].

In the conjunctiva map biopsy should be obtained from 17 specific sites, including four clock hours of the limbus, three each from the upper and lower forniceal conjunctiva, three from the upper and lower tarsal conjunctiva, and one from the caruncle (Fig. 7.7) [12, 16]. Following a thorough examination of all biopsies, cryotherapy can be considered for addressing pagetoid disease. Mitomycin-C is recommended in cases with limited involvement, while cases with diffuse pagetoid spread or associated orbital involvement may necessitate orbital exenteration. Although orbital exenteration is now less frequently performed, it remains a suitable option for advanced and diffuse SGC with orbital invasion in the absence of metastasis.

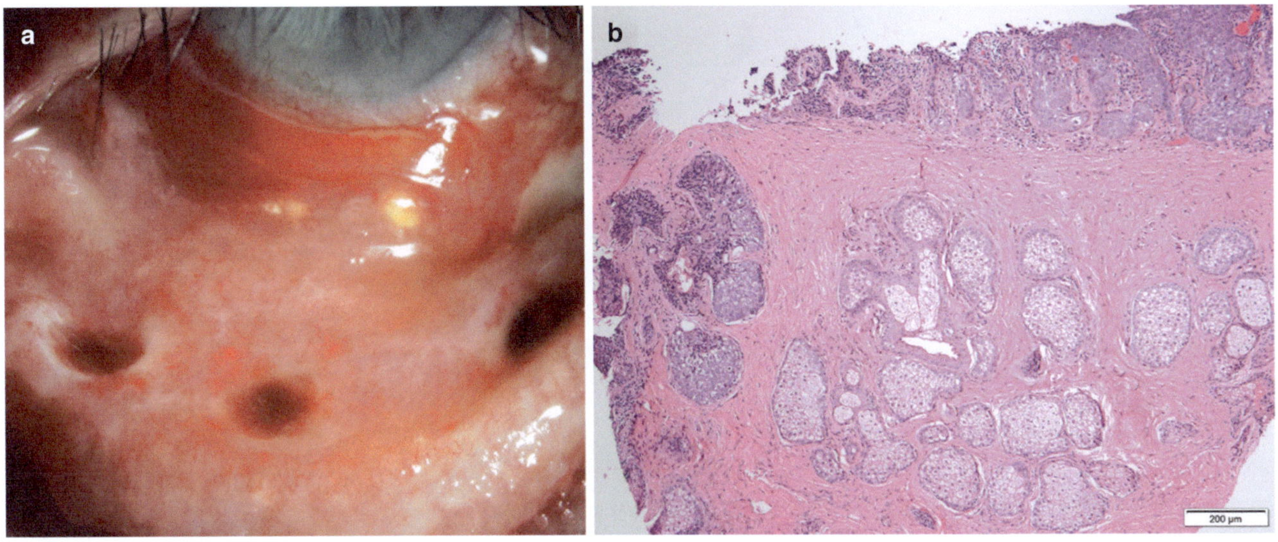

Fig. 7.7 Punch biopsies of the inferior tarsal conjunctiva that include tarsus with sebaceous glands (**a**) were positive for carcinomatous involvement (**b**)

7.10.2 Cryotherapy

As the removal of wide margins is not possible in the case of conjunctival lesions, supplemental treatment by double freeze-thaw cycle cryotherapy is indicated. Combination therapy with cryotherapy, topical chemotherapy, [31–33] and radiotherapy [34] can also be used in advanced cases [1].

7.10.3 Topical Chemotherapy

Topical chemotherapy with mitomycin C drops has been found to be effective as an alternative to complete conjunctivectomy or exenteration in selected case [34–36].

7.10.4 Sentinel Lymph Node Biopsy

The technique of sentinel node biopsy or at least strict regional lymph node surveillance was suggested as a useful method for SGC of the eyelid and conjunctiva [35, 36] especially for patients with eyelid sebaceous carcinoma of 10 mm or more in greatest dimension, tumors that involves full thickness of the eyelid, with invasion of adjacent ocular or orbital structures, with perineural invasion, when enucleation, exenteration, or bone resection is required for its complete resection, or when tumor is not resectable (Chap. 10) [37]. Localized regional lymph node metastasis is treated by lymph node dissection or by a combination of chemotherapy and radiotherapy [38].

7.10.5 Radiotherapy

In the past irradiation was considered as not highly effective in the management of SGC; it has been advocated only in selected cases. However, newer studies are suggesting that radiation therapy is a safe and effective treatment for patients with sebaceous carcinoma of the eyelid. It appears to contribute to prolonged survival as a result of good tumor control, and it also facilitates functional and cosmetic preservation of the eyelid [39, 40]. Postoperative radiation therapy after radical surgery is suggested for adequate disease control in advanced disease (Figs. 7.8 and 7.9) [41, 42].

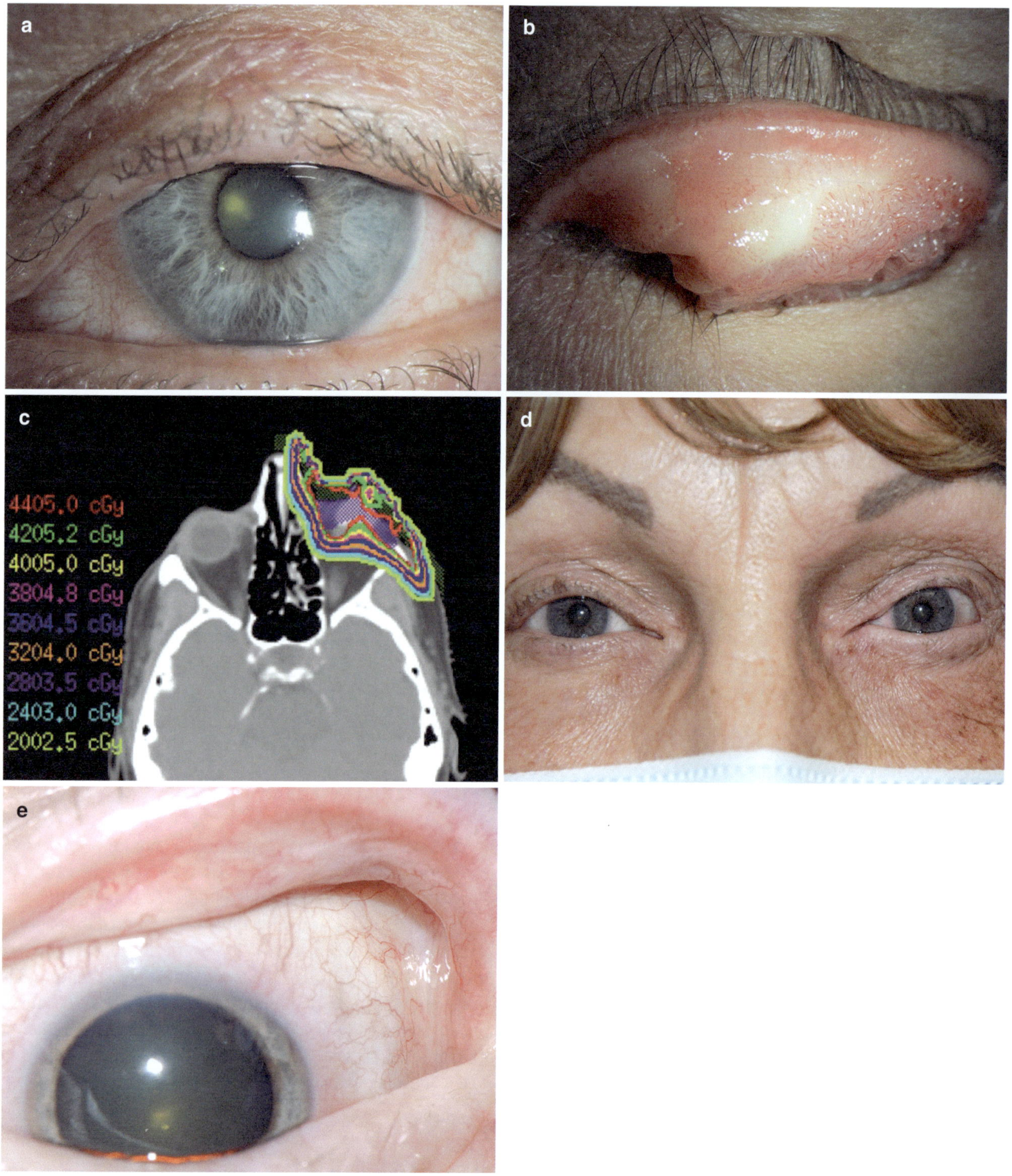

Fig. 7.8 A year old woman with upper eyelid bump noted for approximately two years. The growth was not obvious on external examination (**a**) until the lid was everted (**b**) revealing papillomatous mass involving the upper lid up to the fornix and extending to eyelid margin laterally. The lesion was excised and sebaceous gland carcinoma was confirmed with negative deep margin, but the lateral margin was positive. Adjuvant EBRT 40 Gy in 15 fractions was prescribed. 9 MeV electrons were delivered to the left eyelid using 5 mm bolus and a daily eye shield for posterior structure sparing with an En-Face technique to the total dose (**c**). Sentinel lymph node biopsy was negative. Other than mild dryness managed by artificial tears and a few episodes of trichiasis (epilated), at 4 year visit patient remains recurrence free (**d**) without metastasis (negative CT neck soft tissues). The anterior segment examination was unremarkable mild radiation cataract causing visual acuity of 20/40 (**e**)

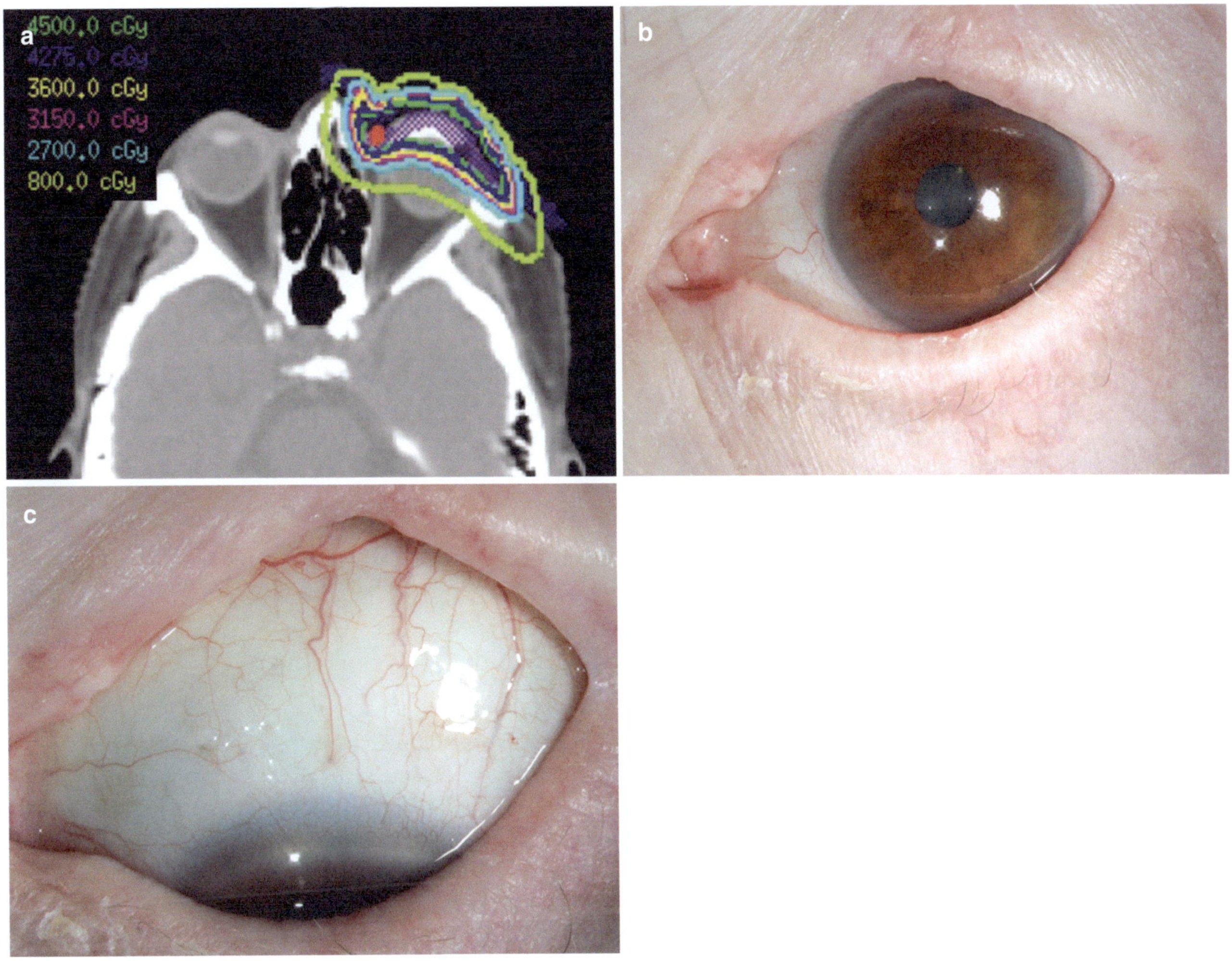

Fig. 7.9 A 65-year-old woman with invasive sebaceous carcinoma of the left upper eyelid resected with MOHS (positive margin) and followed by adjuvant EBRT 45 Gy in 25 fractions. 6 MeV electrons were delivered to the left eyelid using 5 mm bolus and a daily eye shield for posterior structure sparing with an En-Face technique to the total dose (**a**). Sentinel lymph node biopsy was negative. Subsequently had marginal recurrences (×2) that required excision about 2 and 2.9 years after radiation and conjunctival recurrence treated by excision and cryotherapy 3.4 years after radiation. Conjunctival map biopsies excluded widespread pagetoid extension. At 4 year post radiation, there was absence of local recurrence (**b**, **c**) and systemic metastasis (CT neck soft tissue). Patient was managing well with artificial tears and scleral contact lens for lid lag and dry eye

7.10.6 Systemic Chemotherapy

Regional spread to lymph nodes and hematogenous metastasis to distant organs is treated by chemotherapy [1, 4, 5, 16, 22].

7.11 Prognosis

7.11.1 Prognostic Factors

The visual prognosis varies with the extent of the disease and the type of treatment employed [6, 16]. Various factors have been associated with a worse prognosis, including vascular, lymphatic, and orbital invasion; involvement of both upper and lower eyelids; poor differentiation; multicentric origin; duration of symptoms more than 6 months; tumor diameter exceeding 10 mm; a highly infiltrative pattern; pagetoid invasion; and hyperexpression of tumor suppressor gene p53 [43].

According to the applied practical review of the American Joint Committee on Cancer (AJCC) 7th edition [34, 44], primary SGC is classified, like all other carcinomas of the eyelids, into stages I, II, III, and IV (Box 5.2), according to the various parameters of the primary tumor (T category), regional lymph nodes (N category), and metastases (M category). These include the size of the primary tumor; adjacent invasion; complete resection that requires enucleation, exen-

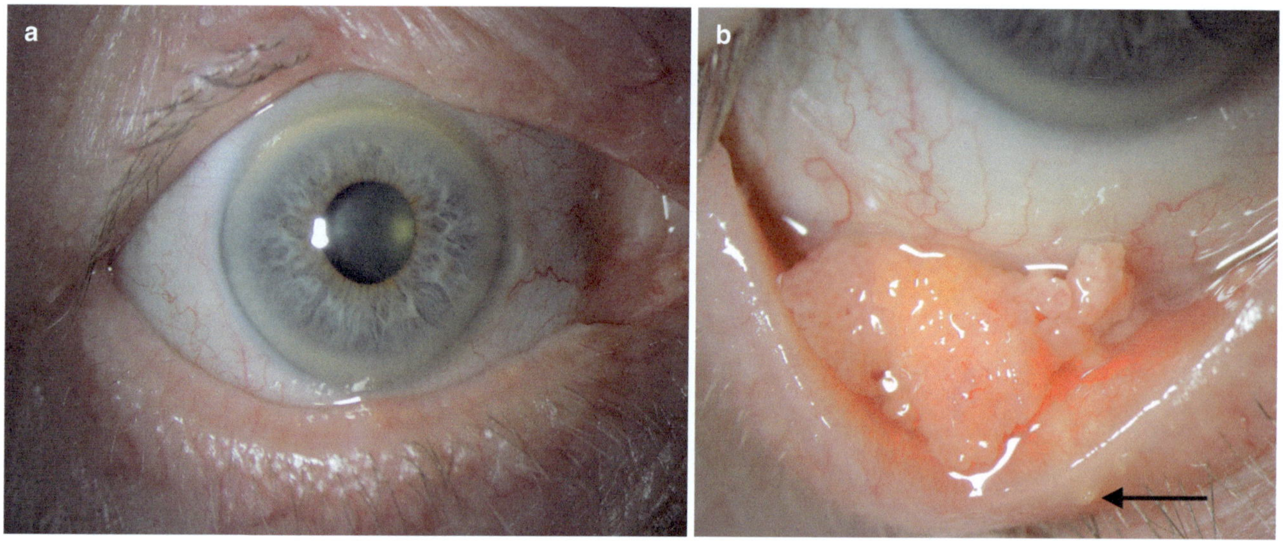

Fig. 7.10 An 80-year-old man had sebaceous gland carcinoma of the right upper eyelid. After wide excision, multiple map biopsies were negative, and sentinel lymph node biopsy was negative 6 months ago (**a**). After 6 months, he was resented with distant local recurrence appearing as a yellowish papillomatous mass in the inferior fornix (**b**)

teration, or bone resection; involvement of regional lymph nodes; extensive invasion making the tumor not resectable; and evidence of distant metastasis. It was found that the T category correlates well with outcomes in patients with sebaceous carcinoma of the eyelid [37, 44].

All patients with SGC should be followed regularly because of the risk of recurrence as well as the potential for metastasis and mortality.

7.11.2 Local Growth

Regardless of its origin, SGC can show direct local extension beyond its original site and involve the entire eyelid, the adjacent eyelid, and invade the orbital soft tissues, lacrimal secretory system, lacrimal excretory system, and the cranial cavity (Fig. 7.10). Such local growth is more likely to occur in neglected or recurrent cases [5, 6].

7.11.3 Local Recurrence

Despite radical surgery like orbital exenteration with extended neck dissection, locoregional failure rate may be high, and the 5-year local recurrence rates following wide excision have ranged from 9 to 36% [37]. Adequate disease control must be achieved by combined modality approach of radical surgery followed by postoperative radiation therapy [45].

7.11.4 Metastasis

The most common path of metastasis of eyelid SGC is via the lymphatic channels to regional lymph nodes, which occurs in about 30% of cases. From the upper eyelid, it tends to metastasize to preauricular and parotid nodes, which are the most common sites of metastasis, and from the lower lid region, it tends to metastasize to the submandibular and cervical nodes [5, 12, 16]. Advanced cases of eyelid SGC occasionally exhibit distant metastasis, probably by hematogenous spread, mainly to the liver, lung, bone, and brain [5, 22].

Periocular sebaceous carcinomas had a higher incidence of regional or distant metastases at presentation compared with extraocular head and neck sites. Lymph node metastasis was found to be associated with p21 downregulation, and therefore, it was suggested that p21 immunoreactivity should be used as a tool for prediction of nodal metastasis in sebaceous carcinoma of the eyelid [43].

7.11.5 Mortality

The 5-year tumor-related death rate was estimated in the past to be as high as 30% [29] and 50–67% [42], for patients presenting with lymph nodal metastases [46]. However, increased awareness and earlier aggressive treatment have markedly improved this to less than 10% (Table 7.2) [2, 46].

Table 7.2 Survival rates with eyelid sebaceous gland carcinoma

First author	Year	Country	Cases	Mortality rate (%)	Follow-up (years)
Boniuk	1968	USA	88	30	5
Ni	1979	China	100	41	5–15
Ni	1982	China	82	24	4
Rao	1982	USA	104	22	5
Doxanas	1984	USA	40	15	Not available
Zurcher	1998	England	43	9	3
Muqit	2004	Scotland	32	3	5

Reproduced with permission from Muqit et al. [1]

References

1. Shields JA, Demirci H, Marr BP, et al. Sebaceous carcinoma of the ocular region: a review. Surv Ophthalmol. 2005;50:103–22. https://doi.org/10.1016/j.survophthal.2004.12.008.
2. Kass LG, Hornblass A. Sebaceous carcinoma of the ocular adnexa. Surv Ophthalmol. 1989;33:477–90. https://doi.org/10.1016/0039-6257(89)90049-0.
3. Sargen MR, Mai Z-M, Engels EA, et al. Ambient ultraviolet radiation and sebaceous carcinoma incidence in the United States, 2000-2016. JNCI Cancer Spectr. 2020;4:20. https://doi.org/10.1093/jncics/pkaa020.
4. Margo CE, Mulla ZD. Malignant tumors of the eyelid: a population-based study of non-basal cell and non-squamous cell malignant neoplasms. Arch Ophthalmol. 1998;116:195–8. https://doi.org/10.1001/archopht.116.2.195.
5. Song X, Jia R, Fan X. An update on eyelid sebaceous cell carcinoma. Int Ophthalmol Clin. 2019;59:1–11. https://doi.org/10.1097/IIO.0000000000000272.
6. Khan JA, Doane JF, Grove AS. Sebaceous and meibomian carcinomas of the eyelid. Recognition, diagnosis, and management. Ophthalmic Plast Reconstr Surg. 1991;7:61–6. https://doi.org/10.1097/00002341-199103000-00008.
7. Shields JA, Demirci H, Marr BP, et al. Sebaceous carcinoma of the eyelids: personal experience with 60 cases. Ophthalmology. 2004;111:2151–7. https://doi.org/10.1016/j.ophtha.2004.07.031.
8. Dasgupta T, Wilson LD, Yu JB. A retrospective review of 1349 cases of sebaceous carcinoma. Cancer. 2009;115:158–65. https://doi.org/10.1002/cncr.23952.
9. Wick MR, Goellner JR, Wolfe JT, Su WP. Adnexal carcinomas of the skin. II. Extraocular sebaceous carcinomas. Cancer. 1985;56:1163–72. https://doi.org/10.1002/1097-0142(19850901)56:5<1163::aid-cncr2820560533>3.0.co;2-a.
10. Shields CL, Shields JA, White D, Augsburger JJ. Types and frequency of lesions of the caruncle. Am J Ophthalmol. 1986;102:771–8. https://doi.org/10.1016/0002-9394(86)90407-1.
11. Magazin M, Dalvin LA, Salomao DR, et al. Sebaceous carcinoma of the eyelid: proposed nomenclature for multifocal and multicentric disease. Ophthalmic Plast Reconstr Surg. 2023;39:117–22. https://doi.org/10.1097/IOP.0000000000002281.
12. Dowell-Esquivel C, Lee R, DiCaprio RC, Nouri K. Sebaceous carcinoma: an updated review of pathogenesis, diagnosis, and treatment options. Arch Dermatol Res. 2023;316:55. https://doi.org/10.1007/s00403-023-02747-7.
13. Shields JA, Shields CL. Sebaceous carcinoma of the glands of Zeis. Ophthalmic Plast Reconstr Surg. 1988;4:11–4. https://doi.org/10.1097/00002341-198801130-00002.
14. Herman DC, Chan CC, Bartley GB, et al. Immunohistochemical staining of sebaceous cell carcinoma of the eyelid. Am J Ophthalmol. 1989;107:127–32. https://doi.org/10.1016/0002-9394(89)90210-9.
15. Cavanagh HD, Green WR, Goldberg HK. Multicentric sebaceous adenocarcinoma of the meibomian gland. Am J Ophthalmol. 1974;77:326–32. https://doi.org/10.1016/0002-9394(74)90738-7.
16. Gniesmer S, Sonntag SR, Schiemenz C, et al. Diagnosis and treatment of malignant eyelid tumors. Die Ophthalmol. 2023;S1:33–9. https://doi.org/10.1007/s00347-023-01945-y.
17. Sinard JH. Immunohistochemical distinction of ocular sebaceous carcinoma from basal cell and squamous cell carcinoma. Arch Ophthalmol. 1999;117:776–83. https://doi.org/10.1001/archopht.117.6.776.
18. Asadi-Amoli F, Khoshnevis F, Haeri H, et al. Comparative examination of androgen receptor reactivity for differential diagnosis of sebaceous carcinoma from squamous cell and basal cell carcinoma. Am J Clin Pathol. 2010;134:22–6. https://doi.org/10.1309/AJCP89LYTPNVOBAP.
19. Fan YS, Carr RA, Sanders DSA, et al. Characteristic Ber-EP4 and EMA expression in sebaceoma is immunohistochemically distinct from basal cell carcinoma. Histopathology. 2007;51:80–6. https://doi.org/10.1111/j.1365-2559.2007.02722.x.
20. Ansai S, Takeichi H, Arase S, et al. Sebaceous carcinoma: an immunohistochemical reappraisal. Am J Dermatopathol. 2011;33:579–87. https://doi.org/10.1097/DAD.0b013e31820a2027.
21. Sramek B, Lisle A, Loy T. Immunohistochemistry in ocular carcinomas. J Cutan Pathol. 2008;35:641–6. https://doi.org/10.1111/j.1600-0560.2007.00871.x.
22. Cicinelli MV, Kaliki S. Ocular sebaceous gland carcinoma: an update of the literature. Int Ophthalmol. 2019;39:1187–97. https://doi.org/10.1007/s10792-018-0925-z.
23. Yunoki T, Tabuchi Y, Hayashi A. Expression of anti-apoptotic protein BAG3 in human sebaceous gland carcinoma of the eyelid. Anticancer Res. 2017;37:1931–4. https://doi.org/10.21873/anticanres.11532.
24. McCluggage WG. Recent developments in vulvovaginal pathology. Histopathology. 2009;54:156–73. https://doi.org/10.1111/j.1365-2559.2008.03098.x.
25. Stanoszek LM, Wang GY, Harms PW. Histologic mimics of basal cell carcinoma. Arch Pathol Lab Med. 2017;141:1490–502. https://doi.org/10.5858/arpa.2017-0222-RA.
26. Cho KJ, Khang SK, Koh JS, et al. Sebaceous carcinoma of the eyelids: frequent expression of c-erbB-2 oncoprotein. J Korean Med Sci. 2000;15:545–50. https://doi.org/10.3346/jkms.2000.15.5.545.
27. Gill M, Garg S, Kalra R, Sen R. Sebaceous carcinoma of the eyelid diagnosed on fine needle aspiration cytology. J Cytol. 2012;29:75–6. https://doi.org/10.4103/0970-9371.93231.
28. Arathi C, Vijaya C. Scrape cytology in the early diagnosis of eyelid sebaceous carcinoma. J Cytol. 2010;27:140–2. https://doi.org/10.4103/0970-9371.73301.
29. Kwitko ML, Boniuk M, Zimmerman LE. Eyelid tumors with reference to lesions confused with squamous cell carcinoma. I. Incidence and errors in diagnosis. Arch Ophthalmol. 1963;69:693–7. https://doi.org/10.1001/archopht.1963.00960040699003.

30. Cook BE, Bartley GB. Treatment options and future prospects for the management of eyelid malignancies: an evidence-based update. Ophthalmology. 2001;108:2088–98. https://doi.org/10.1016/s0161-6420(01)00796-5.
31. Tumuluri K, Kourt G, Martin P. Mitomycin C in sebaceous gland carcinoma with pagetoid spread. Br J Ophthalmol. 2004;88:718–9. https://doi.org/10.1136/bjo.2003.034215.
32. Rosner M, Hadar I, Rosen N. Successful treatment with mitomycin C eye drops for conjunctival diffuse intraepithelial neoplasia with sebaceous features. Ophthalmic Plast Reconstr Surg. 2003;19:477–9. https://doi.org/10.1097/01.IOP.0000092801.56423.AD.
33. Shields CL, Naseripour M, Shields JA, Eagle RC. Topical mitomycin-C for pagetoid invasion of the conjunctiva by eyelid sebaceous gland carcinoma. Ophthalmology. 2002;109:2129–33. https://doi.org/10.1016/s0161-6420(02)01239-3.
34. Yen MT, Tse DT, Wu X, Wolfson AH. Radiation therapy for local control of eyelid sebaceous cell carcinoma: report of two cases and review of the literature. Ophthalmic Plast Reconstr Surg. 2000;16:211–5. https://doi.org/10.1097/00002341-200005000-00008.
35. Nijhawan N, Ross MI, Diba R, et al. Experience with sentinel lymph node biopsy for eyelid and conjunctival malignancies at a cancer center. Ophthalmic Plast Reconstr Surg. 2004;20:291–5. https://doi.org/10.1097/01.IOP.0000131733.36054.36.
36. Tryggvason G, Bayon R, Pagedar NA. Epidemiology of sebaceous carcinoma of the head and neck: implications for lymph node management. Head Neck. 2012;34:1765–8. https://doi.org/10.1002/hed.22009.
37. Esmaeli B, Nasser QJ, Cruz H, et al. American Joint Committee on Cancer T category for eyelid sebaceous carcinoma correlates with nodal metastasis and survival. Ophthalmology. 2012;119:1078–82. https://doi.org/10.1016/j.ophtha.2011.11.006.
38. Murthy R, Honavar SG, Burman S, et al. Neoadjuvant chemotherapy in the management of sebaceous gland carcinoma of the eyelid with regional lymph node metastasis. Ophthalmic Plast Reconstr Surg. 2005;21:307–9. https://doi.org/10.1097/01.iop.0000169426.57497.24.
39. Owen JL, Kibbi N, Worley B, et al. Sebaceous carcinoma: evidence-based clinical practice guidelines. Lancet Oncol. 2019;20:e699–714. https://doi.org/10.1016/S1470-2045(19)30673-4.
40. Aronow ME, Singh AD. Radiation therapy: conjunctival and eyelid tumors. Dev Ophthalmol. 2013;52:85–93. https://doi.org/10.1159/000351062.
41. Hata M, Koike I, Omura M, et al. Noninvasive and curative radiation therapy for sebaceous carcinoma of the eyelid. Int J Radiat Oncol Biol Phys. 2012;82:605–11. https://doi.org/10.1016/j.ijrobp.2010.12.006.
42. Deo SVS, Shukla NK, Singh M, et al. Locally advanced sebaceous cell carcinoma (T3) of eyelid: incidence and pattern of nodal metastases and combined modality management approach. Orbit. 2012;31:150–4. https://doi.org/10.3109/01676830.2011.648799.
43. Kiyosaki K, Nakada C, Hijiya N, et al. Analysis of p53 mutations and the expression of p53 and p21WAF1/CIP1 protein in 15 cases of sebaceous carcinoma of the eyelid. Invest Ophthalmol Vis Sci. 2010;51:7–11. https://doi.org/10.1167/iovs.09-4127.
44. Droll L, Seigler D, Esmaeli B. Prospective collection of data using the 7th edition of the AJCC Cancer Staging Manual for cancers of the eyelid, orbit, and conjunctiva. Ophthalmic Plast Reconstr Surg. 2011;27:142. https://doi.org/10.1097/IOP.0b013e3181f2a02c.
45. Callahan EF, Appert DL, Roenigk RK, Bartley GB. Sebaceous carcinoma of the eyelid: a review of 14 cases. Dermatologic Surg. 2004;30:1164–8. https://doi.org/10.1111/j.1524-4725.2004.30348.x.
46. Muqit MMK, Roberts F, Lee WR, Kemp E. Improved survival rates in sebaceous carcinoma of the eyelid. Eye. 2004;18:49–53. https://doi.org/10.1038/sj.eye.6700523.

Cutaneous Melanoma

8

Jacob Pe'er and Robert Folberg

8.1 Introduction

Cutaneous melanoma of the eyelid is a rare tumor, representing fewer than 1% of all malignant neoplasms of the eyelid skin [1], 1% of all skin melanomas [2], and 7% of cutaneous malignant melanomas of the head and neck region [3]. Many primary melanomas of the eyelid involve the mucosal surfaces of the palpebral and bulbar conjunctiva. In these cases, one must manage not only the eyelid but also the conjunctival component of the lesion. One may argue reasonably that primary conjunctival melanomas may affect the eyelid secondarily.

This chapter, therefore, focuses on the rare subset of melanomas confined to the eyelid skin. Our knowledge of such tumors is based on one large surveillance, epidemiology and end results (SEER) database [4–6] and a few case series and case reports. We describe and discuss the epidemiology, etiology, clinical behavior, prognosis, and the appropriate management of these malignancies.

8.2 Epidemiology

Most of the reported cases of cutaneous melanoma of the eyelid are of white patients from series in North America, Australia, and Europe [7–13]. Still, eyelid skin melanoma is also reported in an Asian series of eyelid tumors [14, 15]. According to the SEER database, the incidence of these tumors rose in four decades five times, from about 0.2 cases per million in the 1970s to about 1 case per million in the 2010s, with an average annual percent change of about 1.2% [4, 5]. In this database, male subjects showed a higher average incidence rate than female subjects, although in several small series, the incidence was similar in men and women [10–12]. Eyelid cutaneous melanomas are tumors of adults and older people, with a peak incidence in the sixth and seventh decades of life [10–13, 16].

8.3 Etiology and Pathogenesis

Ultraviolet radiation most likely contributes to the etiology of eyelid melanoma. These malignancies appear mostly in fair-skinned elderly adults, and the histological findings of solar elastosis in most cases of cutaneous melanomas. The higher incidence of the tumor in the lower eyelid and the relatively frequent association with basal cell carcinoma support this pathogenesis [10, 12, 13, 17, 18].

Ten cases of cutaneous melanoma were reported in the eyelids and periorbital region in patients with oculodermal melanocytosis (nevus of Ota) [19]. This is a relatively high incidence of this rare tumor in a relatively rare condition; thus, oculodermal melanocytosis may be considered a risk factor for the development of eyelid cutaneous melanoma. Preexisting pigmented lesions that show a sudden or gradual increase in size were seen in most patients in one series [9].

8.4 Clinical Features

Eyelid cutaneous melanoma arises most frequently in the lower eyelid, many times from a preexisting longstanding pigmented lesion that increases in size gradually. However, a newly acquired pigmented lesion is also typical (Fig. 8.1)

J. Pe'er (✉)
Division of Ophthalmology, Hadassah Medical Center, and Faculty of Medicine, Hebrew University of Jersalem, Jerusalem, Israel
e-mail: peer@hadassah.org.il

R. Folberg
Oakland University William Beaumont School of Medicine, Rochester, MI, USA

EyeCare Partners Innovation Center, Ballwin, MO, USA

B. C. K. Patel et al. (eds.), *Clinical Ophthalmic Oncology*, https://doi.org/10.1007/978-3-031-72328-5_8

[12]. In one series [10], the three most frequently listed clinical characteristics of the melanoma were pigmentation, documented growth, and ulceration or hemorrhage. Other suspicious signs are irregular borders and variegated shades of brown, red, white, blue, or dark black color. Cutaneous melanoma can be amelanotic (Fig. 8.2).

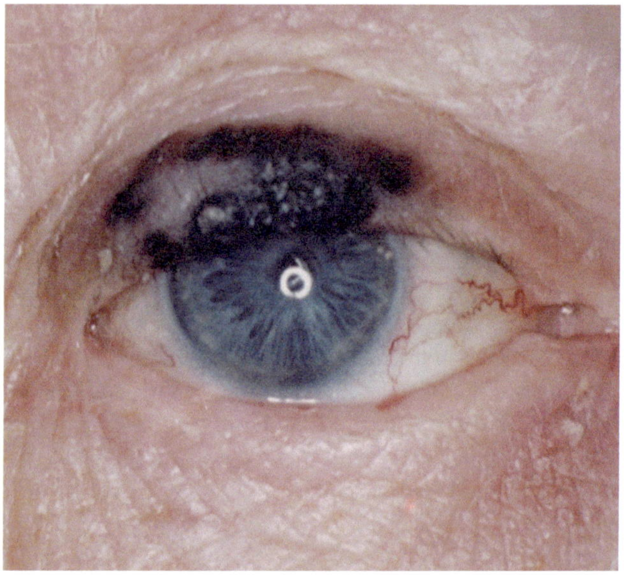

Fig. 8.1 Large cutaneous melanoma of right upper eyelid with involvement of the eyelid margin (Photograph courtesy of Dr. Peter A. Martin)

Most eyelid melanomas evolve through the lentigo maligna precursor lesion [13, 17, 18, 20]. Lentigo maligna is a slowly developing non-palpable pigmented macule, usually on the exposed cutaneous surface of elderly patients (Fig. 8.3). It gradually enlarges in size over time, while some areas may undergo regression. The lesions change shape and size and may change color from tan to brown to black. When there is progression to lentigo maligna melanoma, the invasive areas are usually marked by small nodular formations. They are generally dark brown or black, although invasion may occur without any obvious clinical changes. Theoretically, eyelid melanomas may evolve through dysplastic nevi that affect the eyelid or as melanomas of the superficial spreading type. Nodular melanomas are exceptionally rare among these already rare tumors, and small, heavily pigmented nodules at the eyelid margin may well represent pigmented basal cell carcinomas.

The classification of cutaneous melanomas is evolving. The fifth edition of the WHO Classification of Tumors [21] points to nine "families" of melanomas. This classification attempts to merge etiology (UV radiation exposure), genetic mutational pathways, with clinical and histological features of the "classical" approach cited in the previous paragraph. Three families are associated with exposure to UV radiation. Superficial spreading melanoma is classified as a low-CSD (low cumulative sun damage) lesion, unlike lentigo maligna melanoma, a high-CSD lesion.

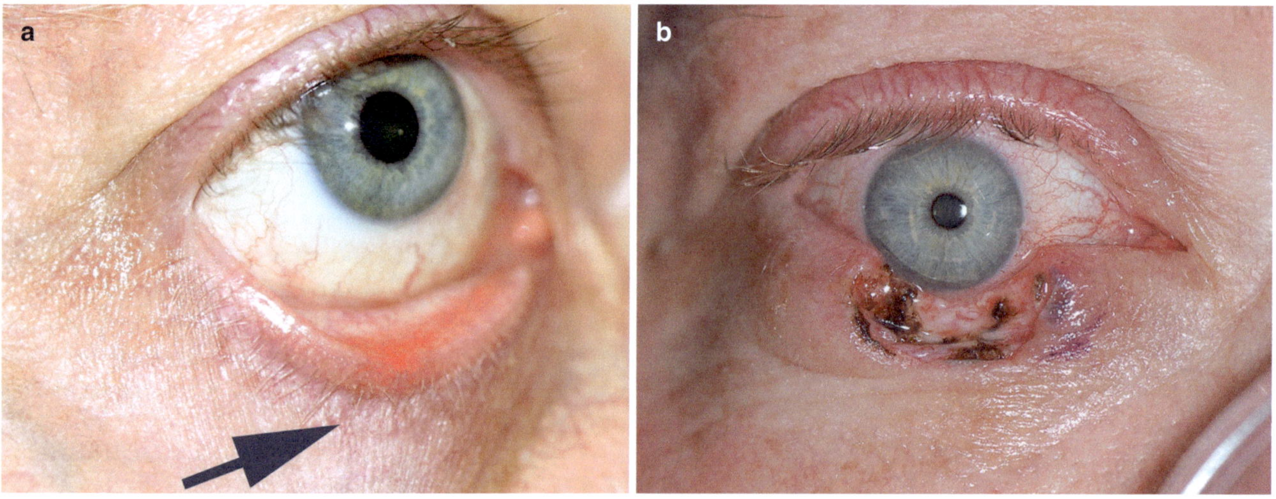

Fig. 8.2 Amelanotic melanoma of the right lower eyelid (**a**). Defect after slow Mohs resection of amelanotic melanoma of the right lower eyelid (**b**). Courtesy of Bhupender C. Patel, MD Salt Lake City, Utah, USA)

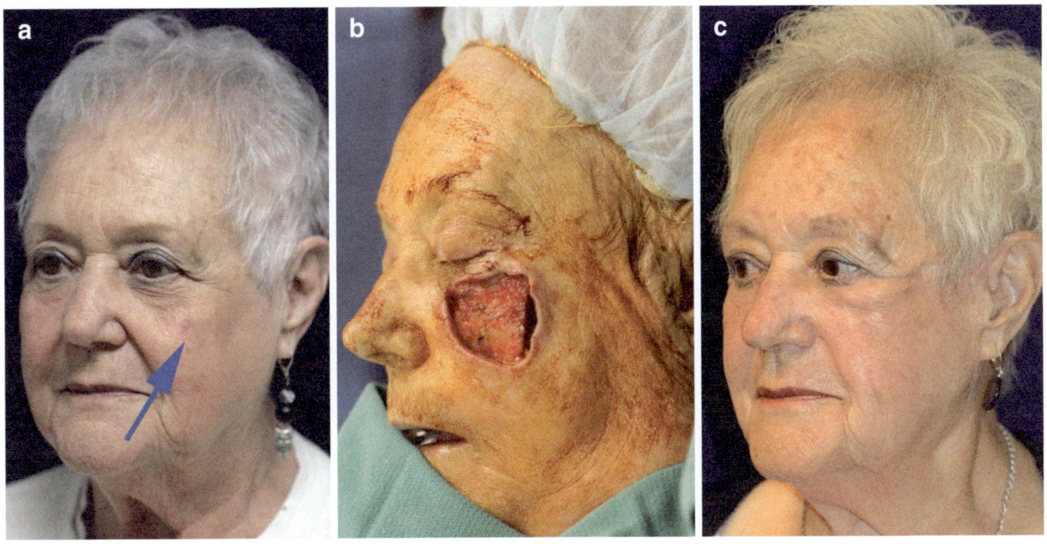

Fig. 8.3 Melanoma arising in lentigo maligna affecting the left lower eyelid and cheek (**a**, left). Defect after slow-Mohs resection (**b**, Middle). Three years after repair of defect and no recurrence of tumor (**c**, Right). Courtesy of Bhupender C. Patel, MD Salt Lake City, Utah, USA)

Desmoplastic melanoma, reported in the eyelid skin [22], is a third "family" of lesions associated with UV radiation as a mutagen (Fig. 8.4). Six melanoma lesion families lack a clear relationship to UV radiation. Among these are mucosal and uveal melanomas.

Eyelid melanoma can often involve the eyelid margins. In such cases, the mucocutaneous junction may be breeched and the palpebral conjunctiva may be affected. It is often difficult to know whether the melanoma originates in the skin or in the conjunctiva. Such cases have a worse prognosis; some relate this to the conjunctival involvement that may grow unseen for many years [11].

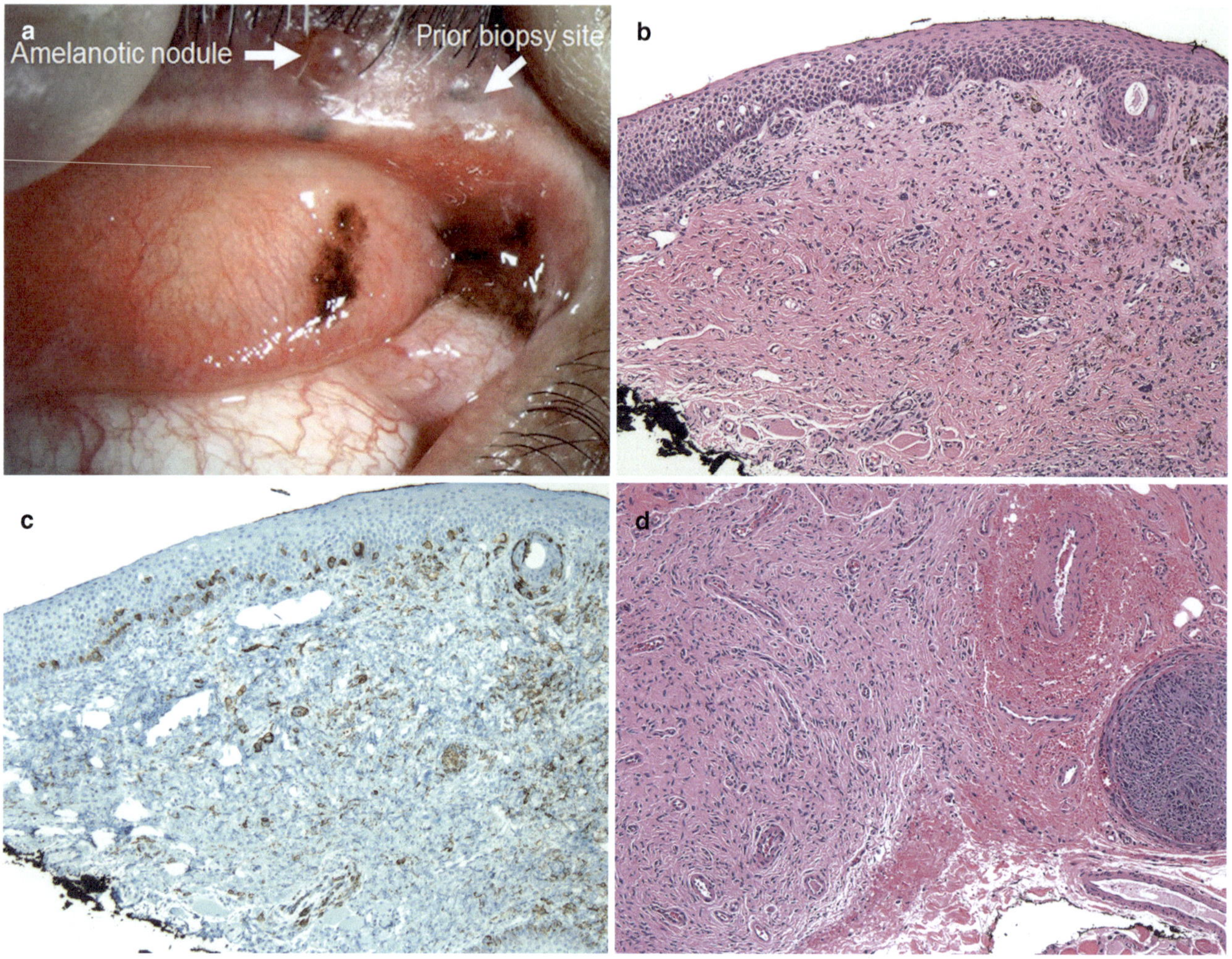

Fig. 8.4 A 56-year-old woman with neurofibromatosis type 1 (NF1) presented with a left upper eyelid amelanotic nodule with adjacent eyelid margin hyperpigmentation. External photograph of the patient's everted left upper eyelid. (**a**) Noted within the photograph is an amelanotic nodule (large arrow) next to the prior shave biopsy site (small arrow). Also visible within the photograph are hyperpigmented lesions within the palpebral conjunctiva resembling primary acquired melanosis PAM. Initial biopsy specimen demonstrates atypical, but relatively paucicellular, dermal infiltrate embedded in a fibrous stroma (**b**, hematoxylin and eosin stain 10×). The overlying epidermis reveals scattered atypical, vacuolated cells with pagetoid spread. HMB-45 immunostain highlights both the dermal and epidermal components of the melanoma (**c**). Full thickness eyelid excision and conjunctival map biopsy identified desmoplastic melanoma of the eyelid. Left side of photomicrograph shows neurofibroma. Right side shows neurotrophic spread by melanoma, characteristic of desmoplastic melanoma (**d**, hematoxylin and eosin, 10×). In addition to invasive conjunctival melanoma conjunctival melanoma in situ was identified on map biopsy. Note full-thickness proliferation of atypical, vacuolated cells (**e**, hematoxylin and eosin, 20×), characteristic of melanoma in situ. HMB-45 immunostain of the conjunctival map biopsy confirms melanocytic differentiation (**f**, 20×). Sentinel lymph node biopsy was negative. Following surgical excision for the eyelid melanoma, she was treated with and topical mitomycin C for the conjunctival melanoma. The patient has been tumor-free without evidence of recurrence free for more than 10 years (**g**). Reproduced with permission from Rubinstein TJ, Plesec TP, Singh AD. Desmoplastic melanoma of the eyelid and conjunctival melanoma in neurofibromatosis type 1: A clnical pathological correlation. Surv Ophthalmol. 2015;60:72-7

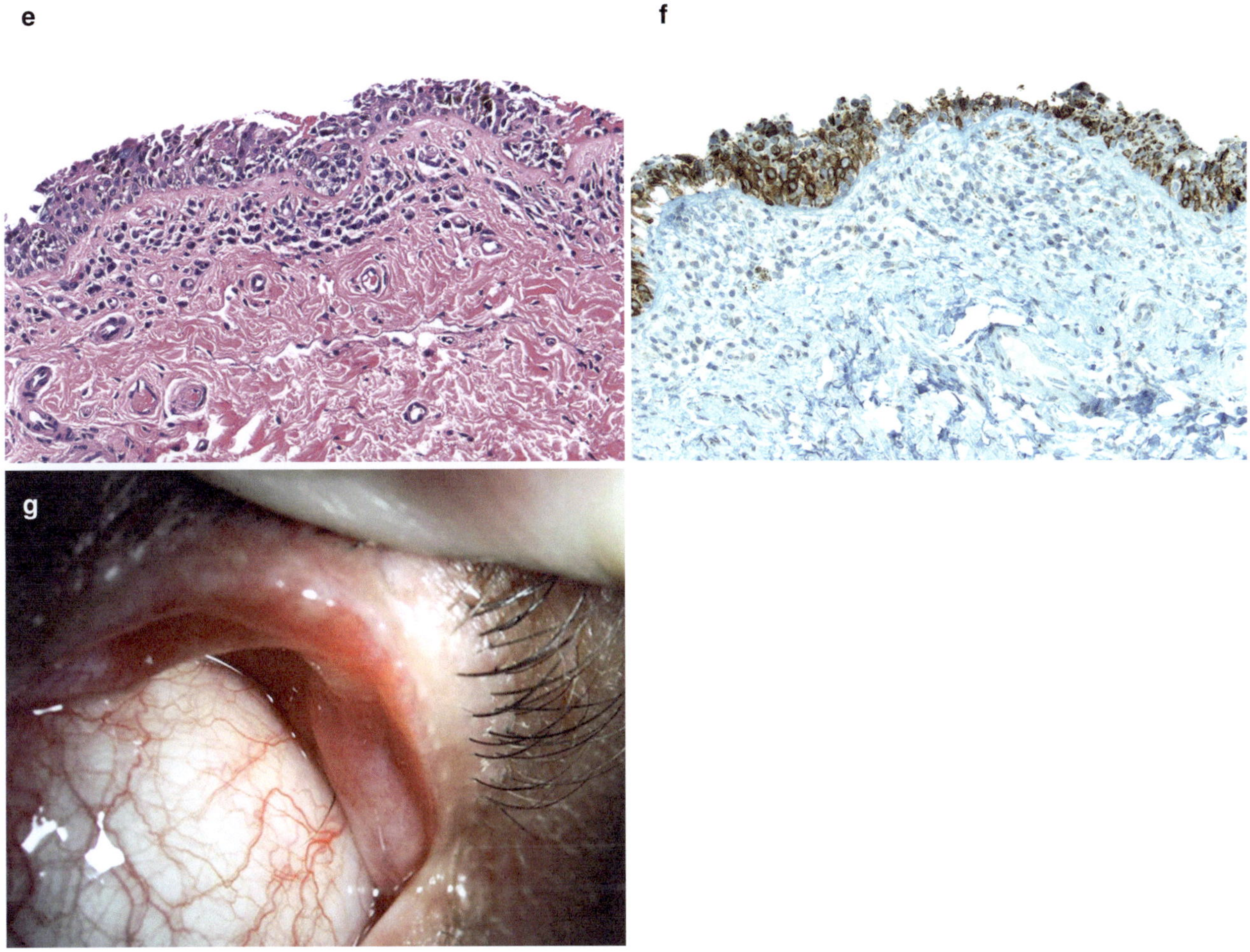

Fig. 8.4 (continued)

8.5 Diagnosis and Differential Diagnosis

The clinical examination of pigmented periocular lesions requires the ophthalmologist to provide an exceptional level of illumination (beyond that typically available in ophthalmic examining lanes that are used for refraction, slit-lamp examination, and funduscopy). One should be prepared to turn the room lights up to maximum level and to cast additional illumination on the affected area by a dedicated light near the examination chair. Magnification may help the ophthalmologist to detect subtle changes in a lesion's color and texture, and the lens used for indirect ophthalmoscopy may be especially useful in this setting. Ophthalmologists should also not overlook the utility of the slit lamp in examining the eyelids for malignancies of all types, not only pigmented eyelid lesions. The slit lamp provides exceptional magnification and illumination, critical to achieving a focused clinical differential diagnosis. Recently reported promising techniques include reflectance confocal microscopy, impedance spectroscopy, and digital epi-luminescence microscopy, have advantages over clinical inspection [23–26]. However, these instruments are not widely available and have not replaced standard examination.

Most nevi of the eyelid margin are nodular, reflecting the space-occupying characteristics of the intradermal collection of nevus cells. Lesions with a roughened or exaggerated skin texture are more likely to be of epithelial origin, even if pigmented. Thus, melanocytes may generate pigmentation within seborrheic keratosis. These lesions should never be mistaken for melanomas because (a) the precursor lesions of most melanomas in the periocular skin are flat (pigmented seborrheic keratosis is elevated), and (b) seborrheic keratosis features an irregular surface texture, while invasive melanoma typically produces a smooth nodular surface in the context of an otherwise flat precursor lesion in which skin markings are unaffected.

As mentioned above, basal cell carcinomas may be pigmented by the generation of excess melanin pigment in an otherwise "mundane" basal cell carcinoma of the nodular type. Such lesions are rare and may be mistaken for malignant melanomas of the nodular type. The treatment of pigmented nodular lesions of the eyelid involves total resection, so the initial treatment of these lesions is identical regardless of the eventual histological diagnosis. Spitz nevi may be confused clinically and histologically for melanomas of the nodular type on and around the eyelid (Chap. 4).

8.6 Histopathologic and Molecular Features

Lentigo maligna is remarkable for epidermal atrophy in the context of effacement of the rete and solar elastosis. Upon this background, one may encounter atypical melanocytes populating the basal layers of the epidermis and along adnexal structures such as the pillar units of the eyelash. Ophthalmologists should realize that in the terminology of contemporary dermatopathology, these lesions may be called "melanoma in situ," meaning that atypical melanocytes are within the epidermis, confined above the epidermal basement membrane.

Any breach of the epidermal basement membrane by atypical melanocytes renders the lesion a malignant melanoma. Should the invasive component arise in the context of an intradermal melanocytic lesion featuring melanocytes in a pagetoid distribution, one might then state that the melanoma is of a superficial spreading type. The type of melanoma (lentigo maligna melanoma or superficial spreading melanoma) does not influence the clinical behavior of the lesion.

The primary prognostic parameter for melanomas of the eyelid skin is the depth of invasion measured by a calibrated ocular micrometer from the top of the granular layer of the epidermis to the point of deepest invasion into the dermis, as was described by Breslow [27]. Other prognostic factors of importance in cutaneous melanoma at different body sites include the presence of ulceration (a poor prognostic sign), which is seldom seen in primary eyelid melanomas. Cell type, so significant among the histological characteristics of uveal melanoma, does not appear to play an independent role in this histological prognosis of eyelid melanomas.

Immunohistochemical markers such as S-100, HMB-45, MART-1/Melan A, SOX10 and others, have been used for many years in anatomic pathology diagnosis of melanoma. However, most of melanocytic markers have limited influence on differentiation between benign and malignant forms of the disease [28]. Ki-67 antigen, a marker of the proliferation portion of the cell cycle, shows low proliferation index in nevi and high in melanoma. Molecular pathology tests have been used for investigating genetic changes of melanoma; the most commonly used is BRAF mutation that has importance in targeted therapies. However, the application of genomic analysis in the diagnosis and prognosis of melanoma is still evolving [28].

Recently, preferentially expressed antigen in melanoma (PRAME) expression by immunohistochemistry has been used to distinguish cutaneous nevi from melanoma. However, unlike PRAME immunohistochemistry, which can separate uveal melanomas into lower and higher risks for metastasis, PRAME expression in the skin has not been reported to be an independent prognostic marker for cutaneous melanoma [29].

8.7 Treatment

8.7.1 Excision

There is a consensus that complete surgical excision with free surgical margins of healthy skin is the treatment of choice for cutaneous malignant melanoma in general and eyelid melanoma in particular. However, the ideal width of the surgical margins that are necessary in order to prevent recurrences is a matter of controversy. Harris et al. [30] recommended simple excision for in situ melanoma, 1 cm margins for tumors of 1 mm thickness or less, 2 cm margins for tumors of 1–4 mm depth, and at least 2 cm for more than 4 mm depth. However, because of difficulties in eyelid reconstruction, most studies exclude eyelid melanomas from these recommendations. Early diagnosis and treatment are essential in managing eyelid melanomas and especially for adequate functional and cosmetic lid reconstruction. In an extensive series of cutaneous eyelid melanoma from Australia, the authors recommended a surgical excision margin of 3 mm for eyelid melanoma ≤1 mm in Breslow thickness, and 5 mm for melanomas >1 mm in thickness [31].

Several experts have endorsed modified "slow" Mohs' surgery (mapped serial excision) using rush-paraffin sections and delayed repair for lentigo maligna and lentigo maligna melanoma [13, 17, 32–34]. They found that this technique offers a high early cure rate in conjunction with tissue conservation. They also found that the recommendation of 1 cm margins for melanoma of less than 1 mm thick is insufficient for complete excision. Cook and Bartley [1] recommended modified Mohs' technique using frozen tissue as treatment of choice. However, frozen tissue sections for melanoma are controversial because of freeze artifacts that make accurate interpretation difficult. A recent survey of 44 cases did not find that margins of excision have a statistically significant effect on local, regional, or distant recurrence [35]. A recent study comparing wide local excision and Mohs micrographic surgery, limited to the American Joint Committee on Cancer (AJCC) stage T1, demonstrated no significant difference in all-cause or cause-specific survival for patients treated with these two techniques [36].

Resection of periorbital and eyelid melanomas is challenging because of the important anatomic structures in this region [37]. The challenge lies in the need to provide the best functional and aesthetic results and resecting the primary lesion to effect the cure and protect the eye. The surgeon should not compromise the adequate margins to facilitate periorbital reconstruction without therapeutic compromise. The type of reconstruction performed depends on the size of the surgical defect and its location (e.g., primary closure, full-thickness skin grafts, upper lid mucocutaneous flaps, cheek advancement flaps, cervico-facial flaps, inferiorly-based nasolabial flaps, trans conjunctival flaps, frontalis muscle flaps, and medial transposition Z-plasty) (Chap. 11) [37]. The needs of most patients can be met by one procedure [38], but in complex cases two or more procedures are required. In an extensive series of eyelid melanoma, more than a third of the patients require more than one excision to achieve clear margins, supporting delayed reconstruction for eyelid melanoma [39].

8.7.2 Palliative Therapy

Primary use of nonsurgical ablation in cutaneous melanoma is not recommended [31]. Treatment methods such as cryotherapy, radiotherapy, topical treatment with azelaic acid, and curettage electrodissection are associated with high recurrence rates. In addition, these techniques do not provide tissue for histologic assessment of tumor thickness, the single most significant prognostic parameter in the management of melanoma. Cryotherapy and external beam radiation can be used as adjuvant therapy, although according to one study [12], adjuvant radiotherapy did not add at all to cure; thus radiotherapy is at best palliative. One group reported a successful treatment with brachytherapy, using Iodine-125 applicator in eyelid malignant melanoma [40], and another group using Ru-106 applicator (unpublished data). Recently treatment of eyelid lentigo maligna melanoma by topical Imiquimod 5% cream was reported to be an effective option as primary adjuvant therapy [41, 42].

8.7.3 Chemotherapy and Immunotherapy

In advanced metastatic cutaneous melanoma, chemotherapy has been used with limited success, mostly increasing survival but not curing the disease. Immunotherapy has been introduced in recent years for treating metastatic cutaneous melanoma. In recent years, immunotherapy has become a cornerstone in the treatment of advanced cases of melanoma, intending to modulate the host immunity against the tumor [43]. Currently the leading drugs for immune checkpoint inhibitors therapy for cutaneous melanoma are Ipilimumab (yervoy), Pembrolizumab (keytruda) and Nivolumab (opdivo) [44]. Adjuvant immunotherapy can be used in after complete surgical excision in patients with a high risk diseases unrespectable disease or metastatic disease. Several case series have reported a combination of radiation therapy and immunotherapy, suggesting a biologic interaction between these two methods [45].

8.7.4 Sentinel Lymph Node Biopsy

The elective lymph node dissection in patients with periocular melanoma is controversial [37, 46]. The procedure is probably not indicated for lesions less than 1.0 mm thick and may offer only a slight advantage for lesions thicker than 4.0 mm (Chap. 12). It is currently recommended to perform elective lymph node dissection for melanomas of "intermediate" thickness (1–4 mm), which may have generated occult nodal metastases. Sentinel lymph node mapping using lymphoscintigram has been advocated in order to locate suspicious involved lymph nodes and prevent unnecessary lymph node dissection. The technique has evolved into intraoperative lymphatic mapping and facilitates selective sentinel lymphadenectomy [47]. When positive, fine-needle aspiration biopsy or excision of the node should be performed for histologic confirmation of the metastatic disease. In those patients with histologic confirmation of nodal metastases but no evidence of distant metastases, parotidectomy or modified neck dissection is performed [37] (Chap. 12). Histologic features associated with a positive sentinel lymph node include greater tumor thickness, a greater number of mitotic figures and ulceration [46].

8.8 Prognosis

8.8.1 Prognostic Factors

Aage, gender, and histologic type are not of prognostic value [47]. Location of the tumor in the upper or lower lid and in the canthi does not affect prognosis. Nevertheless, melanoma's location in the lid margin involving the mucocutaneous junction is associated with higher mortality [8]. The involvement of the palpebral conjunctiva in such cases may explain this association. The status of the excision margins in cutaneous eyelid melanoma is not associated with local, regional, or distant recurrence [37]. In a large study, positive regional lymph node status was the most important prognostic factor for invasive melanoma survival [48].

8.8.2 Recurrence

Local recurrence of eyelid cutaneous melanoma is common, ranging from 7% to 78%, depending on the technique and extent of excision [44]. Local recurrence is not rare also when melanomas are completely excised [12]. Regional lymph node metastases were also reported in patients with completely-excised eyelid melanoma. In large series, local recurrence occurred in 21%, nodal metastasis in 11%, and distant metastasis in 4% [31]. In another series, regional lymph node metastasis was found in 29% of eyelid skin melanoma [44].

8.8.3 Mortality

The mortality rate from eyelid cutaneous melanoma varies significantly in various series, ranging from 7 to 58% [8, 10, 13]. The wide variation in the reported mortality may reflect the relative rarity of primary melanoma confined to the skin of the eyelid, and the high mortality in a series from a major tertiary cancer center is likely explained by a selection bias with more advanced cases treated in this setting [12]. The time from diagnosis to death ranges from 8 months to 14 years [47]. The late recurrence in many patients reinforces the need for long-term follow-up of patients treated for cutaneous eyelid melanoma.

References

1. Cook BE Jr, Bartley GB. Treatment options and future prospects for the management of eyelid malignancies: an evidence-based update. Ophthalmology. 2001;108(11):2088–100.
2. Rodriguez-Sains RS, Jakobiec FA, Iwamoto T. Lentigo maligna of the lateral canthal skin. Ophthalmology. 1981;88(12):1186–92.
3. Batsakis J. Tumors of the head and neck. Baltimore: Williams and Wilkins; 1974.
4. Shan Y, Xu Y, Lu Y, et al. Epidemiology and survival outcomes for eyelid primary malignant melanoma: an analysis of 1397 cases in the SEER database. J Ophthalmol. 2020;2020:4858636.
5. Brunetti P, Margo CE, French DD. Incidence of cutaneous melanoma of eyelid analysis of surveillance, epidemiology, and end results database. Ocul Oncol Pathol. 2021;7:66–9.
6. Go CC, Kim DH, Go BC, et al. Clinicopathologic characteristics and prognostic factors impacting survival in melanoma of the eyelid. Am J Ophthalmol. 2022;234:71–80.
7. Naidoff MA, Bernardino VB, Clark WH. Melanocytic lesions of the eyelid skin. Am J Ophthalmol. 1976;82(3):371–82.
8. Garner A, Koornneef L, Levene A, et al. Malignant melanoma of the eyelid skin: histopathology and behaviour. Br J Ophthalmol. 1985;69(3):180–6.
9. Zoltie N, O'Neill TJ. Malignant melanomas of eyelid skin. Plast Reconstr Surg. 1989;83(6):994–6.
10. Grossniklaus HE, McLean IW. Cutaneous melanoma of the eyelid. Clinicopathologic features. Ophthalmology. 1991;98(12):1867–73.
11. Tahery DP, Goldberg R, Moy RL. Malignant melanoma of the eyelid. A report of eight cases and a review of the literature. J Am Acad Dermatol. 1992;27(1):17–21.
12. Vaziri M, Buffam FV, Martinka M, et al. Clinicopathologic features and behavior of cutaneous eyelid melanoma. Ophthalmology. 2002;109(5):901–8.
13. Chan FM, O'Donnell BA, Whitehead K, et al. Treatment and outcomes of malignant melanoma of the eyelid: a review of 29 cases in Australia. Ophthalmology. 2007;114(1):187–92.
14. Wang JK, Liao SL, Jou JR, et al. Malignant eyelid tumours in Taiwan. Eye. 2003;17(2):216–20.
15. Takamura H, Yamashita H. Clinicopathological analysis of malignant eyelid tumor cases at Yamagata University Hospital: statistical comparison of tumor incidence in Japan and in other countries. Jpn J Ophthalmol. 2005;49(5):349–54.
16. Oliver JD, Boczar D, Sisti A, et al. Eyelid melanoma in the United States: a national cancer database analysis. J Craniofac Surg. 2019;30:2412–5.
17. Then SY, Malhotra R, Barlow R, et al. Early cure rates with narrow-margin slow-Mohs surgery for periocular malignant melanoma. Dermatologic Surg. 2009;35(1):17–23.
18. Kostopoulos E, Champsas G, Konofaos P, et al. Eyelid melanoma: our experience a propos of 23 cases. Ann Chir Plast Esthet. 2012;57(2):158–63.
19. Patel BC, Egan CA, Lucius RW, et al. Cutaneous malignant melanoma and oculodermal melanocytosis (nevus of Ota): report of a case and review of the literature. J Am Acad Dermatol. 1998;38:862–5.
20. Demirci H, Johnson TM, Frueh BR, et al. Management of periocular cutaneous melanoma with a staged excision technique and permanent sections: the square procedure. Ophthalmology. 2008;115(12):2295–300.
21. Lazar AJ, Scolyer RA, de la Fouchandière A, Gerami P, Massi D. Melanocytic neoplasms. In: Elder DE, Barnhill RL, Bastian BC, editors. WHO classification of tumours. Skin tumours. 5th ed. Geneva: WHO; 2022.
22. Rubinstein TJ, Plesec TP, Singh AD. Desmoplastic melanoma of the eyelid and conjunctival melanoma in neurofibromatosis type 1: a clinical pathological correlation. Surv Ophthalmol. 2015;60:72–7.
23. Ahlgrimm-Siess V, Laimer M, Rabinovitz HS, et al. Confocal microscopy in skin cancer. Curr Dermatol Rep. 2018;7:105–18.
24. Annessi G, Bono R, Abeni D. Correlation between digital epiluminescence microsopy parameters and hitopathological changes in lentigo maligna and solar lentigo: a dermoscopic index in the diagnosis of lentigo maligna. J Am Acad Deramatol. 2017;76:234–43.
25. Mohr P, Birgersson U, Berking C, et al. Electric impedance spectroscopy as a potential adjunct diagnoaia tool for cutaneous melanoma. Skin Res Technol. 2013;19:75–83.
26. Serban ED, Farnetani F, Pellacani G, et al. Role of in-vivo reflectance confocal microscopy in analysis of melanocytic lesions. Acta Dermatovenerol Croat. 2018;26:64–7.
27. Breslow A. Thickness, cross-sectional areas and depth of invasion in the prognosis of cutaneous melanoma. Ann Surg. 1970;172(5):902–8.
28. Mancera N, Smalley KSM, Margo EM. Melanoma of the eyelid and periocular skin: histopathologic classification and molecular pathology. Surv Ophthalmol. 2019;62:272–88.
29. Parra O, Ma W, Li Z, et al. PRAME expression in cutaneous melanoma does not correlate with disease-specific survival. J Cutan Pathol. 2023;50(10):903–12. https://doi.org/10.1111/cup.14495.
30. Harris MN, Shapiro RL, Roses DF. Malignant melanoma. Primary surgical management (excision and node dissection) based on pathology and staging. Cancer. 1995;75(2):715–25.
31. Harish V, Bond JS, Scolyer RA, et al. Margins of excision and prognostic factors for cutaneous eyelid melanomas. J Plast Reconstr Aesthet Surg. 2013;66:1066–73.
32. Malhotra R, Chen C, Huilgol S, et al. Mapped serial excision for periocular lentigo maligna and lentigo maligna melanoma. Ophthalmology. 2003;110(10):2011–8.
33. Boulos PR, Rubin PA. Cutaneous melanomas of the eyelid. Semin Ophthalmol. 2006;21(3):195–206.

34. Bladen JC, Malhotra R, Litwin A. Long-term outcomes of margin-controlled excision for eyelid melanoma. Eye. 2023;37:1009–13.
35. Esmaeli B, Youssef A, Naderi A, et al. Margins of excision for cutaneous melanoma of the eyelid skin: the Collaborative Eyelid Skin Melanoma Group report. Ophthalmic Plast Reconstr Surg. 2003;19(2):96–101.
36. Ramachandran V, Phan K. Mohs micrographic surgery versus wide local excision for eyelid melanoma: an analysis of a national database. J Plast Reconstr Aesthet Surg. 2022;75:4410–5.
37. Glat P, Longaker M, Jelks EB, et al. Periorbital melanocytic lesions: excision and reconstruction in 40 patients. Plast Reconstr Surg. 1998;102(1):19–27.
38. Pinto V, Zannetti G, Vilani R, et al. Long term cosmetic and functional results of one stage reconstruction for lower eyelid malignant melanoma: a single center experience of eleven patients. J Maxillofac Oral Surg. 2018;17:625–9.
39. Yin VT, Warneke CL, Merritt HA, Esmaeli B. Number of excisions required to obtain clear surgical margins and prognostic value of AJCC T category for patients with eyelid melanoma. Br J Ophthalmol. 2014;98:1681–5.
40. Stanowsky A, Krey HF, Kopp J, et al. Irradiation of malignant eyelid melanoma with Iodine-125 plaque. Am J Ophthalmol. 1990;110(1):44–8.
41. Elia MD, Lally SE, Hanlon AM, et al. Periocular melanoma in situ treated with imiquimod. Opthal Plast Reconstr Surg. 2016;32:371–3.
42. Neumann I, Patalay R, Kaushik M, et al. Treatment of periocular lentigo maligna with topical 5% Imiquimod: a review. Eye. 2023;37:408–14.
43. Sanlorenzo M, Vujic I, Posch C, et al. Melanoma immunotherapy. Cancer Biol Ther. 2014;15:665–74.
44. Lu JE, Chang JR, Berry JL, et al. Clinical update on checkpoint inhibitor therapy for conjunctival and eyelid melanoma. Int Ophthalmol Clin. 2020;60:77–89.
45. Barker CA, Postow MA. Combinations of radiation therapy and immunotherapy for melanoma: a review of clinical outcomes. Int J Radiat Oncol Biol Phys. 2014;88:986–97.
46. Pfeiffer ML, Ozgur OK, Myers JN, et al. Sentinel lymph node biopsy for ocular adnexal melanoma. Acta Ophthalmol. 2017;95:e323–8.
47. Esmaeli B, Wang B, Deavers M, et al. Prognostic factors for survival in malignant melanoma of the eyelid skin. Ophthalmic Plast Reconstr Surg. 2000;16(4):250–7.
48. Behbahani S, Malerba S, Maniar A, et al. Outcomes and predictors of survival in cutaneous melanoma of the eyelid: an analysis of the national cancer database. J Am Acad Dermatol. 2021;84:1753–8.

Eyelid Adnexal Tumors

9

Martina C. Herwig-Carl and Karin U. Loeffler

9.1 Introduction

Eyelid adnexal tumors are frequent and comprise a large variety of different entities because the lid is rich in adnexal structures such as hairs (lashes) and glands. Overall, benign adnexal lesions of the eyelids are much more frequent than the malignant lesions [1–3]. In a series of 864 eyelid lesions that were biopsied, 82% were benign [1]. It is reassuring to note that the accuracy of clinically suspected malignant eyelid tumors is reported in the 90% range [1, 2].

Among benign lesions of the eyelid, adnexal tumors are frequent and display a variety of clinical as well as histologic features. Most commonly, they originate from sweat glands or hair follicles. Malignant neoplasms are rare but can occur, and excision and histopathologic evaluation are therefore recommended even for less suspicious tumors (Box 9.1).

Box 9.1
- Eyelid adnexal tumors are frequent and comprise a large variety of different entities.
- Most commonly these lesions arise from sweat glands or hair follicles.
- Histology can provide further information with regard to the origin of the lesion and its dignity.

M. C. Herwig-Carl (✉)
Department of Ophthalmology, University Clinic Bonn, Bonn, NRW, Germany
e-mail: martina.herwig-carl@ukbonn.de

K. U. Loeffler
Division of Ophthalmic Pathology, Department of Ophthalmology, University Clinic Bonn, Bonn, NRW, Germany

9.2 Etiopathogenesis

The eyelid adnexal tumors may be classified as cystic lesions as well as benign and malignant tumors arising from sweat glands, hair follicles, sebaceous glands, and accessory lacrimal glands (Table 9.1). All glands can, particularly in cases of duct obstruction, lead to retention cysts. Epidermal inclusion cysts and epidermoid cysts may occur following trauma, surgery, and inflammatory processes. Otherwise, the precise etiology of most adnexal tumors of the eyelids is still unknown.

Table 9.1 Classification of eyelid adnexal tumors

Types	Subtypes	
Cystic lesions	Benign	Epidermal inclusion cyst
		Retention cyst
		Trichilemmal cyst
Sweat gland tumors	Benign	Apocrine hidrocystoma
		Eccrine hidrocystoma
		Syringoma
		Eccrine spiradenoma
		Pleomorphic adenoma
		Syringocystadenoma papilliferum
	Malignant	Sweat gland adenocarcinoma
		Mucinous sweat gland adenocarcinoma
		Apocrine gland adenocarcinoma
Hair follicle tumors	Benign	Trichoepithelioma
		Trichofolliculoma
		Trichoadenoma
		Trichilemmoma
		Pilomatrixoma
	Malignant	Carcinoma of hair follicles
		Pilomatrix carcinoma
Sebaceous gland tumors	Benign	Sebaceous gland hyperplasia
		Sebaceous gland adenoma
		Sebaceous epithelioma
		Nevus sebaceous of Jadassohn
	Malignant	Sebaceous epithelioma
		Sebaceous gland carcinoma

B. C. K. Patel et al. (eds.), *Clinical Ophthalmic Oncology*, https://doi.org/10.1007/978-3-031-72328-5_9

9.3 Clinical Findings

Benign lesions usually respect the anatomical structures and occur as slowly growing, well-confined tumors with a smooth surface. As with all malignant tumors, clinical symptoms include progressive growth, recurrence after incomplete excision, infiltrative growth, and destruction of adjacent tissue (loss of eyelashes). Ulceration and hemorrhage can be present in advanced stages. Pain is an uncommon presenting feature in this location.

9.4 Treatment, Follow-up, and Prognosis

Management is similar in the majority of these tumors; benign lesions are excised for histologic confirmation, and malignant tumors are removed surgically with a tumor-free margin confirmed by histopathologic evaluation. Follow-up and the prognosis depend on the dignity and on the—extremely rare—development of metastases.

9.5 Cystic Lesions

9.5.1 Epidermal Inclusion Cysts or Epidermoid Cysts

Epidermal inclusion cysts or epidermoid cysts usually occur as smooth dome-shaped nodules of varying size (Fig. 9.1a), frequently revealing a punctum or pore. Occasionally, they appear pigmented. The characteristic feature is a cystic space filled with keratin, lined by regular keratinizing stratified squamous epithelium (Fig. 9.1b). In the case of keratin extrusion after cyst rupture, a marked inflammatory reaction can

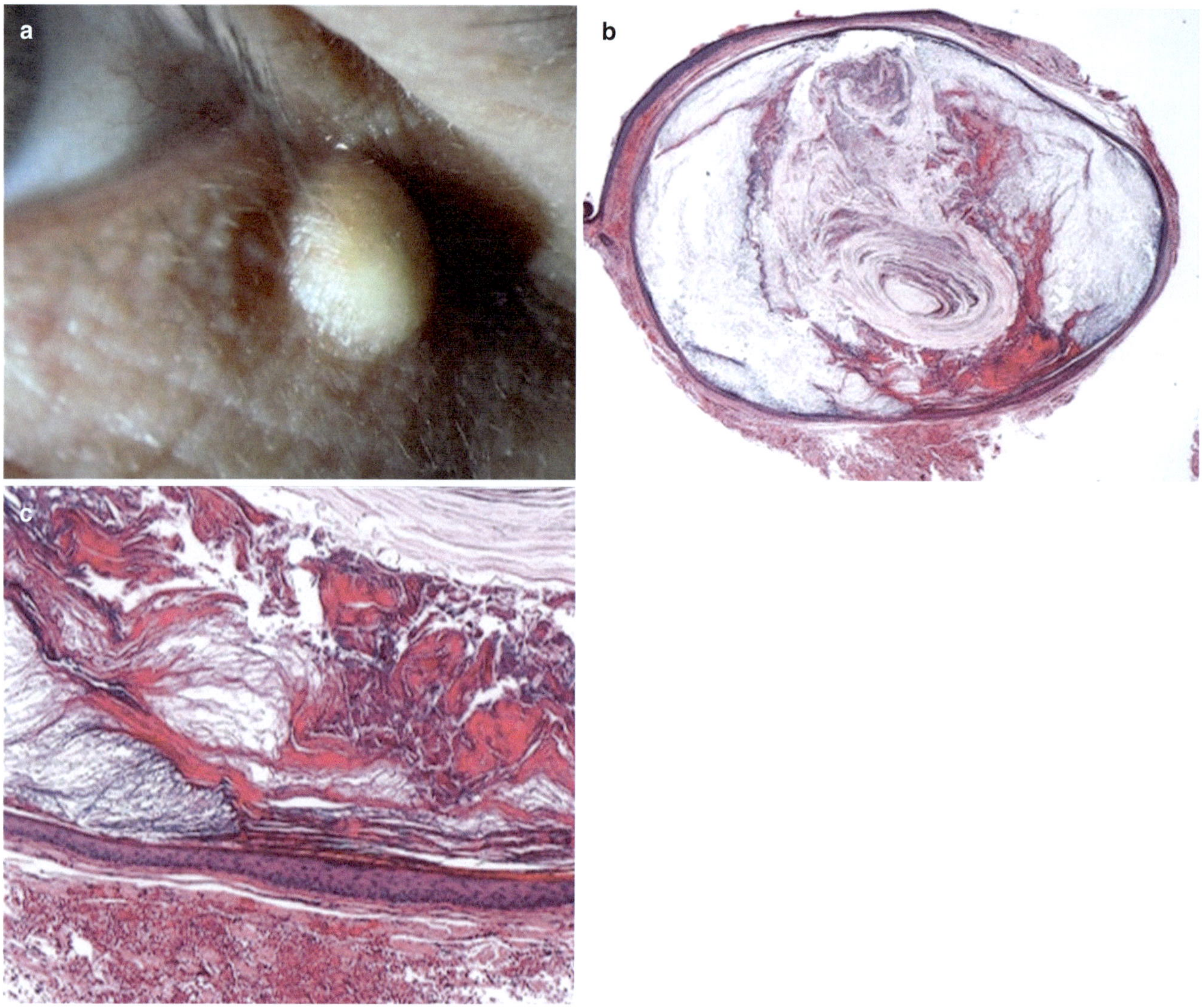

Fig. 9.1 Epidermoid cyst. Yellowish dome-shaped lesion at the lower eyelid (**a**). The cyst is filled with keratin (**b**) and lined by a keratinized squamous epithelium (**c**)

develop. Milia are miniature variants of epidermal cysts. Histologically, comedonal cyst is similar to an epidermoid cyst in that the lining consists of keratinizing stratified squamous epithelium. Clinically, a comedonal cyst is characterized as "blackhead" (comedo with opening onto the surface) or "whitehead" (comedo with blocked opening).

A "sebaceous" *cyst* is a clinical misnomer, as, despite the yellowish color of many cysts, histologic findings do not qualify any of these lesions as sebaceous. Clinically, the term is used most often for epidermoid or trichilemmal cyst.

9.5.2 Retention Cysts

Retention cysts can develop from all glands with the sudoriferous cyst, originating from sweat glands, as the most frequent type. The typical lining consists of a layer of nonkeratinizing glandular epithelium and a thin layer of myoepithelial cells.

9.5.3 Trichilemmal (Pilar) Cysts

Trichilemmal (pilar) cysts occur frequently in the scalp and appear as intradermal yellowish-smooth intradermal swelling. The cyst lining is composed of basophilic cells surrounded by a rim of fibrous tissue. Toward the lumen, the cells develop into squamous epithelium with pale and fairly high keratocytes that abruptly turn into keratin without a granular layer. Sometimes calcification occurs, and often cholesterol clefts are seen.

9.6 Sweat Gland Tumors

9.6.1 Benign Tumors

There are two types of sweat glands: eccrine and apocrine. Eccrine sweat glands are widely distributed in the body, and each gland consists of a single duct with a coiled deeper component [4]. By contrast, the apocrine sweat glands are limited to the special regions such as axilla, nipple, external ear, external genitalia, and the eyelids [4]. The apocrine glands and their ductal openings are closely associated with eyelashes [5]. Apocrine hidrocystoma and eccrine hidrocystoma represent the majority of the benign sweat gland tumors. In contrast to apocrine hidrocystoma, the eccrine hidrocystoma does not involve the eyelid margin. This is due to the fact that the eccrine sweat glands are distributed throughout the eyelid skin and are not confined to the eyelid margin unlike the apocrine glands [5].

9.6.1.1 Apocrine Hidrocystoma

Apocrine hidrocystoma (cystadenoma, apocrine tubular adenoma, cyst of Moll) is usually a solitary nodule affecting mostly the head (cheek) or neck in middle-aged people of either sex. It presents as a translucent or bluish-black nodule up to about 1 cm in diameter involving the eyelid margin (Fig. 9.2a) [6]. In rare instances, it can occur as multiple lesions [7, 8] and can be a feature of Schopf-Schulz-Passarge syndrome [8, 9]. Histopathology reveals an unilocular or multilocular cystic space (Fig. 9.2b) that is lined by a single or double layer of epithelial cells, surrounded by an outer layer representing myoepithelial cells, while the inner layer frequently shows the typical decapitation secretion. In some areas, epithelial proliferations can be found (Fig. 9.2c).

9.6.1.2 Eccrine Hidrocystoma

A typical *eccrine hidrocystoma* of the eyelid manifests in an adult as a solitary clear cystic lesion (Smith and Chernosky type) [10], although cases with simultaneous bilateral involvement (Robinson type) [11] have also been reported (Fig. 9.3a). The tumor is usually located along the medial or lateral aspect of the eyelid. On average, eccrine hidrocystoma measures 4 mm in the largest dimension, and it is rare for them to be larger than 10 mm [12]. Histologically, this tumor probably just represents a markedly dilated sweat gland duct with a presumably functional pathogenesis (Fig. 9.3b). Myoepithelial cells and decapitation secretion are absent (Fig. 9.3c).

9.6.1.3 Syringoma

Syringomas are common lesions on the upper eyelids, especially in females. They usually present as multiple small asymptomatic nodules (2–3 mm) but show a wide variety of clinical pictures (Fig. 9.4a) [13]. Histology shows interconnecting eccrine ducts and strands, lined by two layers of flattened cuboidal cells and sometimes giving rise to the characteristic tadpole configuration (Fig. 9.4b). Intracellular glycogen accumulation can cause a clear cell variant.

9.6.1.4 Eccrine Spiradenoma

Eccrine spiradenomas are uncommon tumors presenting as a mostly tender or painful subcutaneous nodule of fairly characteristic histology. Sharply demarcated aggregations of basaloid cells without connection to the dermis are arranged in a rosette-like fashion. Two types of tumor cells can be distinguished: the more peripheral small basophilic cells with round and hyperchromatic nuclei and the more central cells with larger oval nuclei and a pale-staining eosinophilic cytoplasm. Due to a rich vascular supply, this tumor can resemble an angioma, hemangiopericytoma, or glomus tumor.

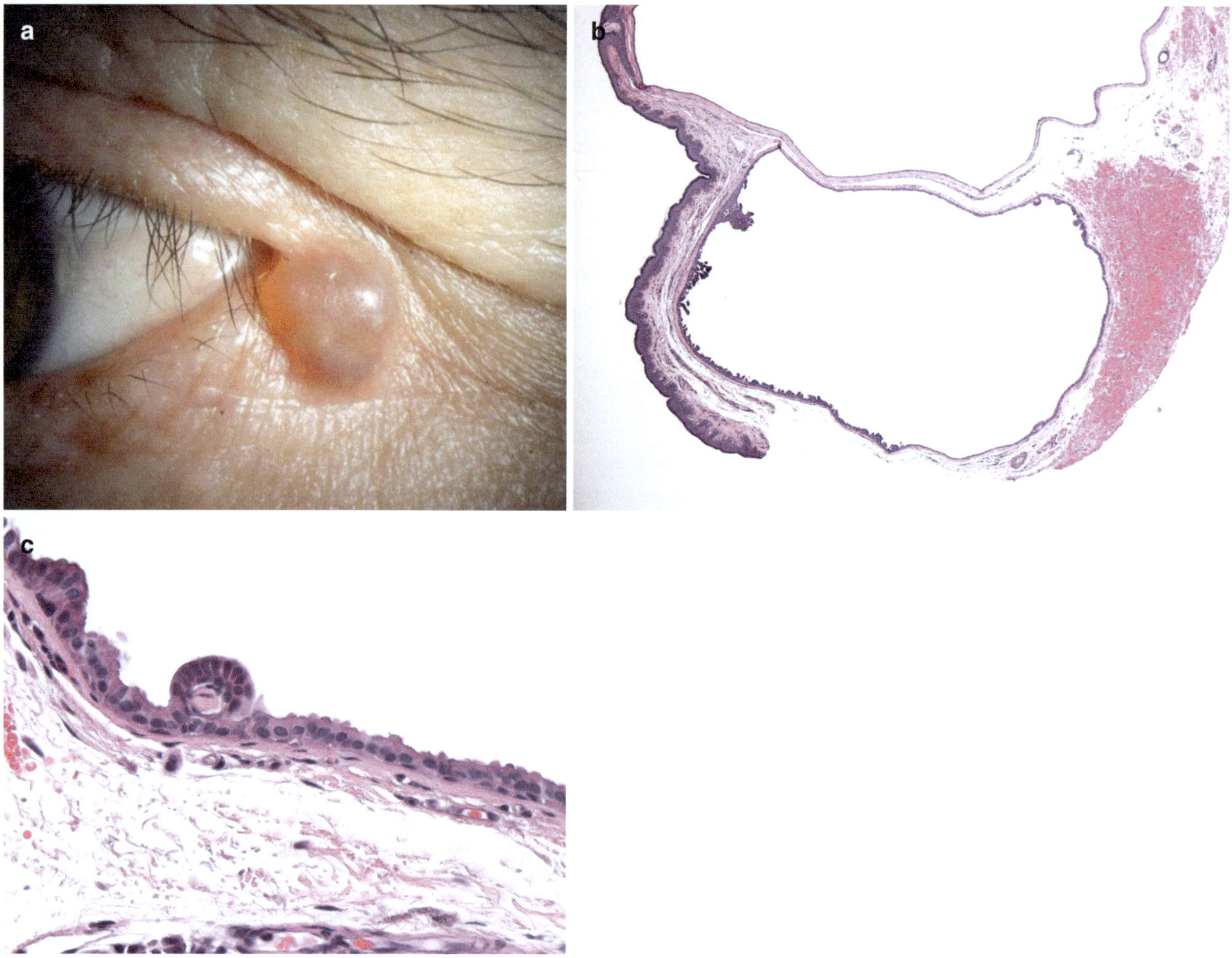

Fig. 9.2 Apocrine hidrocystoma. Note bluish color of the cystic lesion involving the eyelid margin (**a**). Histology shows cyst lined by a single to double layer of epithelial cells, surrounded by flattened myoepithelial cells. Proliferations of the epithelial lining are characteristic. Typical decapitation secretion is also found (**b**). Note focal epithelial proliferation (**c**)

9.6.1.5 Pleomorphic Adenomas (Benign Mixed Tumor)

Pleomorphic adenomas (benign mixed tumor) usually occur in the lacrimal or salivary glands but can also occur in accessory lacrimal glands of the eyelid. This lesion presents as a slowly growing either firm or cystic subcutaneous nodule, usually solitary and asymptomatic. Histologically, it is multilobulated and composed of a mixture of epithelial glandular elements embedded in myxoid stroma [14]. The stromal component can become very prominent, sometimes exhibiting a chondroid (pseudocartilaginous) and/or hyalinized appearance [15].

9.6.1.6 Syringocystadenoma Papilliferum

Syringocystadenoma papilliferum is usually a solitary lesion that presents as a grey to dark-brown papillary or warty excrescence which is clinically often mistaken for basal cell carcinoma or cyst [16]. Although it can grow in an endophytic or exophytic fashion, histopathology characteristically shows superficially located papillae communicating with duct-like structures in the deeper aspect. The lining consists of the typical double-layered epithelium with flattened myoepithelial cells at the outer zone and tall columnar cells at the inner zone [17]. Further entities such as eccrine acrospiroma, eccrine cylindroma, eccrine spiradenocylindromas, and apocrine adenomas exist.

9.6.2 Malignant Tumors

9.6.2.1 Sweat Gland Adenocarcinomas (Malignant Syringoma)

Sweat gland adenocarcinomas (malignant syringoma) most frequently affect the nasolabial and periorbital region and present nonspecifically as a slowly growing plaque-like lesion, sometimes associated with hyperkeratosis [18].

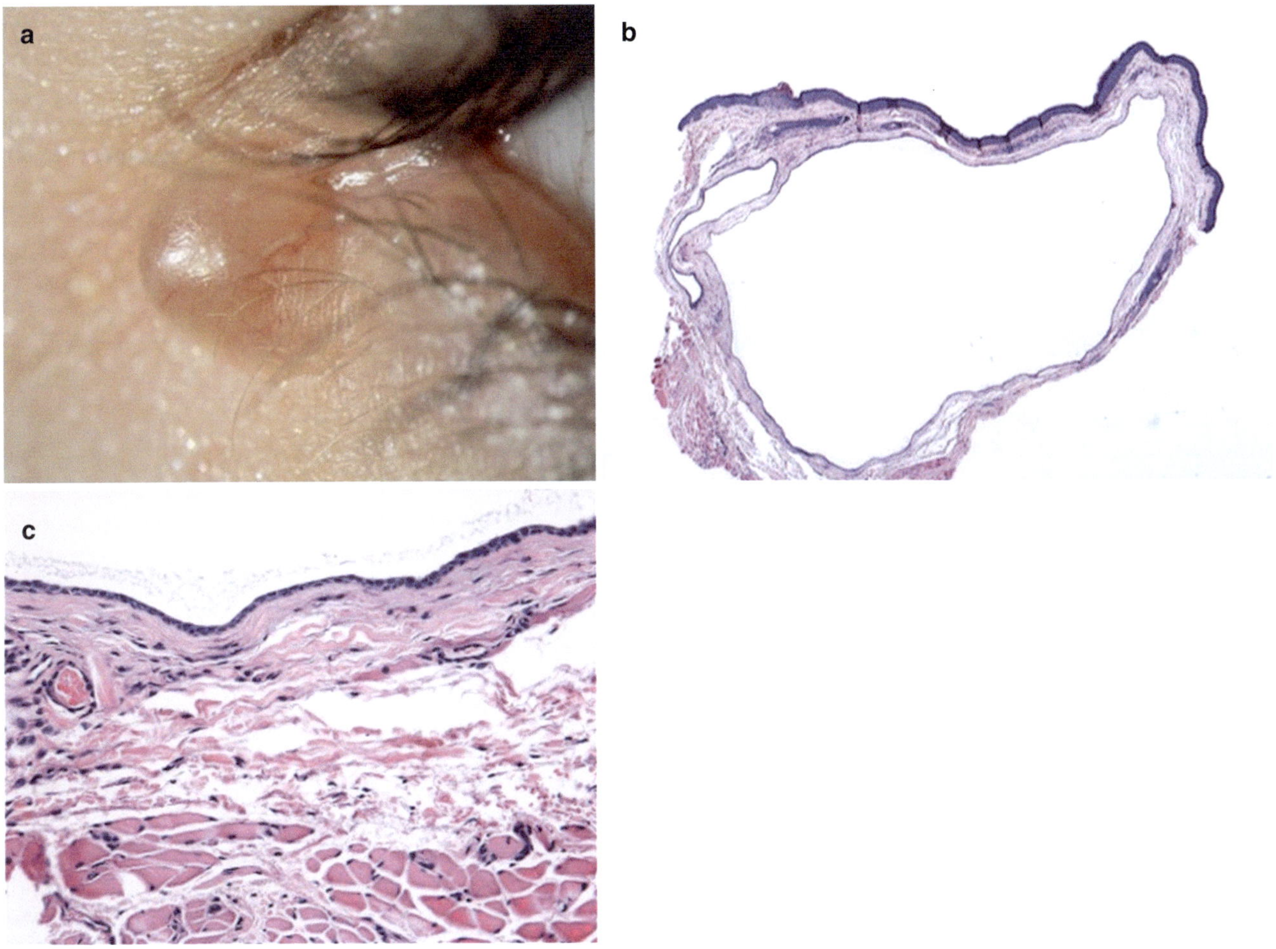

Fig. 9.3 Eccrine hidrocystoma. Note the gap between the tumor and the eyelid margin (**a**). There is the absence of papillary projections into the cystic cavity (**b**). The lining cuboidal epithelium is double layered and the cells lack decapitation (**c**)

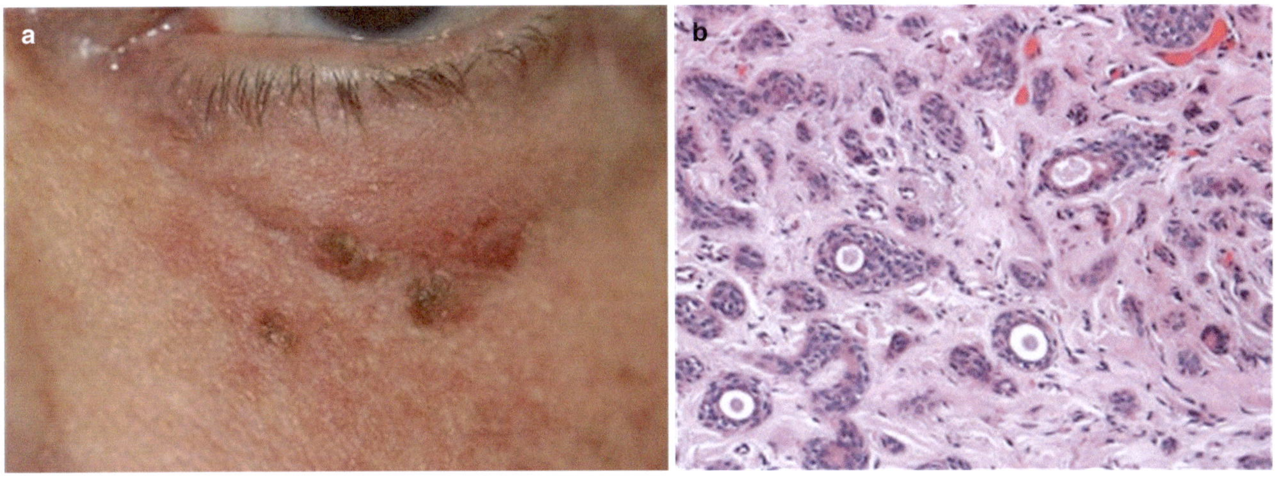

Fig. 9.4 Syringoma. Multiple syringomas of the lower eyelid in an older woman (**a**). The histopathology shows interconnecting eccrine ducts and stands which may present in a comma-shaped fashion (**b**)

Typically, the margins are not well delineated, and sometimes pain can be present due to perineural infiltration. Histology shows various features including small- to medium-sized squamous microcysts, solid strands of cells with ductular lumina, and small solid infiltrative strands, all embedded in a dense fibrous stroma.

9.6.2.2 Mucinous Sweat Gland Adenocarcinoma

Mucinous sweat gland adenocarcinoma is rare and shows a predilection for the eyelid and presents as a slowly growing flesh-colored, erythematous, or bluish nodule [19]. It is locally aggressive and frequently recurs, but distant metastases are uncommon. Histology shows islands of tumor cells embedded in an abundant pool of mucin, separated by fibrous septae. The tumor cells are cuboidal with a pink-staining, sometimes vacuolated cytoplasm and round nuclei. Often a glandular differentiation is present, and sometimes light- and dark-cell forms can be distinguished. Immunohistochemistry supports an eccrine derivation.

9.6.2.3 Apocrine Gland Adenocarcinoma (Carcinoma of the Glands of Moll)

Apocrine gland adenocarcinoma (carcinoma of the glands of Moll) is rare and most documented cases have affected the axilla. Fewer than ten cases have been described to arise from the glands of Moll in the eyelid [20]. The clinical appearance is of a reddish cystic nodular lesion located at the lid margin with a smooth surface (Fig. 9.5a). The tumor cells reveal a variably glandular, papillary, or diffuse growth, sometimes with cyst formation and necrosis, and decapitation secretion is a typical feature (Fig. 9.5b). Occasionally, intracytoplasmic diastase-resistant, periodic acid-Schiff-positive granules, and intracytoplasmic iron can be demonstrated while glycogen is negative. Normal apocrine glands are often found in close proximity to the tumor, and occasionally a preexisting apocrine adenoma may be evident. Since primary cutaneous apocrine carcinoma is indistinguishable from metastatic mammary ductal apocrine carcinoma, a careful breast assessment should be advised especially in cases where the diagnosis is questionable [21].

9.7 Hair Follicle Tumors

9.7.1 Benign Tumors

9.7.1.1 Trichoepithelioma

Trichoepithelioma is a hamartomatous lesion that may be solitary, multiple, or even familial [22]. The typical histologic appearance shows numerous horn cysts, partially within nests of basaloid cells that are sometimes difficult to distinguish from basal cell carcinoma. There can be continuity with the epidermis while ulceration is exceedingly rare. In trichoepithelioma, however, the perilobular connective tissue is more conspicuous and is frequently associated with the formation of papillary mesenchymal bodies [23]. Occasionally, a foreign body giant cell reaction to free keratin and calcification is seen. Trichoepithelioma shows less follicular differentiation than trichofolliculoma [24].

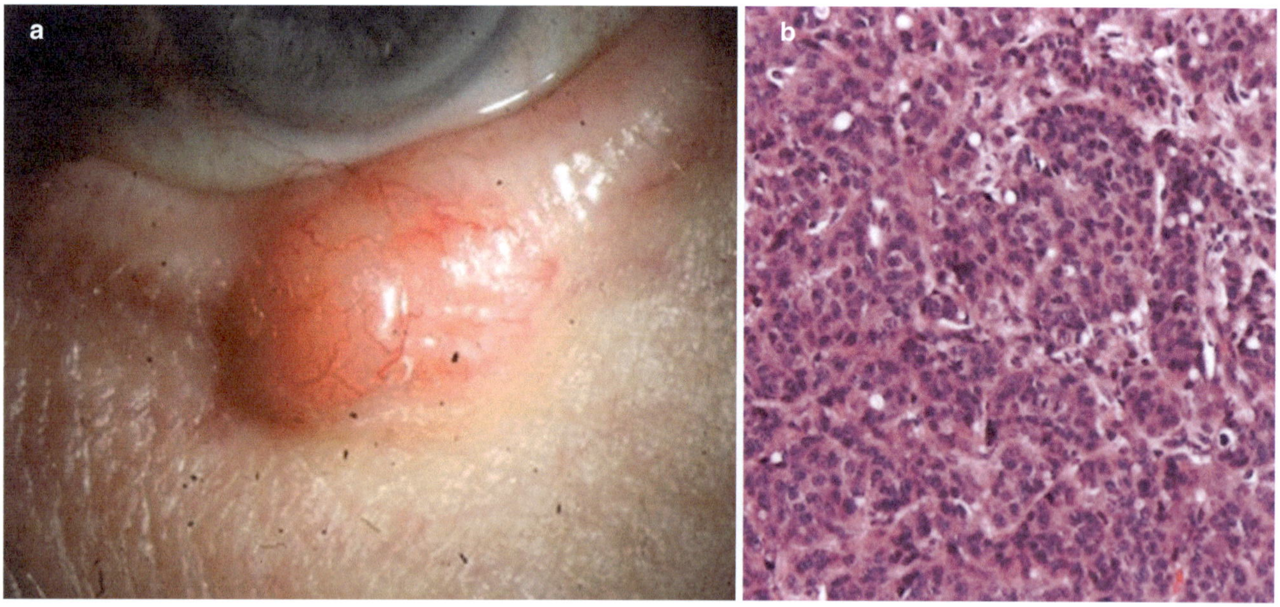

Fig. 9.5 Carcinoma of the glands of Moll in the eyelid. A reddish cystic nodular lesion located at the lid margin (**a**). Histologically, there is a papillary growth of tumor cells with mitotic figures and atypia (**b**)

9.7.1.2 Trichofolliculoma

Trichofolliculoma is a hamartoma presenting as a single dome-shaped papule with a central pore. Characteristic is the presence of one or more silky white threadlike hairs growing out of this opening [25]. A wide age range is affected, although lesions are very rare in children. Histologically, this tumor consists of a cystic cavity (dilated hair follicle) lined by stratified squamous epithelium usually continuous with the surface epithelium. Arising from its wall are numerous hair follicles. Abortive pilar differentiation, small primitive sebaceous acini, keratocysts, stromal granulomatous inflammation surrounding hair shaft fragments, and focal calcification are additional features. A variant of trichofolliculoma with numerous additional sebaceous glands is called sebaceous trichofolliculoma. A trichoepithelioma with prominent desmoplastic stroma is categorized as desmoplastic trichoepithelioma.

9.7.1.3 Trichoadenoma

Trichoadenoma is a rare tumor that occurs as a solitary asymptomatic soft or firm nodule of varying size and yellowish or erythematous color [26]. Under a normal epidermis, there is a well-defined fibroepithelial tumor composed of keratinous cysts and a conspicuous fibrovascular stroma. The cysts are lined by keratinizing epithelium including a granular layer. Sometimes solid epithelial islands are also present, but evidence of hair follicle formation is lacking.

9.7.1.4 Trichilemmoma

Trichilemmoma may be solitary or multiple and presents as a small warty or smooth skin-colored papule on the face of older adults (Fig. 9.6) [27]. Solitary trichilemmoma represents a proliferation of the follicular outer root sheath with close-set lobules connecting with the epidermis. There is usually peripheral nuclear palisading, but pleomorphism and mitoses tend to

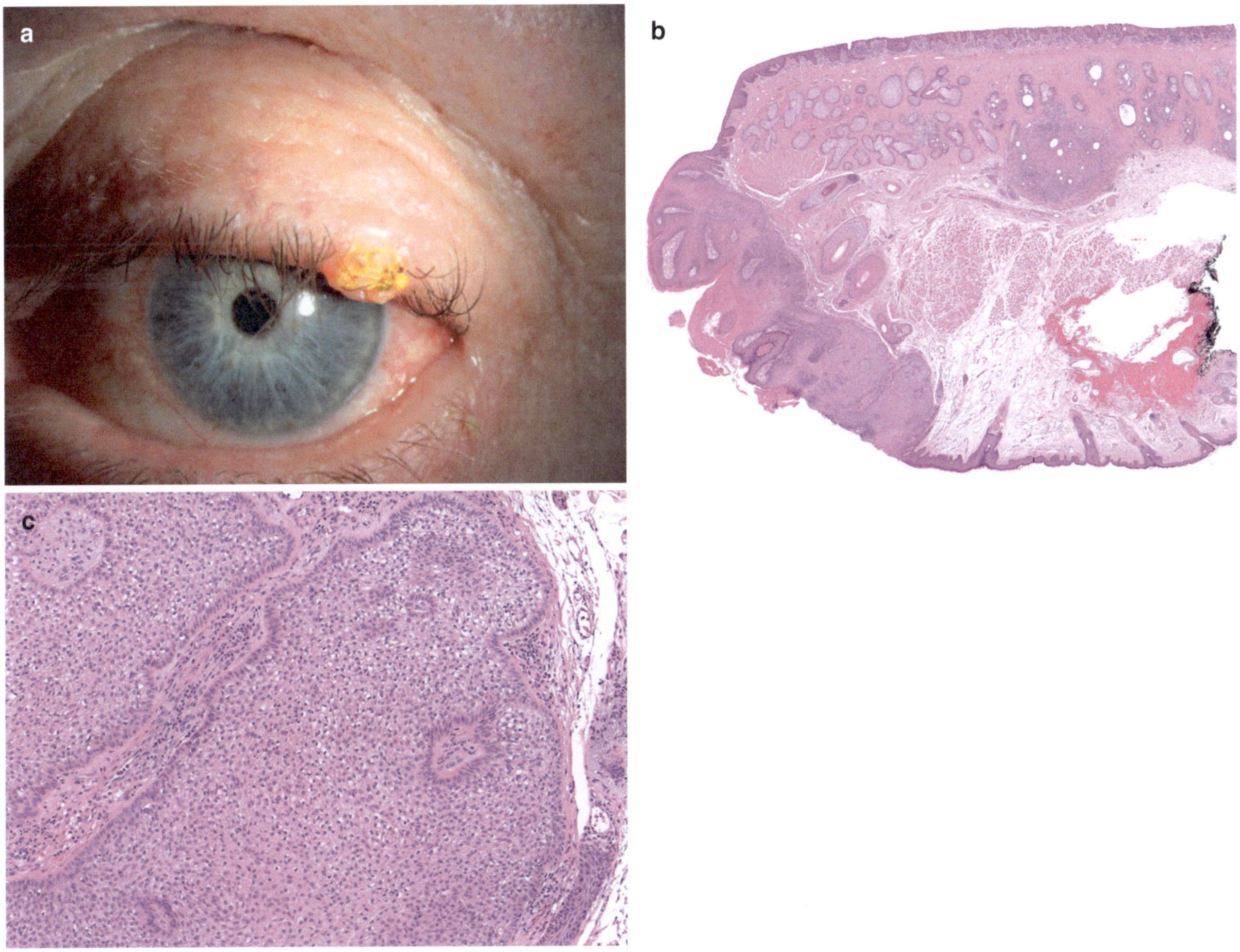

Fig. 9.6 Trichilemmoma. A 71-year-old man with nodular lesion arising from anterior lamella along lash line (**a**). A full thickness wedge excision was performed. Skin at eyelid margin shows epidermal proliferation with parakeratotic surface (**b**, H&E 1.6×) (note unrelated chalazion on conjunctival side). Higher power shows monomorphic cells with cytoplasmic clearing/vacuolation and peripheral nuclear palisading (**c**, H&E 12×). Courtesy of Gabrielle A. Yeaney, MD Division of Ocular Pathology, Diagnostics Institute, Cleveland Clinic, Cleveland, OH, USA

be absent. Intracellular glycogen can result in a conspicuous clear cell component. Another typical feature is a dense PAS-positive mantle surrounding individual tumor lobules. A variant with marked keratinization, squamous eddies, and surface hyperkeratosis and parakeratosis is called keratinizing trichilemmoma [24]. Associated with the presence of multiple trichilemmomas is the rare autosomal dominant condition called Cowden's (multiple hamartoma) disease [28].

9.7.1.5 Pilomatrixoma (Calcifying Epithelium of Malherbe)

Pilomatrixoma (calcifying epithelium of Malherbe) usually presents as a solitary lesion but can rarely be part of an autosomal dominantly inherited disorder or a systemic disease such as dystrophia myotonia or Gardner's syndrome [29]. It is a slowly growing hard nodule of bluish or reddish tint and frequently located subcutaneously beneath the eyebrow (Fig. 9.7a). Most often teenagers and older adults in the sixth and seventh decades are affected [30]. Histology reveals a well-circumscribed tumor consisting of two different cell populations: small basophilic basaloid cells and the characteristic and diagnostic pale-pinkish ghost cells (Fig. 9.7b). Frequently, calcification and a foreign body giant cell reaction are encountered, and occasionally melanin pigment is found. Even bone formation and amyloid deposition may be features. Mitoses are seen in early lesions but are not abnormal and simply indicate a rapid growth phase (Fig. 9.8) [31].

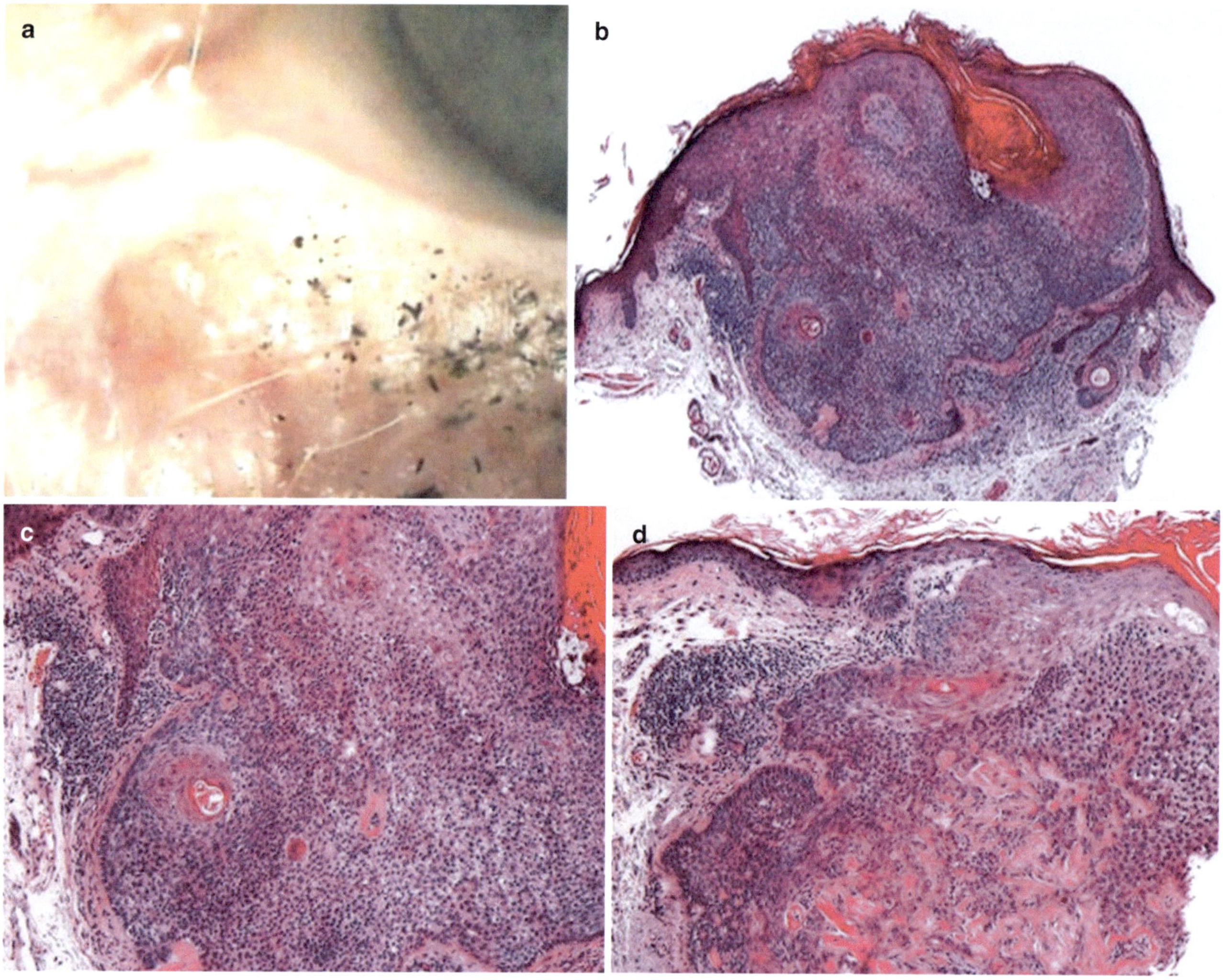

Fig. 9.7 Trichilemmoma of the lower eyelid. A solitary papule is located (clinically suspicious for basal cell carcinoma) at the eyelid margin of an older lady (**a**). The lesion shows a lobular architecture, peripheral pallisading, and a surrounding hyline membrane. Adjacent to the lesion are hair follicles (**b**). The cells show a clear cell component (**c**). Sclerotic stroma is also occasionally present (**d**)

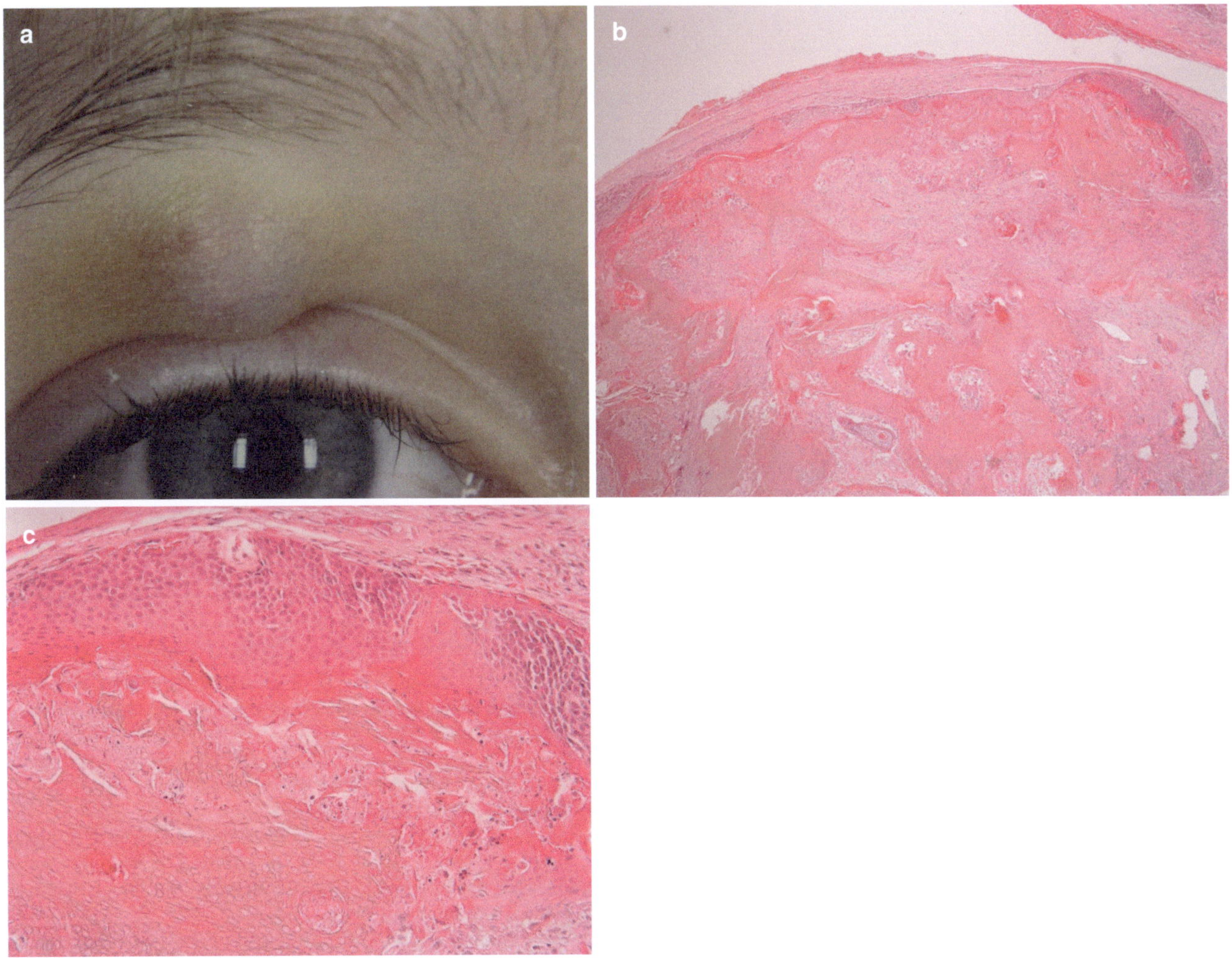

Fig. 9.8 Pilomatrixoma. Bluish-reddish nodule on the upper lid (**a**). Histology shows an epithelioid island surrounded by pinkish ghost/shadow cells and inflammation (**b**)

9.7.2 Malignant Tumors

9.7.2.1 Carcinoma of Hair Follicles (Trichilemmal Carcinoma)

Carcinoma of hair follicles (trichilemmal carcinoma) is a rare tumor that is found predominantly on sun-exposed skin of the elderly. The clinical presentation ranges from papule or a nodule to plaque that often ulcerates. Usually, the lesion is erythematous or flesh colored and measures between 5 and 20 mm in diameter. Despite a histologically worrying picture, recurrences and metastases are absent.

9.7.2.2 Pilomatrix Carcinomas

This rare tumor has been described in middle-aged patients [32]. However, only a few cases have been observed in the ocular adnexa [33].

9.8 Sebaceous Gland Tumors

9.8.1 Benign Tumors

9.8.1.1 Sebaceous Gland Hyperplasia

Sebaceous gland hyperplasia usually presents as a yellowish umbilicated papule 1–2 mm in size on the face of older adults. Clinically, it can be mistaken for basal cell carcinoma. Histopathologically, regular mature but hyperplastic sebaceous glands are seen that are situated rather superficially in the dermis while the epidermis is normal (Fig. 9.9).

9.8.1.2 Sebaceous Gland Adenoma

Sebaceous gland adenomas are rare and present as tan, yellow, or reddish papules/nodules about 5 mm in diameter, most frequently located on the face of older people (mean

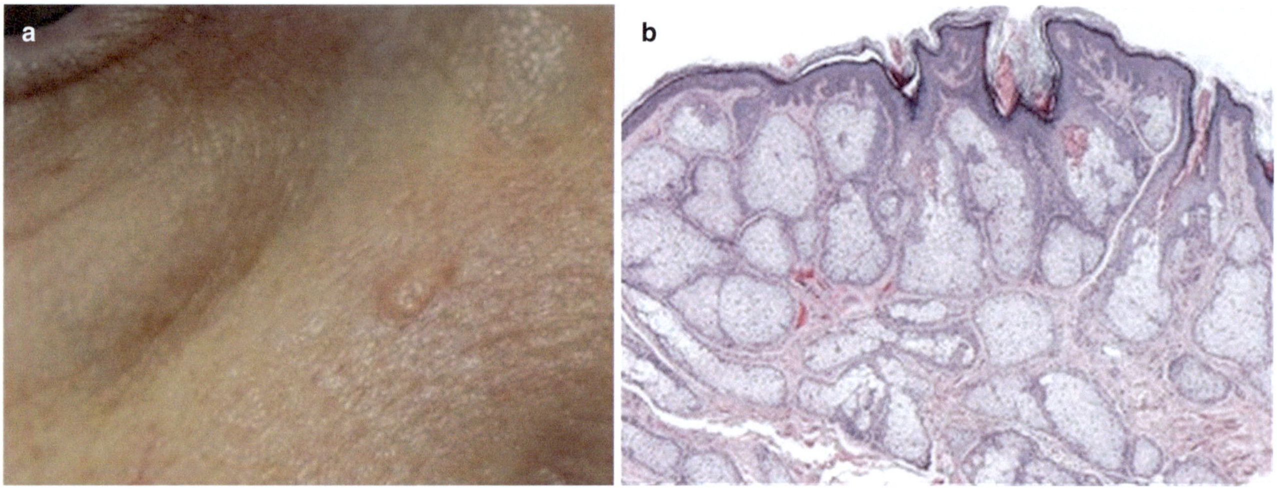

Fig. 9.9 Sebaceous gland hyperplasia. Yellowish papule with a central umbilication (**a**). The histologic picture shows conglomerates of regular sebaceous glands (**b**)

age: 60 years). Clinically, they can easily be misdiagnosed as basal cell carcinoma. Sebaceous gland adenoma in a younger person can be an indication for the Muir-Torre syndrome (Chap. 11) [34].

9.8.1.3 Sebaceous Epithelioma/Sebaceoma

Eyelid sebaceous epithelioma, or sebaceoma, is a rare entity [35]. It clinically appears as a nodular tumor, e.g., on the eyelid margin [36]. Histologically basaloid cells and vacuolated sebaceous cells without cellular atypia are found. Cells with sebaceous differentiation can be highlighted immunohistochemilly by adipophilin staining. Sebaceomas can be also associated with Muir-Torre syndrome [37]. Some authors consider this lesion a variant of basal cell carcinoma, i.e., a basal cell carcinoma with sebaceous differentiation [38].

9.8.1.4 Nevus Sebaceous of Jadassohn

Nevus sebaceous of Jadassohn is a complex choristoma comprising abnormalities of the hair follicles, sweat glands, sebaceous glands, and epidermis [39]. All of these tissues can proliferate and can constitute the major part of the tumor. Malignant transformation of any of the components is possible, with basal cell carcinoma being the most frequent [40].

9.8.2 Malignant Tumors

9.8.2.1 Sebaceous Gland Carcinoma

Sebaceous gland carcinoma is covered in a separate chapter (Chap. 6).

References

1. Kersten RC, Ewing-Chow D, Kulwin DR, Gallon M. Accuracy of clinical diagnosis of cutaneous eyelid lesions. Ophthalmology. 1997;104(3):479–84.
2. Margo CE. Eyelid tumors: accuracy of clinical diagnosis. Am J Ophthalmol. 1999;128(5):635–6.
3. Deprez M, Uffer S. Clinicopathological features of eyelid skin tumors. A retrospective study of 5504 cases and review of literature. Am J Dermatopathol. 2009;31(3):256–62.
4. Warwick R, Williams PL. Gray's anatomy, vol. 35. Edinburgh: Longman Group Ltd; 1973. p. 1168–9.
5. Warwick R. Eugene Wolf's anatomy of the and orbit, vol. 7. London: H.K. Lewis & Co. Ltd; 1976. p. 195–7.
6. Smith JD, Chernosky ME. Apocrine hidrocystoma (cystademnoma). Arch Dermatol. 1974;109(5):700–2.
7. Sacks E, Jakobiec FA, McMillan R. Multiple bilateral apocrine cystadenomas of the lower eyelids. Light and electron microscopic studies. Ophthalmology. 1987;94(1):65–71.
8. Alessi E, Gianotti R, Coggi A. Multiple apocrine hidrocystomas of the eyelids. Br J Dermatol. 1997;137(4):642–5.
9. Verplancke P, Driessen L, Wynants P, Naeyaert JM. The Schopf-Schulz-Passarge syndrome. Dermatology. 1998;196(4):463–6.
10. Smith JD, Chernosky ME. Hidrocystomas. Arch Dermatol. 1973;108(5):676–9.
11. Robinson R. Hidrocystoma. J Cutan Genitourinary Dis. 1893;11:293–303.
12. Singh AD, McCloskey L, Andrew M, Parsons. Eccrine hidrocystoma of the eyelid. Eye. 2005;19:77–9.
13. Lee SJ, Cho S, Cho SB. Syringomas versus sebaceous gland prominence of the eyelids. J Cosmet Laser Ther. 2011;13(3):130–1.
14. Alyahya GA, Stenman G, Persson F. Pleomorphic adenoma arising in an accessory lacrimal gland of Wolfring. Ophthalmology. 2006;113(5):879–82.
15. Jordan DR, Nerad JA, Patrinely JR. Chondroid syringoma of the eyelid. Can J Ophthalmol. 1989;24(1):24–7.
16. Barbarino S, McCormick SA, Lauer SA, Milman T. Syringocystadenoma papilliferum of the eyelid. Ophthalmic Plast Reconstr Surg. 2009;25(3):185–8.

17. Behera M, Chatterjee S. A case of syringocystadenoma papilliferum of eyelid with literature review. Indian J Ophthalmol. 2015;63(6):550–1.
18. Esmaeli B, Ramsay JA, Chorneyko KA. Sclerosing sweat-duct carcinoma (malignant syringoma) of the upper eyelid: a patient report with immunohistochemical and ultrastructural analysis. Ophthalmic Plast Reconstr Surg. 1998;14(6):441–5.
19. Boynton JR, Markowitch W. Mucinous eccrine carcinoma of the eyelid. Arch Ophthalmol. 1998;116(8):1130–1.
20. Paridaens D, Mooy CM. Apocrine sweat gland carcinoma. Eye. 2001;15(2):253–4.
21. Hunold AC, Herwig MC, Holz FG. Pigmented tumour of the eyelid with unexpected findings. Case Rep Pathol. 2012;2012:471368.
22. Aurora AL. Solitary trichoepithelioma of the eyelid. Indian J Ophthalmol. 1974;22(2):32–3.
23. Brooke JD, Fitzpatrick JE, Golitz LE. Papillary mesenchymal bodies: a histologic finding useful in differentiating trichoepitheliomas from basal cell carcinomas. J Am Acad Dermatol. 1989;21(3):523–8.
24. Tellechea O, Cardoso JC, Reis JP. Benign follicular tumors. An Bras Dermatol. 2015;90(6):780–96; quiz 97–8.
25. Carreras B Jr, Lopez-Marin I Jr, Mellado VG, Gutierrez MT. Trichofolliculoma of the eyelid. Br J Ophthalmol. 1981;65(3):214–5.
26. Shields JA, Shields CL, Eagle RC Jr. Trichoadenoma of the eyelid. Am J Ophthalmol. 1998;126(6):846–8.
27. Hidayat AA, Font RL. Trichilemmoma of eyelid and eyebrow. A clinicopathologic study of 31 cases. Arch Ophthalmol. 1980;98(5):844–7.
28. Bardenstein DS, McLean IW, Nerney J, Boatwright RS. Cowden's disease. Ophthalmology. 1988;95(8):1038–41.
29. Boniuk M, Zimmerman LE. Pilomatrixoma (benign calcifying epithelioma) of the eyelids and eyebrow. Arch Ophthalmol. 1963;70:399–406.
30. Yap EY, Hohberger GG, Bartley GB. Pilomatrixoma of the eyelids and eyebrows in children and adolescents. Ophthalmic Plast Reconstr Surg. 1999;15(3):185–9.
31. Herwig MC, Vogel A, Holz FG, Loffler KU. Pilomatrixoma of the ocular adnexae: clinical and histologic analysis (13 cases). Klin Monatsbl Augenheilkd. 2009;226(5):404–8.
32. Jones C, Twoon M, Ho W. Pilomatrix carcinoma: 12-year experience and review of the literature. J Cutan Pathol. 2018;45(1):33–8.
33. Cahill MT, Moriarty PM, Mooney DJ, Kennedy SM. Pilomatrix carcinoma of the eyelid. Am J Ophthalmol. 1999;127(4):463–4.
34. Singh AD, Mudhar H, Bhola R. Sebaceous adenoma of the eyelid in Muir-Torre syndrome. Arch Ophthalmol. 2005;123:562–5.
35. Mittal R, Tripathy D. Sebaceoma of the eyelid: a rare entity. Can J Ophthalmol. 2014;49(3):e78–80.
36. Yonekawa Y, Jakobiec FA, Zakka FR, Fay A. Sebaceoma of the eyelid. Ophthalmology. 2012;119(12):2645.
37. Abbas O, Mahalingam M. Cutaneous sebaceous neoplasms as markers of Muir-Torre syndrome: a diagnostic algorithm. J Cutan Pathol. 2009;36(6):613–9.
38. McKee PH. Sebaceous epithelioma pathology of the skin with clinical correlations. London: Mosby; 1996.
39. Traboulsi EI, Zin A, Massicotte SJ. Posterior scleral choristoma in the organoid nevus syndrome (linear nevus sebaceus of Jadassohn). Ophthalmology. 1999;106(11):2126–30.
40. Cribier B, Scrivener Y, Grosshans E. Tumors arising in nevus sebaceus: a study of 596 cases. J Am Acad Dermatol. 2000;42(2):263–8.

Eyelid Stromal Tumors

10

Geeta K. Vemuganti, Gabrielle Yeaney, and Arun D. Singh

10.1 Introduction

Eyelid stromal tumors could be considered under several distinct categories based on the tissue of origin: fibrous tissue tumors; fibrohistiocytic tumors; lipomatous tumors; smooth muscle tumors; skeletal muscle tumors; vascular tumors; perivascular tumors; neural tumors; lymphoid, plasmacytic, and leukemic tumors; cartilage and bone tumors; secondary tumors; metastatic tumors; and hamartomas, choristomas, and other miscellaneous lesions. Some of the inflammatory and infective conditions such as chalazion, pyogenic granuloma, verruca vulgaris, and molluscum contagiosum may manifest with features clinically simulating tumors. This chapter describes the salient features and management of common eyelid stromal tumors. It would be worthwhile to mention here that further information on clinical classification of tumors of the eye could be obtained from the 8th edition of TNM which encompasses several important changes over the previous 7th edition. It is also important to note that the 5th edition of WHO blue book on classification of tumors takes into consideration the tumors of oculo-adenexal soft tissue/bone tumors and hematolymphoid tumors into separate chapters similar to the approach to other organ systems. It also elaborates on disease codes, imaging, macroscopic details, cytology, and molecular pathology as applicable [1].

G. K. Vemuganti (✉)
School of Medical Sciences, University of Hyderabad, Hyderabad, India
e-mail: gvmd@uohyd.ac.in

G. Yeaney
Department of Pathology and Laboratory Medicine, Diagnostics Institute, CC Lerner College of Medicine of CWRU, Cleveland Clinic, Cleveland, OH, USA
e-mail: yeaneyg@ccf.org

A. D. Singh
Cole Eye Institute, Cleveland Clinic, Cleveland, OH, USA
e-mail: Singha@ccf.org

10.2 Fibrous Tissue Tumors

Fibrous tissue tumors comprise of several benign lesions (fibroma, keloid, nodular fasciitis, and proliferative fasciitis), fibromatosis, and a malignant tumor (fibrosarcoma).

10.2.1 Fibromas

Fibromas are rare tumors that could be congenital, developmental, or acquired [2]. Congenital fibroma presents as a diffusely infiltrative lower eyelid nodule that recurs following local excision. The histologic and electron-microscopic features point to the hamartomatous origin of this tumor with partial myofibroblastic differentiation [2]. Developmental fibroma has a propensity for involvement of the infraorbital region and lower eyelid and is diffusely infiltrative. Recurrence often follows local excision [3].

A typical fibroma is sparsely cellular with prominent collagen bundles separated by compressed fibroblasts. Rarely it can present as multiple lesions in the eyelid and face [4]. Characteristic feature is lack of inflammation without zonal pattern. Pleomorphic fibroma is a variant with multinucleate giant cells.

10.2.2 Eyelid Keloids

Eyelid keloids are hypertrophic cutaneous scars or nodular outgrowths on the surface or the margin of the eyelid that follow surgical intervention or trauma and could occur de novo. Rarely could keloids arise from the tarsus and simulate a tumor [5].

B. C. K. Patel et al. (eds.), *Clinical Ophthalmic Oncology*, https://doi.org/10.1007/978-3-031-72328-5_10

10.2.3 Nodular Fasciitis

Nodular fasciitis is, in general, a relatively common benign reactive fibroblastic proliferation of the soft tissues with acute manifestations that progress rapidly. Currently it is considered as one of the Usp6 associated neoplasm [6]. Nodular fasciitis of the eyelid is rare and only case reports have been published. It presents with a solitary subcutaneous nodule [7]. Although excisional biopsy is curative, the nodules may often resolve spontaneously [7].

Nodular fasciitis is an infiltrative lesion consisting of proliferation of immature and activated fibroblasts, with slit-like spaces between the cells. Foci of myxoid change, endothelial proliferation, lipid-laden macrophages, multinucleated giant cells, and acute and chronic inflammatory cell infiltration are also seen. Ultrastructurally, the cells show characteristic features of myofibroblasts. Clinical presentation and histologic appearance of a pleomorphic spindle cell neoplasm with frequent mitotic figures may raise concern of a malignant neoplasm and lead to unnecessary and overly aggressive therapy. The lesion is therefore called pseudosarcomatous fasciitis.

10.2.4 Fibromatosis

Fibromatosis could be juvenile or adult onset. Juvenile fibromatoses are a distinct group of benign fibrous lesions with aggressive clinical behavior and predilection to occur in the lower eyelid and inferior orbit [8]. Infiltration of the local tissues including extraocular muscle and periosteum results in incomplete removal and local recurrence (Fig. 10.1).

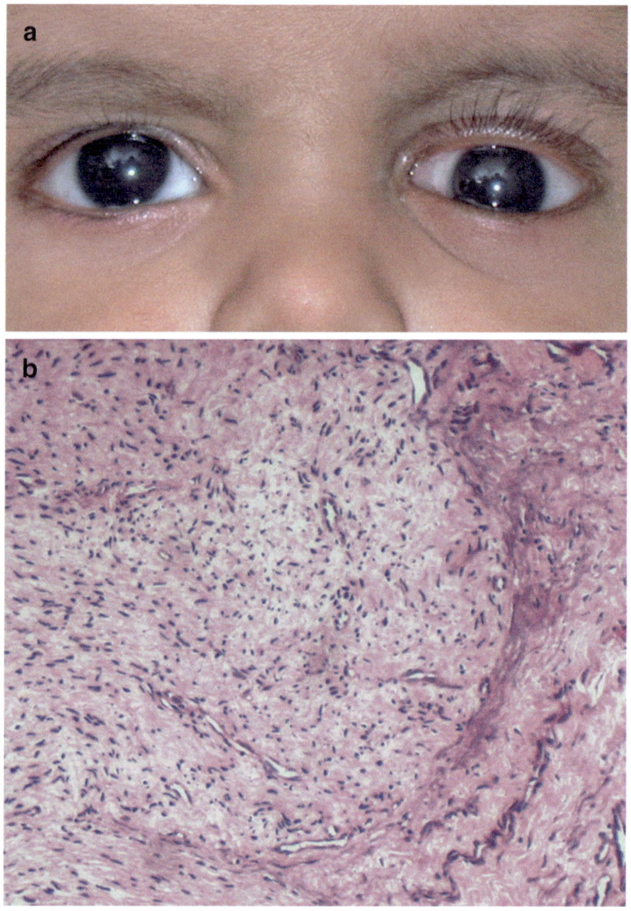

Fig. 10.1 Eyelid fibromatosis. A 6-month-old child with a tethering of the eyelid to a deeper firm mass in the superonasal aspect with consequent lagophthalmos (**a**). Histopathology examination shows infiltrating bundles of spindle cells with lobulated pattern in few areas diagnostic of fibromatosis (**b**, hematoxylin and eosin, original magnification ×200)

10.2.5 Fibrosarcoma

Fibrosarcoma is a highly malignant tumor that can be locally destructive and can metastasize. It manifests as a rapidly progressive poorly circumscribed eyelid nodule or as a second malignant neoplasm in hereditary retinoblastoma survivors with or without prior radiotherapy [9]. Rarely, it could occur in children with local recurrences which could be managed conservatively. Wide surgical excision or orbital exenteration may minimize the risk of local tumor recurrence [9].

The lesion consists of closely packed cells that assume an interlacing woven herringbone pattern. The cells contain a vesicular nucleus with prominent nucleoli, tapering pointed ends with moderate mitotic activity.

10.3 Fibrohistiocytic Tumors

Fibrohistiocytic tumors could be subclassified as benign (xanthelasma, xanthoma, dermatofibroma, xanthogranuloma, juvenile xanthogranuloma, reticulohistiocytoma), intermediate (atypical fibroxanthoma, dermatofibrosarcoma protuberans, angiomatoid fibrous histiocytoma), and malignant (malignant fibrous histiocytoma, malignant fibroxanthoma).

10.3.1 Xanthelasma

Xanthelasma palpebrarum is a common bilateral subcutaneous lesion of the eyelid seen in normolipemic individuals and in those with primary hyperlipemia (types II and III) or secondary hyperlipemia (diabetes mellitus, biliary cirrhosis) [10]. It was found that alteration in apolipoprotein levels in patients with xanthelasma may predispose to cutaneous and systemic depositions of lipids, including atherosclerosis [11]. Xanthelasma manifests as a yellowish-tan soft plaque occurs in the inner canthus in middle-aged individuals (Fig. 10.2). Large nodular xanthelasma is called xanthoma or tuberous xanthoma, which has a known association with Erdheim–Chester disease. Acute-onset eruptive xanthoma occurs in patients experiencing a rapid rise in serum triglyceride levels. Management should include systemic evaluation for the causative etiology and excision or laser [12] or radiofrequency-assisted vaporization of large cosmetically unacceptable lesions [13].

Microscopically, xanthelasma consists of lipid-laden macrophages in the superficial dermis, around blood vessels, and adnexa.

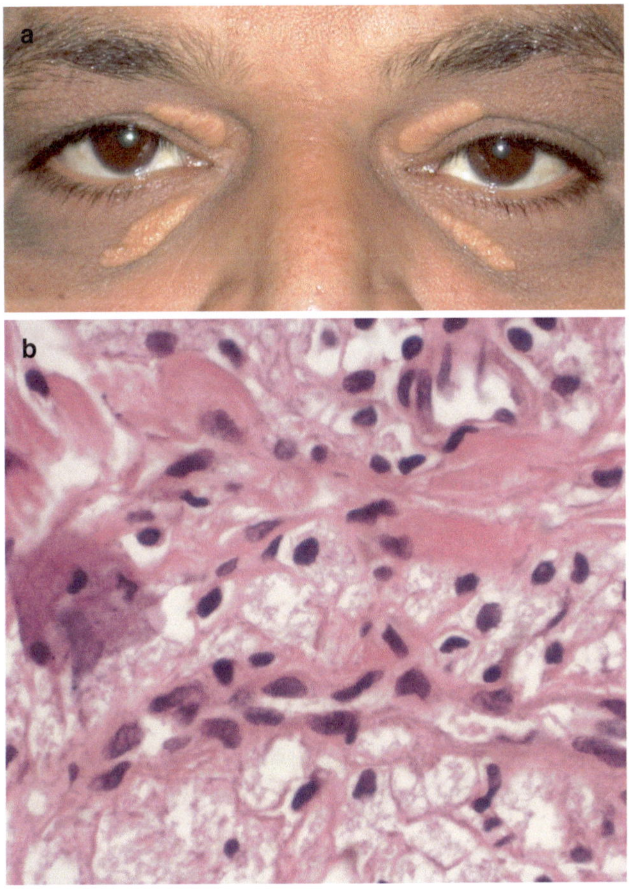

Fig. 10.2 Xanthelasma. Bilateral yellowish placoid lesions clinically diagnostic of xanthelasma (**a**). Sheets of large, foamy lipid-laden cells on histopathology (**b**, hematoxylin and eosin, original magnification × 400)

10.3.2 Xanthogranuloma

Xanthogranuloma is an idiopathic inflammatory granuloma with juvenile and adult variants [14, 15]. Juvenile xanthogranuloma of the eyelid may be a part of systemic affection seen as multiple fleshy superficial eyelid nodules with or without coexisting conjunctival, iris, and orbital involvement. The adult variant may be diffuse and associated with bronchial asthma (Fig. 10.3) [14]. Juvenile xanthogranuloma is known to spontaneously involute, thus qualifying for observation. Systemic corticosteroids are indicated in recalcitrant juvenile xanthogranuloma and as primary therapy for the adult variant [14]. Extensive, cosmetically disfiguring, and steroid-resistant lesions could be excised or treated with systemic chemotherapy or radiotherapy.

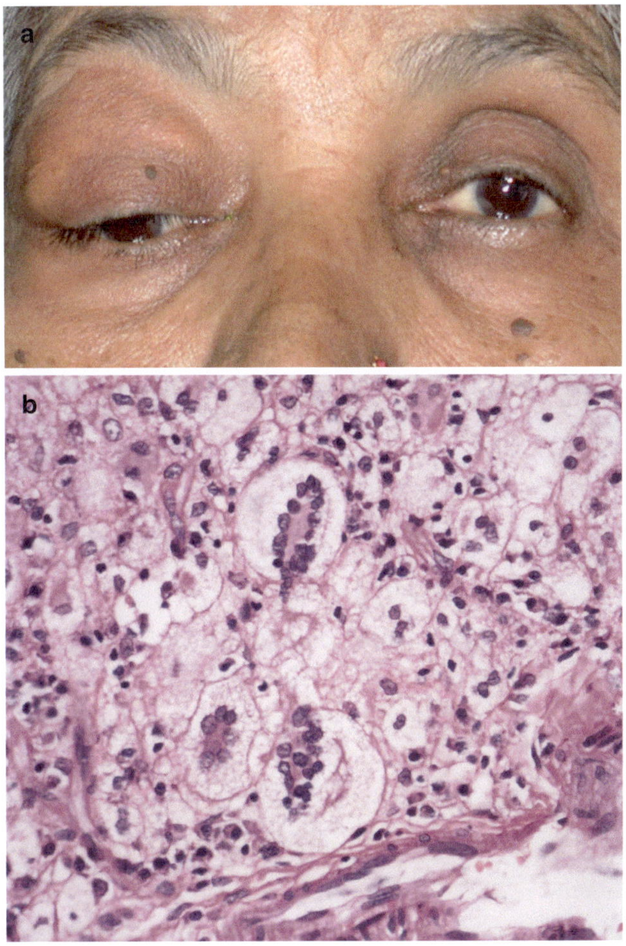

Fig. 10.3 Adult-onset xanthogranuloma presenting as a diffuse eyelid mass with a yellowish haze (**a**). Sheets of foamy histiocytes and classic Touton type of multinucleated giant cells with wreath-like arrangement of the nuclei on histopathology (**b**, hematoxylin and eosin, original magnification ×250)

Xanthogranuloma consists of monomorphic infiltrate of histiocytes, intermixed with lymphocytes and the classic Touton giant cell with a wreath-like arrangement of nuclei and peripheral clear zone.

10.3.3 Dermatofibroma

Dermatofibroma is a nodular painless skin lesion that is typically seen on elbows and legs.

It requires excision with wide margins because of an increased rate of local recurrences [16, 17]. Multiple lesions can be markers of systemic disease such as lupus, HIV, or immunosuppression [18, 19]. It is composed of spindle cell lesion without atypia or mitotic activity demonstrating twisted fascicular pattern (storiform). Immunohistochemistry shows positivity for CD34, factor XIIIa, and CD 163 (Fig. 10.4) [17].

10.3.4 Malignant Fibrous Histiocytoma

Malignant fibrous histiocytoma is now termed as an undifferentiated pleomorphic soft tissue sarcoma that occurs rarely in the eyelid. Malignant fibrous histiocytoma presents as a firm subcutaneous mass, sometimes mimicking a recurrent pyogenic granuloma [20, 21]. Dermatofibrosarcoma protuberans, which manifests as a rapidly growing eyelid nodule, is considered an aggressive form of malignant fibrous histiocytoma. It has tendency for local invasion and is known to metastasize. The mainstay of treatment is complete surgical excision with wide margins. Because of risk of

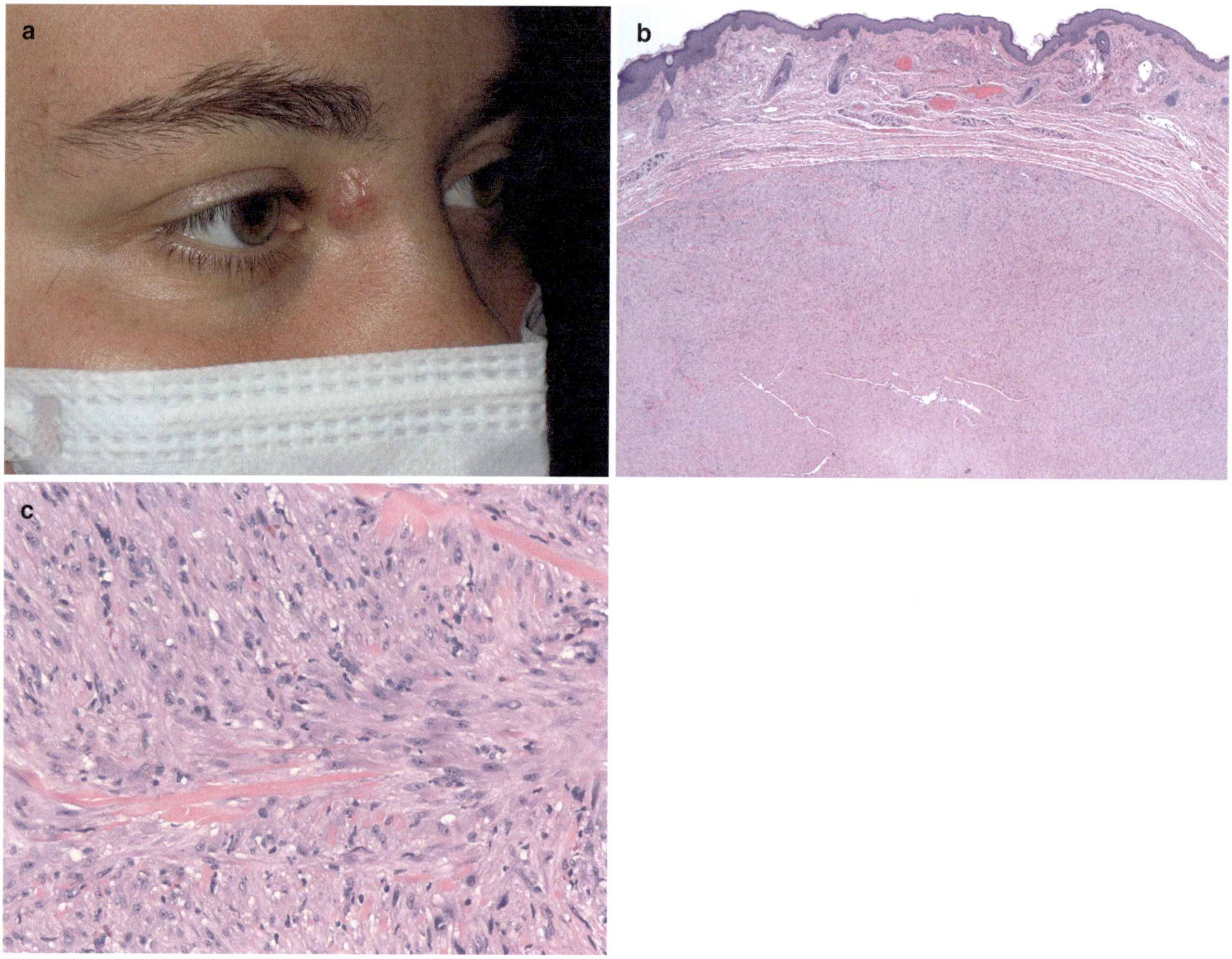

Fig. 10.4 Dermatofibroma. A 23-year-old woman with a history of nodular lesion near medial canthal region for 4 months that recurred with 2 weeks of prior excision (**a**). Dermal spindle cell proliferation arranged in fascicles with intervening fibrous stroma. (**b**, hematoxylin and eosin, original magnification ×20. Cells are elongated with abundant cytoplasm, tapering nuclei, small nucleoli and collagen trapping. (**c**, hematoxylin and eosin, original magnification ×200)

recurrence following excision, consideration should be given to histologic margin control and adjuvant radiotherapy [22].

Malignant fibrous histiocytoma differs from benign variant in exhibiting marked nuclear pleomorphism, high mitotic activity, pericytoma-like areas with foci of xanthoma cells, and multinucleated giant cells.

10.4 Lipomatous Tumors

Lipoma, lipoma variants, and liposarcoma are the lipomatous tumors affecting the eyelid [23].

10.4.1 Lipoma and Lipoma Variants

Lipoma could be congenital or acquired. Nasopalpebral lipoma–coloboma syndrome is an autosomal dominant syndrome characterized by congenital upper eyelid and nasopalpebral lipomas, upper and lower eyelid colobomas, telecanthus, and maxillary hypoplasia [24]. Lipoblastoma is an uncommon benign tumor of adipose tissue that occurs in infants and young children [25]. Intramuscular lipoma of the eyelid manifesting as a slowly growing globular lesion has been described in elderly individuals. Hibernoma is a variant of lipoma that contains embryonal brown fat and is relatively more vascular. If treatment is indicated for cosmetic and functional reasons, complete tumor excision is adequate.

10.4.2 Liposarcoma

Primary liposarcoma is a rare orbital tumor that may involve the eyelid by local extension.

10.5 Smooth Muscle Tumors

Smooth muscle tumors of the eyelid are very rare and could be benign (leiomyoma, angiomyoma) [26] or malignant (leiomyosarcoma) [27].

10.6 Skeletal Muscle Tumors

Rhabdomyoma and rhabdomyosarcoma are the skeletal muscle tumors of the eyelid.

10.6.1 Rhabdomyoma

Rhabdomyoma is a benign tumor of the skeletal muscle and is seen in two forms. The adult form consists of well-differentiated large rounded or polygonal cells with abundant acidophilic cytoplasm containing lipid and glycogen. Some cells appear like spider cells and some may show cross striations. The fetal form is very cellular and consists of immature skeletal muscle fibers and primitive mesenchymal cells. One case of adult-onset rhabdomyoma attributed to chronic irritation by a prosthetic eye has been reported in the literature [28].

10.6.2 Rhabdomyosarcoma

Rhabdomyosarcoma is primarily a malignant orbital tumor with eyelid involvement only in about 3 % of cases [29].

10.7 Vascular Tumors

Benign vascular tumors of the eyelid include nevus flammeus, papillary endothelial hyperplasia, capillary hemangioma, cavernous hemangioma, venous hemangioma, epithelioid hemangioma, arteriovenous malformation, and lymphangioma. Angiosarcoma, lymphangiosarcoma, and Kaposi's sarcoma are the malignant vascular eyelid tumors.

10.7.1 Nevus Flammeus (Port-Wine Stain)

Nevus flammeus is a diffuse congenital vascular malformation of the face, involving the periocular area and eyelid (Fig. 10.5).

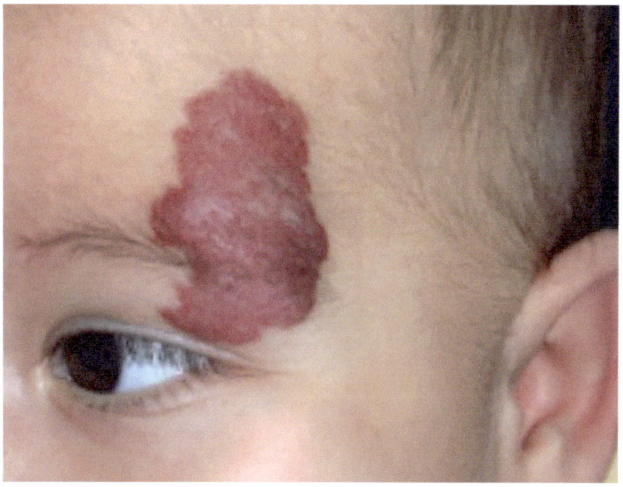

Fig. 10.5 Relatively flat eyelid and forehead hemangioma (port wine stain). Courtesy of Bhupender C. Patel, MD Salt Lake City, Utah, USA)

10.7.2 Pyogenic Granuloma

Papillary endothelial hyperplasia or "pyogenic granuloma" is the most common acquired vascular lesion of the eyelid. It is neither "pyogenic" nor is it a "granuloma." In the recent classification of vascular tumors by International Society for the Study of Vascular Aniomalies (ISSVA), the term pyogenic granuloma (lobular capillary hemangioma) was included under benign vascular tumors [30]. Pyogenic granuloma occurs anywhere in the eyelid, as a rapidly growing, pedunculated reddish-pink mass with or without superficial ulceration and may easily bleed on touch (Figs. 10.6 and 10.7). It usually follows trauma or surgery. Local excision of the lesion is curative [31, 32].

Pyogenic granuloma consists of exuberant mass of proliferating radiating capillaries and edematous stroma with mixed inflammatory infiltrates. Intravascular papillary endothelial hyperplasia is a rare form of "pyogenic granuloma" in which the angiomatous proliferation" is confined entirely within the lumen of a vessel [33]. The repeating units of capillary-sized lobules lined by plump endothelial cells [32].

10.7.3 Capillary (Infantile) Hemangioma

Capillary hemangioma of the eyelid is the most common vascular tumor of the eyelid in children (Fig. 10.8). It is usually congenital in origin and is often sporadic. Occasional reports of acquired capillary hemangiomas have been reported in adults. Newborns of mothers who have undergone amniocentesis and in premature infants are at a risk of developing capillary hemangioma [34]. The pathogenesis of this tumor is not

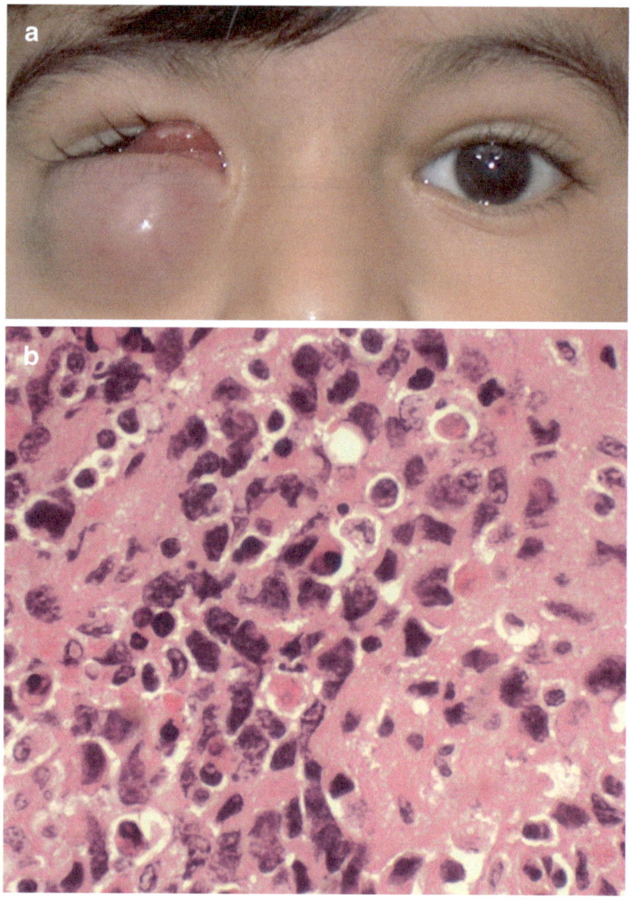

Fig. 10.6 Pyogenic granuloma. The tarsal conjunctiva of the upper eyelid showing a vascular polypoidal reddish-pink mass with superficial ulceration (**a**). Histopathologically, loose edematous stroma with surface necrosis, proliferating blood vessels, and mixed inflammatory infiltrates, characteristic of inflammatory granulation tissue, is present (**b**, hematoxylin and eosin, original magnification ×200)

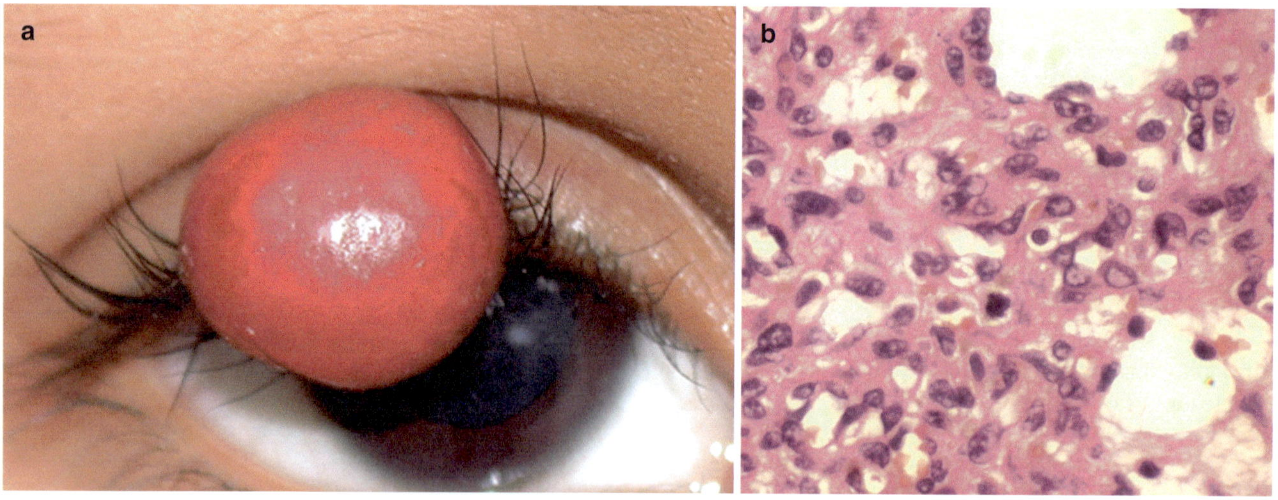

Fig. 10.7 An older child with a large red vascular mass in the upper eyelid (**a**) that was excised. Histopathology shows lobulated appearance with vascular channels lined by plump endothelial cells. Note the presence of a few mitotic figures could be seen in proliferating lesions (**b**, hematoxylin and eosin, original magnification ×400)

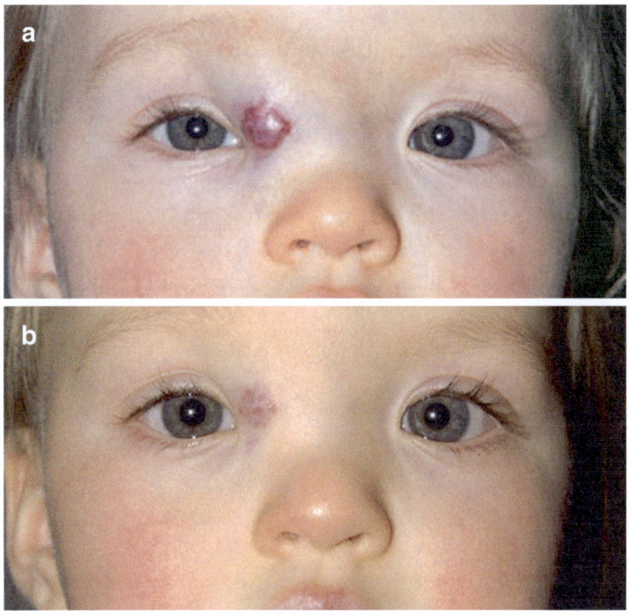

Fig. 10.8 Capillary hemangioma. A 10-month-old female with history of failed intralesional steroid injection. After pediatric cardiology examination, BP, EKG, and echocardiogram, propranolol was started at 1 mg/kg/day in three divided doses daily (**a**, 11/11/2010), with a blood glucose level and repeat blood pressure check after the first dose (blood pressure, taken in the left thigh 87/61; pulse 108; glucose 80; about 2 h after the first increased dose). One week later (11/18/2010), the dosage was doubled to 2 mg/kg/day in three divided doses daily. BP, heart rate, and blood glucose were again checked about 2 h after the first increased dose. No additional testing was performed for increases above 2 mg/kg/day. Her dose was increased to 3 mg/kg/day (12/9/2010). After 3 months of treatment, the infantile hemangioma had shown marked regression (**b**, 2/10/11). The dose was then tapered to 1.5 mg/kg/day (4/13/2011), 1 mg/kg/day (5/25/2011), 0.5 mg/kg/day (6/15/2011), and finally discontinued on 7/1/2011. No regrowth of infantile hemangioma was observed

well understood, but the affected infants have an increased urinary level of basic fibroblastic growth factor, a marker of angiogenesis. Familial congenital capillary hemangioma with autosomal dominant inheritance with incrimination of chromosome 5q has been reported [35]. Congenital capillary hemangioma usually manifests at birth or within the first months of life. There are two distinct clinical variants—superficial and deep. The superficial variant, better known as strawberry hemangioma, appears as a bright red to deep purple, lobulated, spongy, soft eyelid mass that typically blanches on application of direct pressure and engorges when the infant cries or strains. Contiguous conjunctival and orbital extension is known to occur. The superficial variant is localized to the epidermis and dermis, whereas the deep variant lies in the subcutaneous tissue and is bluish or blue gray in color. Congenital capillary hemangioma grows rapidly in size and reaches its final size by 6–12 months of age. It then becomes stable and slowly involutes by 4–7 years of age [36]. About 70% regress by the age of 7 years [36].

Histologically, capillary hemangioma of the eyelid consists of lobules of capillaries separated by sparse fibrous septae. The morphology of the lesion changes with age. An early immature lesion tends to have obliterated lumen with plump endothelial cells and occasional mitotic figures, while in later stages, the lumina increases and the endothelial cells get attenuated, with increasing fibrosis and fat infiltration. The lobular capillary hemangioma show repeating units of various sizes (lobules) consisting of CD34-postive, GLUT-1-negative endothelial cells and SMA-positive pericytes arranged in macro- or microlobules. Some foci may exhibit ectatic vessels or diffuse, nonlobular capillary proliferations [37].

In most instances, congenital capillary hemangioma is a sporadic condition but approximately 20% of patients may manifest it as multiple tumors involving the cutaneous tissue elsewhere, central nervous system, liver, and gastrointestinal tract [34]. Systemic lesions, especially those found in association with Kasabach–Merritt syndrome, could aggressively proliferate and lead to hemorrhage, platelet consumption, disseminated intravascular coagulation, cardiac failure, and death [34].

The main ocular complications are amblyopia and strabismus. Amblyopia could be meridional because of induced astigmatism or because of stimulation deprivation secondary to mechanical ptosis. Because most lesions spontaneously regress, observation, refractive correction, and appropriate amblyopia management are the standard treatment. Active intervention is indicated if the lesion extensively involves the face or is ulcerated with episodes of bleeding and if there is mechanical ptosis with obscuration of pupillary axis or induced astigmatism with amblyopia.

Systemic β-blockers are the first line therapy for the treatment of infantile hemangioma, with very promising results (Fig. 10.8) [38–40]. The dose that has been used is 0.5–2.0 mg/kg/day for several months, with significant reduction in the size of the hemangioma in all babies. Side effects such as bradycardia, hypotension, bronchospasm, hypoglycemia, and electrolyte disturbances have been reported, leading to a reduction in the dose of the drug. A pilot randomized control trial compared efficacy of oral and intralesional propranolol (20 patients randomized to two groups of ten each). Oral propranolol group received dose of 1 mg/kg/day titrated to final dose of 3 mg/kg/day over 1 week which was continued for 6 months and then tapered over 1 week; Group 2 received 3 doses of direct intralesional propranolol hydrochloride 1 mg/ml; 0.2 ml/cm 4–6 weeks apart. Within each group at 6 months, there was a significant reduction in area of involvement and improvement in astigmatism with no statistical difference between the two groups [41]. In another retrospective report, oral propranolol effectiveness was greater in those with segmental and preseptal lesions than in focal and postseptal hemangioma [42].

Topical timolol maleate 0.5% was also found to be effective [43]. In a single-center randomized controlled trial of 42 infants with small (<2 cm) superficial hemangioma located at high-risk areas (tip of ears, tip of nose, eyelids, acral areas, facial areas, scalp, neck, buttocks, perineum and axilla), the patients were either assigned to receive 12 months of topical timolol (study group) or were observed (control group). Mean volume percentage reduction in size was significantly more for the study group at 3, 6, and 12 months. The study result supports early use of topical timolol to reduce the need for further treatment [44].

Alternative treatment modalities include interferon, laser sclerotherapy, and excision of circumscribed anterior lesions. In patients with infantile hemangioma who have failed medical therapy or have residual tumor causing ocular sequelae, adjuvant surgical intervention for soft tissue debulking and ptosis repair can achieve excellent functional and aesthetic outcomes (Fig. 10.9) [45]. A single case of a 71-year-old male in which congenital eyelid hemangioma transformation of into angiosarcoma suggests the need for long-term monitoring [46].

10.7.4 Cavernous Hemangioma

Cavernous hemangioma of the eyelid is a rare, acquired condition and is generally seen in adults (Fig. 10.10) [47]. It may be associated with blue rubber bleb nevus syndrome [48]. The lesions are ill circumscribed and bluish in color and may undergo slow progression. Epithelioid hemangioma also known as angiolymphoid hyperplasia with eosinophilia occurs as a nodular lesion in the eyelid. Kimura disease, which is predominant in Asian population, shares both clinical and histopathologic features with angiolymphoid hyperplasia with eosinophilia and may be clinically indistinguishable [49]. Cavernous hemangioma is composed of large dilated vascular channels filled with blood, hemosiderin-laden macrophages, scattered lymphoplasmacytic infiltrates, and secondary changes such as calcification, phlebolith, and fibrosis.

10.7.5 Arteriovenous Malformations

Arteriovenous malformations, as the name suggests, are communications between arteries and veins that bypass normal capillary beds. In contrast to arteriovenous fistulas, arteriovenous malformations are mainly congenital lesions with multiple large feeding arteries, a central nidus, and numerous dilated draining veins (Fig. 10.11). Rarely, arteriovenous malformations may follow trauma or surgery [50]. While surgical embolization or excision alone may be possible, a combined approach is considered ideal [50].

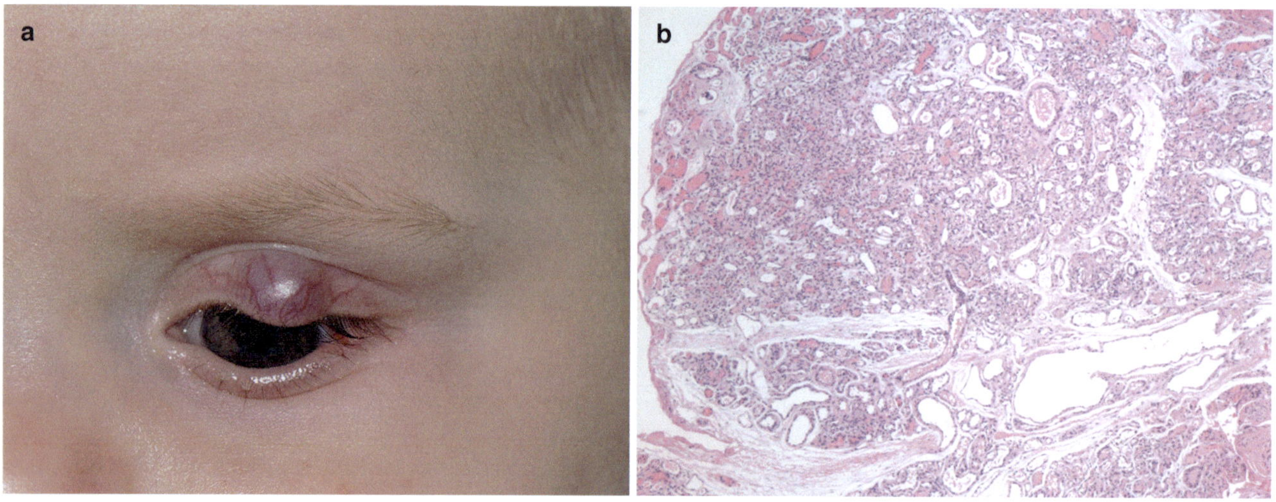

Fig. 10.9 Nodular capillary hemangioma. A 6-month-old child with growing nodular vascular lesion since age 2 months (**a**). No response to topical timolol. Given localized nature of the lesion, it was elected to excise it rather than prescribe oral propranolol. Intraoperatively, the lesion was subcutaneous without visible cutaneous component. Via superior eyelid crease incision submuscular plane was identified. The lesion was circumscribed (6 × 5 × 4 mm), encapsulated, and situated in preaponeurotic space without extension into levator or tarsus. With blunt and sharp dissection and using cautery, the capsule was identified and the hemangioma isolated from surrounding structures. The skin muscle lamina was closed with interrupted 8-0 polygalactin 910 sutures along the lid crease. Histology shows infantile hemangioma with closely approximated lobules of capillaries lined by plump endothelium (**b**, hematoxylin and eosin, original magnification ×40; Immunohistochemistry for GLUT1 positive; not shown)

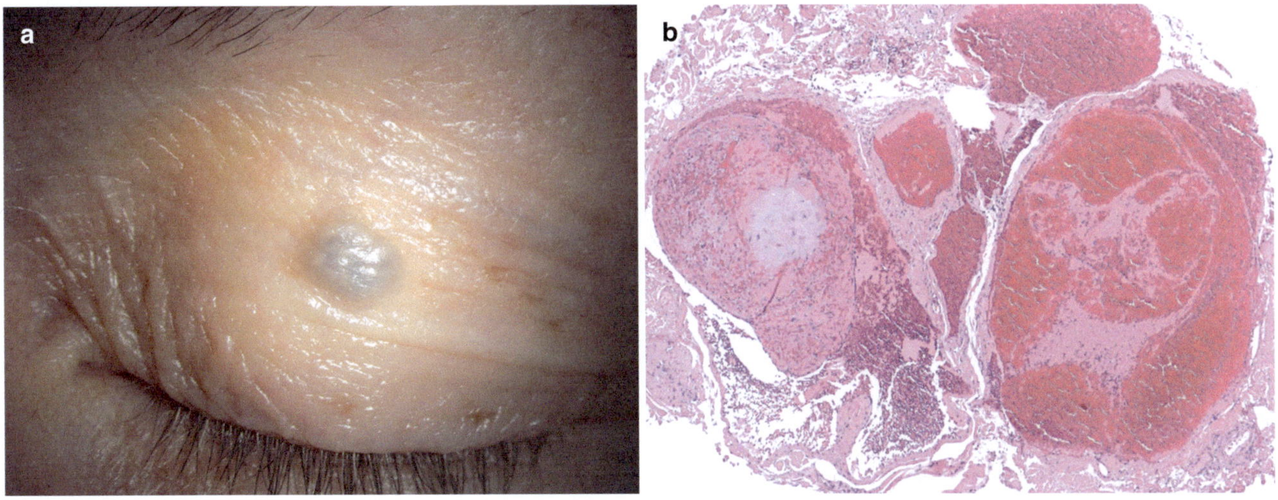

Fig. 10.10 (Cav hemangioma). A 66-year-old female who first noticed the lesion about 6 months ago. No recent change in size, shape, or color. On examination it appeared as a bluish, mobile, firm, subcutaneous nodule (4 × 3 × 2 mm) that could be easily excised (**a**). Histology shows 4–5 variably sized thrombosed thin-walled vessels (**b**, hematoxylin and eosin, original magnification ×40)

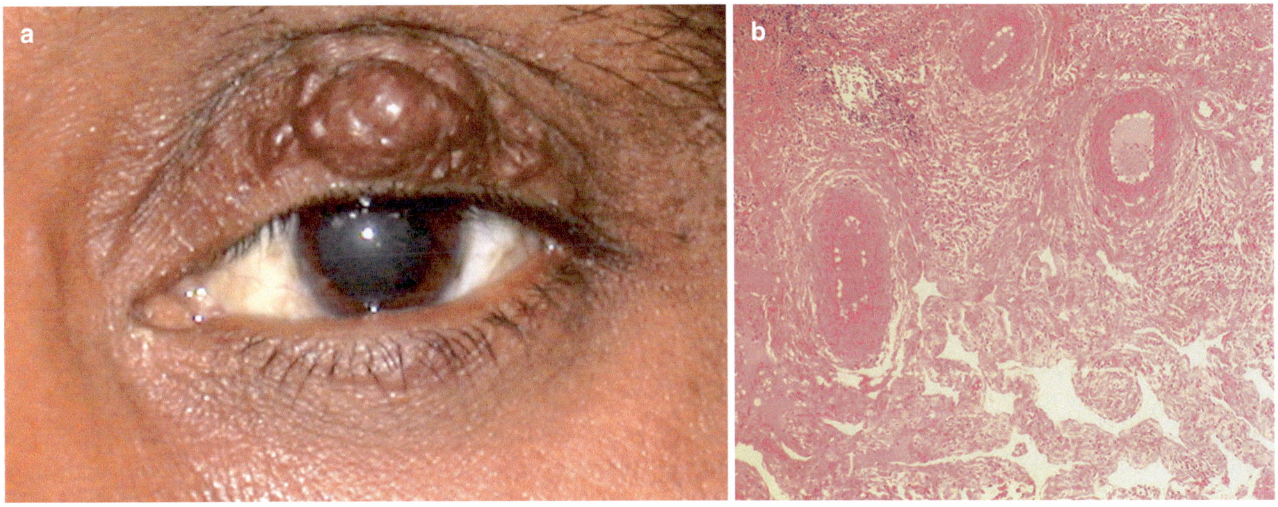

Fig. 10.11 Arteriovenous malformation. A lobulated soft compressible upper eyelid lesion (**a**). Vascular channels of varying sizes including medium-sized feeder vessels on histopathology (**b**, hematoxylin and eosin, original magnification ×200)

10.7.6 Lymphangioma

Lymphangioma commonly manifests in the orbit rather than in the eyelid. Eyelid lesion generally represents the anterior extension of an orbital lymphangioma [51].

10.7.7 Angiosarcoma

Angiosarcoma is an uncommon malignant vascular eyelid tumor. It appears as a raised, reddish-purple, or violaceous subcutaneous placoid lesion, tan colored nodules or a mass that tends to ulcerate and bleed spontaneously or with excessive edema mimicking a Morbihan disease or periorbital hematoma [52–54]. Angiosarcoma most often develops de novo but may arise from preexisting benign vascular tumors such as nevus flammeus or irradiated lymphangioma. It is an aggressive tumor that tends to recur locally and disseminate widely with a 5-year survival ranging from 12 to 29% [55], although patients with isolated eyelid involvement have a much better prognosis [56].

10.7.8 Kaposi's Sarcoma

Kaposi's sarcoma is a malignant vascular tumor that most often presents in the setting of association with acquired immunodeficiency syndrome (AIDS); it is the most common

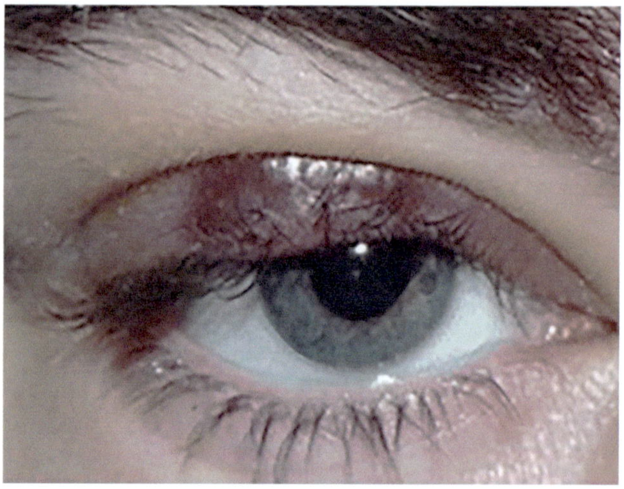

Fig. 10.12 Kaposi Sarcoma. A 32-year-old White man with a 1 month history of enlarging violet-colored mass on the right upper eyelid which had evolved over the course of 1 week. The diagnosis was confirmed with HIV-1 positive testing and histopathology from tissue biopsy. The patient's CD4 count was 23/mm^3 and viral RNA load 427,000/ml. Further systemic evaluation showed a diffuse sarcoma. Reproduced with permission from Sousa Neves F, Braga J, Cardoso da Costa J, Sequeira J, Prazeres S. Kaposi's sarcoma of the conjunctiva and the eyelid leads to the diagnosis of human immunodeficiency virus infection - a case report. BMC Cancer. 2018 Jul 3;18(1):708

malignancy seen in patients with AIDS [57]. However, it can also occur in immunocompetent elderly males as well [58, 59]. The possibility of occult AIDS should be entertained in a young individual with an atypical hordeolum or avascular eyelid mass as Kaposi's sarcoma sometimes mimics these common lesions and represents the initial presenting sign of AIDS [57, 60]. Kaposi's sarcoma appears as a solitary or multifocal, circumscribed, or diffuse smooth blue subcutaneous lesion (Fig. 10.12).

Infection by human herpes virus 8 possibly transforms normal mesenchymal cells to become abnormally sensitive to high levels of cytokines seen in patients with AIDS [57]. Subsequent proliferation and additional mutation result in clinically apparent disease. Histopathologically, Kaposi's sarcoma appears as a network of proliferating endothelial cells that forms slit-like spaces surrounded by spindle-shaped mesenchymal cells and collagen [57]. The tumor cells show immunoreactivity to endothelial markers CD31 and ERG (a subfamily of the ETS family transcription factors) and for human herpes virus HHV-8, which could serve as diagnostic markers [61].

Improvement in immunological status and highly active antiretroviral therapy may result in spontaneous regression of Kaposi's sarcoma. Treatment modalities include local methods such as excision, cryotherapy, and radiotherapy. Systemic chemotherapy is indicated for widespread disease [57]. Second line Paclitaxel given every 2 weeks has reported to show complete response [62].

10.7.9 Perivascular Tumors

Perivascular tumors of the eyelid are very rare and include benign or malignant hemangiopericytoma and glomus tumor.

10.8 Neurogenic Tumors

Neurogenic tumors of the eyelid include a variety of benign (neurofibroma, schwannoma, and neuroglial choristoma) and malignant tumors (malignant peripheral nerve sheath tumor and Merkel cell tumor).

10.8.1 Neurofibroma

Neurofibroma of the eyelid could be plexiform, multifocal, localized, or solitary and constitute nearly 70% of the peripheral nerve sheath tumors of the oculoadenexal region [63].

10.8.2 Schwannoma

Schwannoma (neurilemoma) is one of the common benign peripheral nerve sheath tumors that rarely grow on the eyelid. Clinically it appears as a slow-growing well-defined firm subcutaneous eyelid nodule that could simulate a large chalazion (Fig. 10.13) [64]. Solitary schwannoma lacks systemic association. Multiple lesions, however, are associated with neurofibromatosis type 1 [64].

10.8.3 Merkel Cell Tumor

First described in 1972, Merkel cell tumor is an aggressive primary cutaneous neuroendocrine malignant neoplasm that arises from Merkel cells, which are specialized neuroendocrine receptors of touch located in the eyelid and conjunctiva

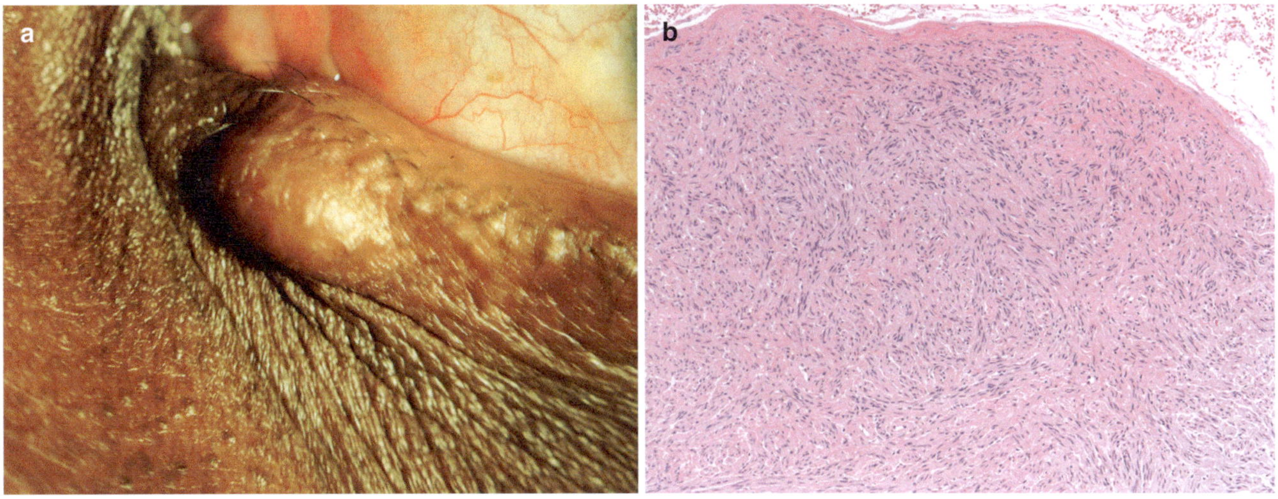

Fig. 10.13 Schwannoma. A 48-year-old man with eyelid cystic lesion (5 × 4 × 2 mm) was present along the medial aspect of the left lower eyelid (**a**). The lesion was excised under local anesthesia was through a 6-mm skin muscle incision made along the inferior aspect of the lesion. The skin flap was reflected and the subcutaneous lesion was excised. The wound could be closed primarily with interrupted 6-0 polygalactin 910 sutures. Histology shows a well circumscribed subcutaneous lesion with fascicles of spindle cells with focal palisading nuclei (**b**, hematoxylin and eosin, original magnification ×200)

[65, 66]. Recent studies have implicated polyoma virus in pathogenesis of Merkel cell carcinoma [67, 68]. A rare occurrence was reported in a patient of chronic rheumatoid arthritis who was treated with tumor necrosis factor (TNF) inhibitors injection (golimumab) for 6 months [69]. Merkel cell tumor is rare, aggressive neuroendocrine malignancy of the skin comprising <3% of malignant eyelid tumors and could be associated with exposure to sun, immunosuppression or viruses [70]. A recent study has shown metastatic potential in 22% of cases specially those with nodal metastasis. It usually occurs in older patients as a painless rapidly progressive vascular purplish-red nodule of the upper eyelid (Fig. 10.14) [65, 66].

On histopathology, the tumor cells are seen to grow in interconnecting sheets and cords (trabecular pattern). The individual cells are uniformly round with scant cytoplasm, large oval nuclei, prominent nucleoli, and abundant mitotic figures. In addition to synaptophysin, CD56, chromogranin and nonspecific enolase, the tumor cells are also immunoreactive for low molecular weight Cytokeratin 20 (CK20), TTF-1 a marker of Merkel cell, which is now considered as a diagnostic feature [71, 72].

Wide surgical excision with tumor-free margins by frozen section control achieves fair local control, although recurrence and metastasis to regional lymph nodes and viscera are not uncommon [65–67, 73]. Adjuvant radiotherapy or cyberknife surgery may help reduce the risk of local recurrence if margins are suspect [74]. Radiation, otherwise, is reserved for recurrent or surgically unresectable tumors [65–67, 73]. Sentinel lymph node biopsy should be considered in cases of Merkel cell tumor of the eyelid (Chap. 21) [75]. Recent evidence points to a clinically meaningful response with the use of immune check point inhibition [76]. As per the AJCC eyelid carcinoma T classification, the disease free state of Merkel Cell Carcinoma correlates with its presentation and is worse for patients with T2b or more extensive tumors. A recent study of 349 cases continues to prove a poor prognosis and death within a year though most of the patients die from reasons other than MCCE [70].

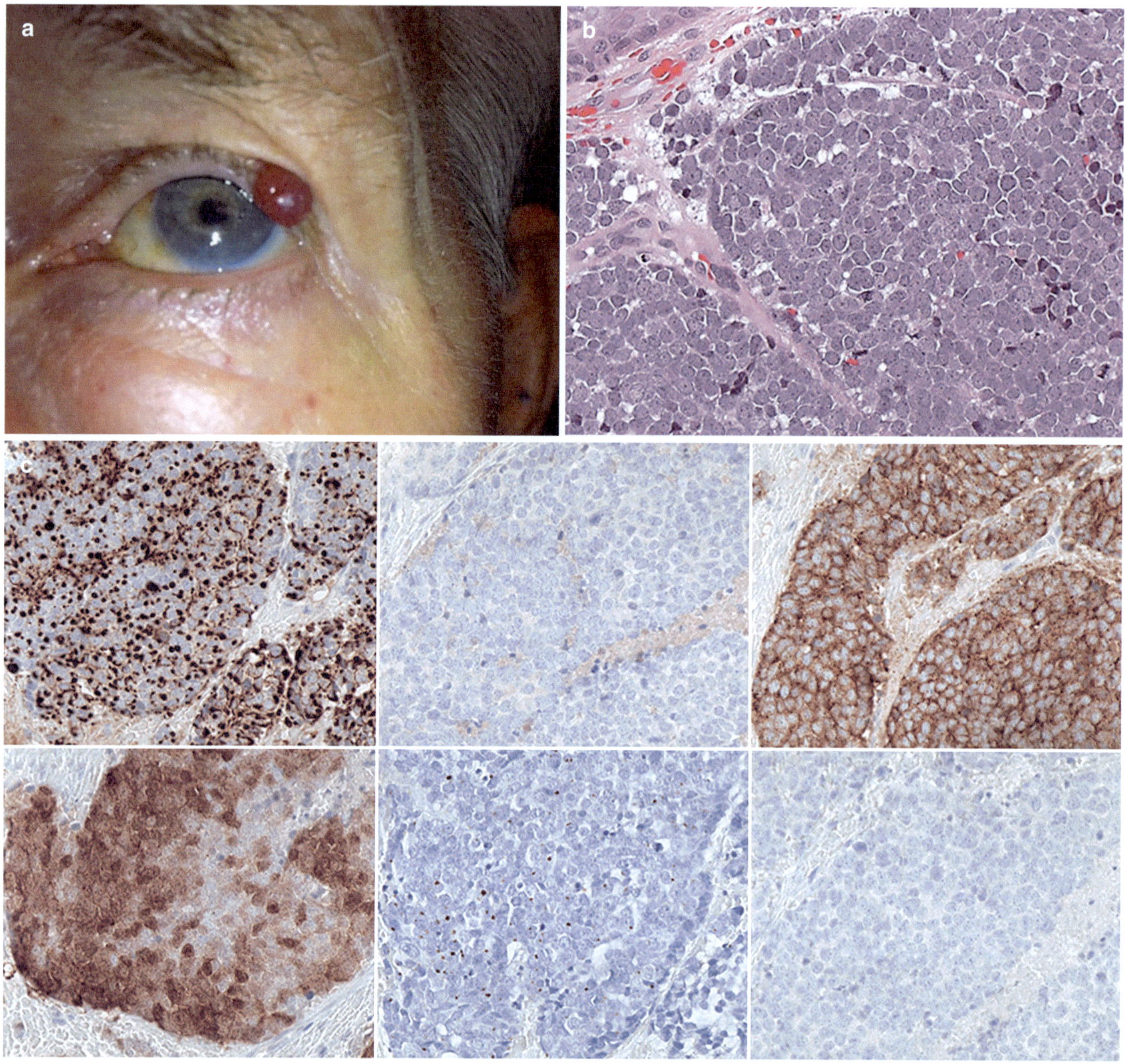

Fig. 10.14 Merkel cell carcinoma. A violaceous nodule involving the margin of the left upper eyelid of an elderly man (**a**). The lesion is characterized by a cellular dermal nodule, sparing the epidermis and exhibiting features of a malignant, undifferentiated, "small blue round cell tumor" (**b**). Immunohistochemical profile of Merkel cell carcinoma. Cytokeratin20 - positive (paranuclear dot pattern) (**c**) (a) cytokeratin7—negative (b), synaptophysin—positive (c), CM2B4—positive (reflecting nuclear expression of Merkel cell polyomavirus) (d), neurofilament—positive (dot-like) (e), thyroid transcription factor protein 1-negative (f). Reproduced with permission from Fleming KE, Ly TY, Pasternak S, Godlewski M, Doucette S, Walsh NM. Support for p63 expression as an adverse prognostic marker in Merkel cell carcinoma: Report on a Canadian cohort. Hum Pathol 2014;45:952-60 and Walsh NM. Merkel cell carcinoma of the eyelid and periocular region: A review. Saudi J Ophthalmol. 2022 Apr 18;35(3):186-192

10.9 Lymphoid, Plasmacytic, and Leukemic Tumors

Lymphoma represents about 13 % of primary malignant eyelid tumors [77]. In a recent multicentric retrospective study, B-cell lymphoma is more common, of which extranodal marginal zone B-cell lymphoma of mucosa-associated lymphoid tissue is the most common type [78], followed by follicular, diffuse large B cell lymphoma, mantle cell lymphoma, and mycoisis fungoidis (Fig. 10.15) [79]. Worst outcomes are reported in DLBCL and MC as compared to the EZML, FL and MF. Recurrence of this malignancy is more closely related to treatment and histopathology than to tumor size or site-specific location. It can either be confined to the eyelid

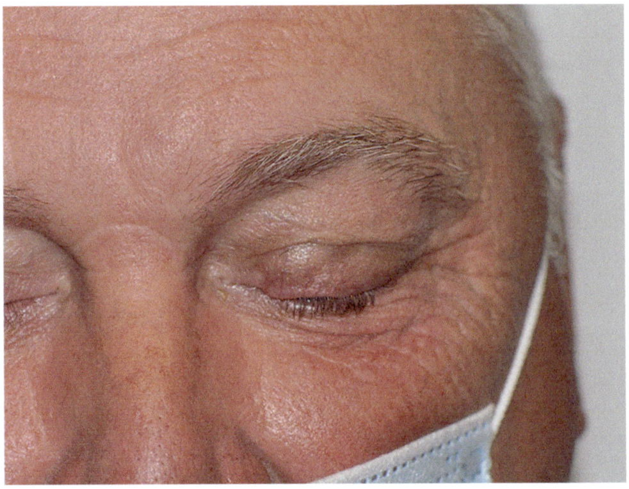

Fig. 10.15 Mantle lymphoma. A 50-year-old man with long standing history of mantle cell lymphoma. He had left upper eyelid infiltration that mimicked chalazion

or have contiguous anterior orbital extension. It manifests as a smooth, firm subcutaneous nodule. In contrast, the less common T-cell lymphoma or mycosis fungoides may present with skin infiltration and ulceration simulating an infectious lesion. Plasmacytoma, a tumor of plasma cell origin, may rarely occur in the eyelid. It could be a primary extramedullary manifestation or with associated multiple myeloma [80]. Leukemic infiltration of the eyelid presenting as a nodular subcutaneous mass or as a diffuse swelling can occur in patients with acute or chronic leukemias [81]. It may even be the primary presentation in the form of granulocytic sarcoma [50]. Relapse of leukemia in the eyelid is also known [81].

Rosai–Dorfman disease is a distinct histiocytic disorder presenting with bilateral, painless, massive cervical lymphadenopathy with a protracted clinical course and in most instances associated with fever, anemia, neutrophilia, elevated erythrocyte sedimentation rate, and polyclonal gammopathy [82]. Eyelid involvement is one of the extranodal manifestations of the disease that is noted in 43% of these patients, presenting as unilateral, bilateral or all four eyelids [83–85]. The other sites involved being skin, nasal cavity and paranasal sinus, orbit, bone, and salivary gland (Fig. 10.16) [86, 87]. The presence of benign histiocytes with emperipolesis, absence of cellular atypia, immunohistochemical profile, and associated clinical features distinguish Rosai–Dorfman disease from other simulating disorder. Management options include observation for mild manifestations with no cosmetic or functional abnormality, surgical excision or debulking, and systemic corticosteroids [87]. Rare occurrence of RDD with MALT lymphoma has been reported recently which could have a bearing on the outcome [88].

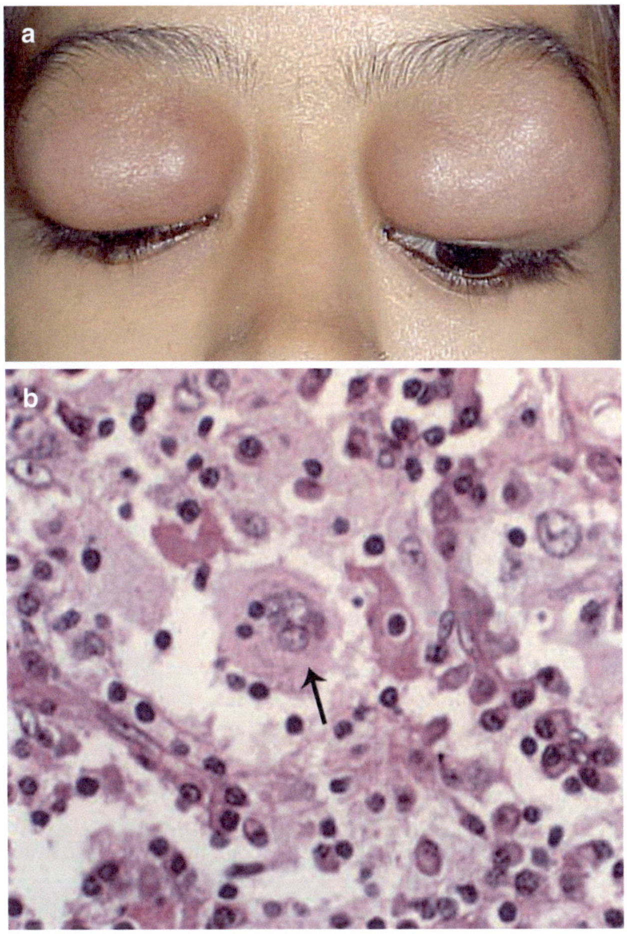

Fig. 10.16 Rosai–Dorfman disease. An 18-year-old girl with bilaterally symmetrical firm eyelid mass and with massive cervical lymphadenopathy and anemia (**a**). Histopathology showing polymorphic population of cells with characteristic histiocytes (arrow) showing lymphophagocytosis (emperipolesis) (**b**, hematoxylin and eosin, original magnification ×400)

10.10 Hamartomas, Choristomas, and Miscellaneous Tumors

Dermoid could involve the eyelid as a contiguous extension of an orbital or a conjunctival lesion. It may, however, primarily involve the eyelid as a very rare manifestation. Cosmetically disturbing and functionally significant dermoids or hamartoma are surgically excised (Fig. 10.17). Ectopic lacrimal gland in the eyelid may present in infancy or early childhood as a cystic mass with or without epiphora [89]. Often it may be a part of a complex choristoma [90]. Heterotopic neuroglial tissue or neuroglial choristoma could manifest as a congenital eyelid mass. Its occurrence is usually associated with other anomalies of cerebral organogenesis [91].

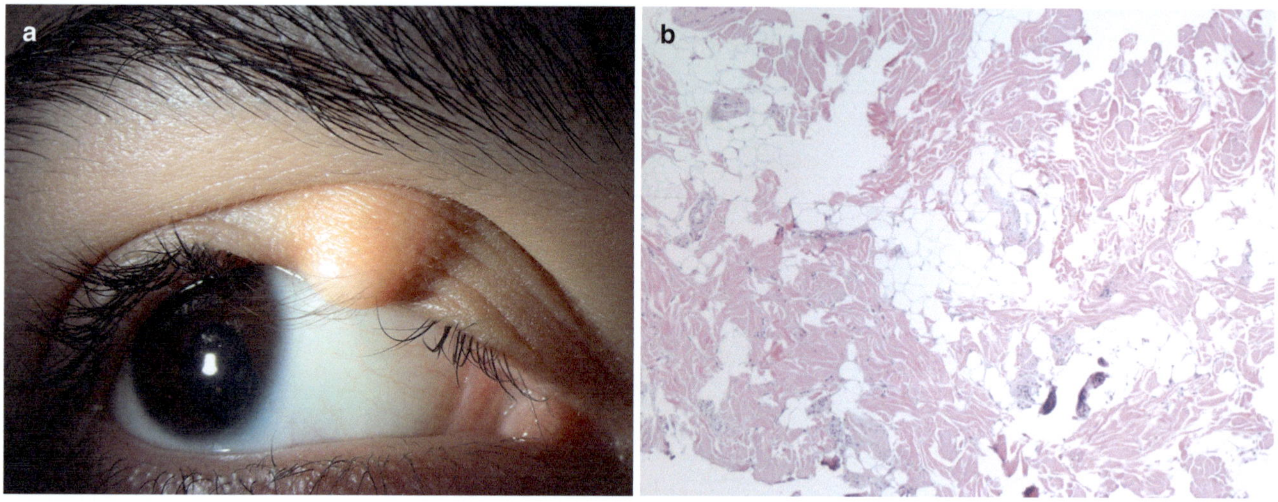

Fig. 10.17 Hamartoma. A 21-year-old female with lid deformity and growth involving right upper eyelid since childhood. Examination showed partial eyelid coloboma with displacement of lashes and a soft nodular lesion (5 × 5 × 4 mm) (**a**). The lesion was partially excised by a skin incision at the superior, temporal, and inferior part of lesion. Only partial excision was done so as to spare the tarsus and the eye lid margin. Portion of the wound was left to heal with secondary intention. Histology highlights benign fibroadipose tissue with clusters of nerve twigs and hair follicles (**b**, hematoxylin and eosin, original magnification ×40)

Phakomatous choristoma or Zimmerman's tumor is a rare congenital hamartoma of lens tissue that probably develops from an abnormal separation or migration of cells from the lens placode into the mesodermal structures of the eyelid [92, 93]. It presents in newborns or young infants as a subcutaneous mass in the medial lower eyelid [93]. Histologically, this lesion comprises of cuboidal cells forming cystic dilated and irregularly branched ducts and cords within a densely fibrotic stroma (Fig. 10.18). Also present are eosinophilic basement membrane-like material, psammoma body-like calcifications, and intraluminal degenerated ghost cells.

10.11 Metastatic Tumors

Eyelid metastasis represents about 1% of all malignant tumors of the eyelid. Rapidly progressive subcutaneous nodule, in a patient with history of prior cancer, should raise the suspicion. The common sources of primary tumor are breast, lung, and cutaneous melanoma.

10.12 Inflammatory and Infective Lesions

Some of the common lesions of inflammatory and infective etiology that often simulate an eyelid tumor include chalazion, pyogenic granuloma, verruca vulgaris, amyloidosis, lipid proteinosis, and molluscum contagiosum.

10.13 Summary

Eyelid stromal tumors manifest with a wide spectrum of clinical features that may often confound even an experienced clinician. Careful attention to clinical history, vital clinical signs, and systemic features may help arrive at a logical differential diagnosis and appropriately manage the patient.

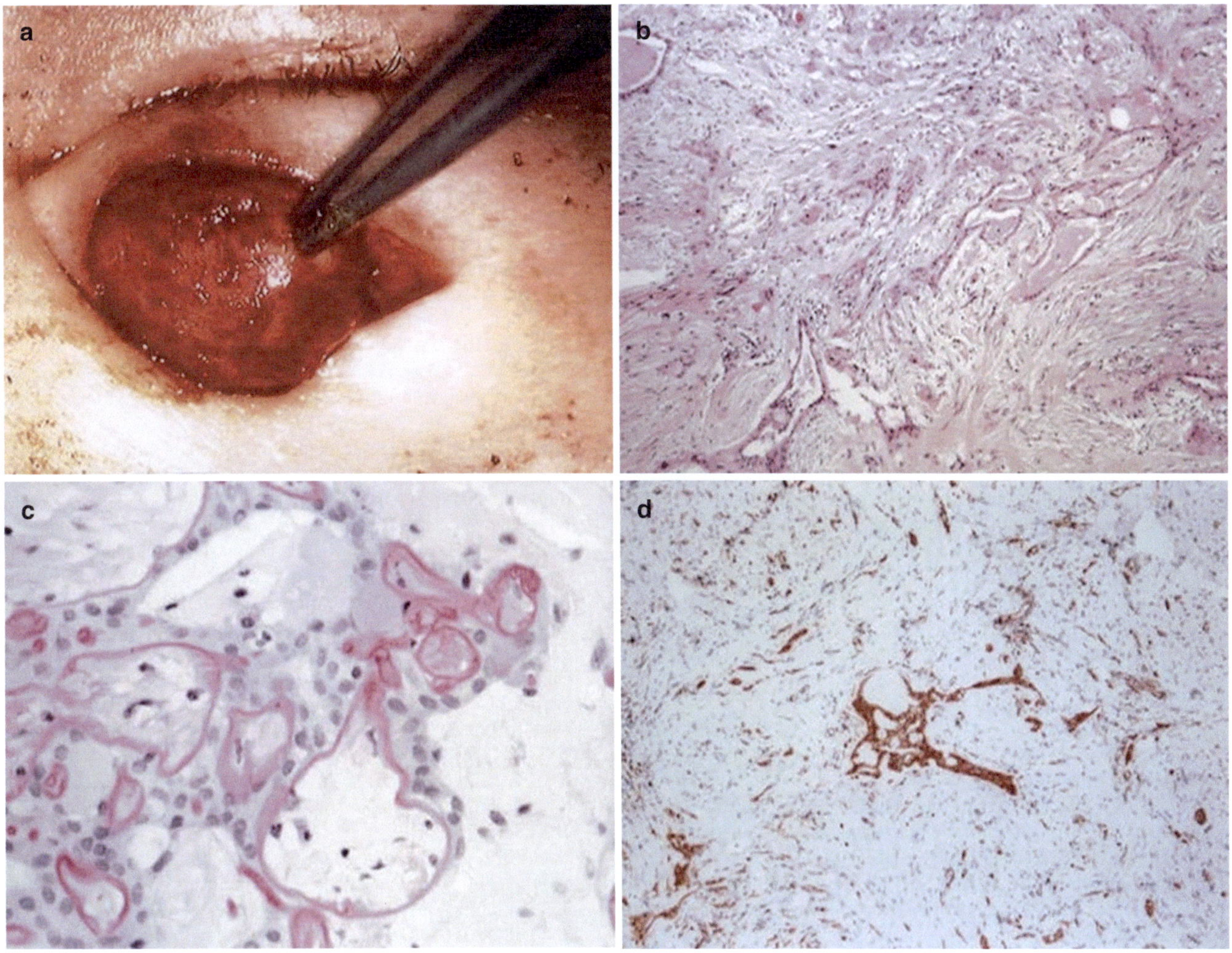

Fig. 10.18 Choristoma. A 12-month-old girl was referred because of a tumor in her left lower eyelid. The mass near the inner canthus had been present since birth and had remained stable since then. The subcutaneous tumor was round, smooth-edged, free from the overlying skin and not sensitive to pressure palpable. No other ocular or systemic abnormalities were detected. The initial clinical diagnosis was dermoid cyst. Excisional biopsy was performed. The tumor was located below the tarsal plate and lateral to the lacrimal sac. The mass was completely excised (**a**). At gross examination, the lesion was pale, firm and round with a homogeneous white cut surface. Histologically, the lesion consisted of cells that were arranged in solid nests, tubules, and cystic formations. These cells were embedded in a densely sclerotic fibrous background. Within the cystic formations, there were eosinophilic material and large ovoid, degenerated cells with abundant eosinophilic foamy cytoplasm (**b**). The epithelial structures were surrounded by thick PAS-positive membranes (**c**). Immunohistochemistry was performed on 4-mm-thick sections from paraffin-embedded tissue. The epithelial cells showed strong immunoreactivity for vimentin (**d**) and negative staining for cytokeratin, glial fibrially acidic protein, epithelial membrane antigen or macrophage marker. Reproduced with permission from Dithmar, S., Schmack, I., Völcker, H.E. *et al.* Phakomatous choristoma of the eyelid. Graefe's Arch Clin Exp Ophthalmol 2004; 242, 40–43

References

1. Milman T, Grossniklaus HE, Goldman-Levy G, et al. The 5th edition of the World Health Organization classification of tumours of the eye and orbit. Ocul Oncol Pathol. 2023;9(3-4):71–95.
2. Witschel H. Congenital solitary fibromatosis of the eyelid (author's transl). Ophthalmologica. 1982;185(1):1–6.
3. Hidayat AA, Font RL. Juvenile fibromatosis of the periorbital region and eyelid. A clinicopathologic study of six cases. Arch Ophthalmol. 1980;98(2):280–5.
4. John M, Chirayath S, Paulson S. Multiple soft fibromas of the lid. Indian J Ophthalmol. 2015;63(3):262–4.
5. D'Hermies F, Dolle C, Verola O, et al. Hypertrophic eyelid conjunctival scar. A tarsal keloid. J Fr Ophtalmol. 2003;26(3):315–8.
6. Hiemcke-Jiwa LS, van Gorp JM, Fisher C, et al. USP6-associated neoplasms: a rapidly expanding family of lesions. Int J Surg Pathol. 2020;28(8):816–25.
7. Hymas DC, Mamalis N, Pratt DV, et al. Nodular fasciitis of the lower eyelid in a pediatric patient. Ophthalmic Plast Reconstr Surg. 1999;15(2):139–42.
8. De Wan J, Evens F, De Mey A. Eyelid tumour and juvenile hyaline fibromatosis. Br J Plast Surg. 2005;58(1):106–11.
9. Weiner JM, Hidayat AA. Juvenile fibrosarcoma of the orbit and eyelid. A study of five cases. Arch Ophthalmol. 1983;101(2):253–9.

10. Griffith DG, Salasche SJ, Clemons DE. Cutaneous abnormalities of the eyelid and face: an atlas with histopathology. New York: McGraw-Hill; 1987.
11. Pandhi D, Gupta P, Singal A, et al. Xanthelasma palpebrarum: a marker of premature atherosclerosis (risk of atherosclerosis in xanthelasma). Postgrad Med J. 2012;88(1038):198–204.
12. Park EJ, Youn SH, Cho EB, et al. Xanthelasma palpebrarum treatment with a 1,450-nm-diode laser. Dermatologic Surg. 2011;37(6):791–6.
13. Dincer D, Koc E, Erbil AH, Kose O. Effectiveness of low-voltage radiofrequency in the treatment of xanthelasma palpebrarum: a pilot study of 15 cases. Dermatologic Surg. 2010;36(12):1973–8.
14. Jakobiec FA, Mills MD, Hidayat AA, et al. Periocular xanthogranulomas associated with severe adult-onset asthma. Trans Am Ophthalmol Soc. 1993;91:99-125; discussion -9.
15. Vick VL, Wilson MW, Fleming JC, Haik BG. Orbital and eyelid manifestations of xanthogranulomatous diseases. Orbit. 2006;25(3):221–5.
16. Mentzel T, Kutzner H, Rutten A, Hugel H. Benign fibrous histiocytoma (dermatofibroma) of the face: clinicopathologic and immunohistochemical study of 34 cases associated with an aggressive clinical course. Am J Dermatopathol. 2001;23(5):419–26.
17. Jakobiec FA, Zakka FR, Tu Y, Freitag SK. Dermatofibroma of the eyelid: immunohistochemical diagnosis. Ophthalmic Plast Reconstr Surg. 2017;33(6):e134–8.
18. Wu PC, Hung YT, Chen WT. Multiple eruptive dermatofibromas associated with altered immunity and systemic lupus erythematosus. Clin Rheumatol. 2023;42(10):2917–8.
19. Ridha Z, Belmesk L, Jfri A, et al. Systemic disease association with multiple eruptive dermatofibromas: a systematic review. J Cutan Med Surg. 2022;26(6):628–9.
20. Khong JJ, Chen CS, James CL, et al. Malignant fibrous histiocytoma of the eyelid: differential diagnosis and management. Ophthalmic Plast Reconstr Surg. 2005;21(2):103–8.
21. Gounder P, Lam M, Vinciullo C, de Sousa JL. Malignant fibrous histiocytoma masquerading as pyogenic granuloma. Orbit. 2017;36(2):122–3.
22. Font RL, Hidayat AA. Fibrous histiocytoma of the orbit. A clinicopathologic study of 150 cases. Hum Pathol. 1982;13(3):199–209.
23. Thyparampil P, Diwan AH, Diaz-Marchan P, et al. Eyelid lipomas: a case report and review of the literature. Orbit. 2012;31(5):319–20.
24. Bock-Kunz AL, Lyon DB, Singhal VK, Grin TR. Nasopalpebral lipoma-coloboma syndrome. Arch Ophthalmol. 2000;118(12):1699–701.
25. Enghardt MH, Warren RC. Congenital palpebral lipoblastoma. First report of a case. Am J Dermatopathol. 1990;12(4):408–11.
26. Jolly SS, Brownstein S, Jordan DR. Leiomyoma of the anterior orbit and eyelid. Can J Ophthalmol. 1995;30(7):366–70.
27. Lin IC, Wu CT, Liao SL, Lin LL. Primary orbital leiomyosarcoma. Ophthalmic Plast Reconstr Surg. 2005;21(6):451–3.
28. Verdolini R, Goteri G, Brancorsini D, et al. Adult rhabdomyoma: report of two cases of rhabdomyoma of the lip and of the eyelid. Am J Dermatopathol. 2000;22(3):264–7.
29. Shields CL, Shields JA, Honavar SG, Demirci H. Clinical spectrum of primary ophthalmic rhabdomyosarcoma. Ophthalmology. 2001;108(12):2284–92.
30. ISSVA Classification for Vascular Anomalies tIW, Melbourne., 2014. Apr LaoFAf, cation-2018.
31. Ferry AP. Pyogenic granulomas of the eye and ocular adnexa: a study of 100 cases. Trans Am Ophthalmol Soc. 1989;87:327–43; discussion 43-7
32. Bejjanki KM, Mishra DK, Kaliki S. Periocular lobular capillary hemangioma in adults: a clinicopathological study. Middle East Afr J Ophthalmol. 2019;26(3):138–40.
33. Werner MS, Hornblass A, Reifler DM, et al. Intravascular papillary endothelial hyperplasia: collection of four cases and a review of the literature. Ophthalmic Plast Reconstr Surg. 1997;13(1):48–56.
34. Shields CL, Shields JA, Minzter R, Singh AD. Cutaneous capillary hemangiomas of the eyelid, scalp, and digits in premature triplets. Am J Ophthalmol. 2000;129(4):528–31.
35. Walter JW, Blei F, Anderson JL, et al. Genetic mapping of a novel familial form of infantile hemangioma. Am J Med Genet. 1999;82(1):77–83.
36. Jackson R. The natural history of strawberry naevi. J Cutan Med Surg. 1998;2(3):187–9.
37. Stagner AM, Jakobiec FA. A critical analysis of eleven periocular lobular capillary hemangiomas in adults. Am J Ophthalmol. 2016;165:164–73.
38. Missoi TG, Lueder GT, Gilbertson K, Bayliss SJ. Oral propranolol for treatment of periocular infantile hemangiomas. Arch Ophthalmol. 2011;129(7):899–903.
39. Snir M, Reich U, Siegel R, et al. Refractive and structural changes in infantile periocular capillary haemangioma treated with propranolol. Eye. 2011;25(12):1627–34.
40. Ni N, Guo S, Langer P. Current concepts in the management of periocular infantile (capillary) hemangioma. Curr Opin Ophthalmol. 2011;22(5):419–25.
41. Mehta A, Bajaj MS, Pushker N, et al. To compare intralesional and oral propranolol for treating periorbital and eyelid capillary hemangiomas. Indian J Ophthalmol. 2019;67(12):1974–80.
42. Bejjanki KM, Akhtar K, Gupta AP, Kaliki S. Effect of oral propranolol on periocular infantile capillary hemangioma: outcomes based on extent of involvement. Middle East Afr J Ophthalmol. 2021;28(1):6–10.
43. Xue K, Hildebrand GD. Topical timolol maleate 0.5% for infantile capillary haemangioma of the eyelid. Br J Ophthalmol. 2012;96(12):1536–7.
44. Cheng J, Lam YY, Fung GPG, et al. Randomised controlled trial: can topical timolol maleate prevent complications for small superficial infantile haemangiomata in high-risk areas? Pediatr Res. 2020;88(5):756–60.
45. Men CJ, Ediriwickrema LS, Paik JS, et al. Surgical intervention of periocular infantile hemangiomas in the era of beta-blockers. Ophthalmic Plast Reconstr Surg. 2020;36(1):70–3.
46. Shalhoub SY. Rare multiple keratocysts of the mandible. Ann Dent. 1987;46(2):52–4.
47. Bajaj MS, Nainiwal SK, Pushker N. Multifocal cavernous hemangioma: a rare presentation. Orbit. 2003;22(3):155–9.
48. McCannel CA, Hoenig J, Umlas J, et al. Orbital lesions in the blue rubber bleb nevus syndrome. Ophthalmology. 1996;103(6):933–6.
49. Hidayat AA, Cameron JD, Font RL, Zimmerman LE. Angiolymphoid hyperplasia with eosinophilia (Kimura's disease) of the orbit and ocular adnexa. Am J Ophthalmol. 1983;96(2):176–89.
50. Hayes BH, Shore JW, Westfall CT, Harris GJ. Management of orbital and periorbital arteriovenous malformations. Ophthalmic Surg. 1995;26(2):145–52.
51. Rootman J, Hay E, Graeb D, Miller R. Orbital-adnexal lymphangiomas: a spectrum of hernodynarnically isolated vascular harnartornas. Ophthalmology. 1986;93(12):1558–70.
52. Ferguson DC, Mawn LA, Al-Rohil RN. Cutaneous angiosarcoma of the eyelid mimicking morbihan disease. Am J Dermatopathol. 2018;40(8):617–20.
53. Lemanski N, Farber M, Carruth BP, Wladis EJ. Primary adnexal angiosarcoma masquerading as periorbital hematoma. Surv Ophthalmol. 2014;59(6):655–9.
54. Guo QY. Atypical lymphocytes in schizophrenic patients. Zhonghua Shen Jing Jing Shen Ke Za Zhi. 1986;19(3):185–7.
55. Conway R, Hammer T, Viestenz A, Holbach L. Cutaneous angiosarcoma of the eyelids. Br J Ophthalmol. 2003;87(4):514–5.

56. Papalas JA, Manavi CK, Woodward JA, et al. Angiosarcoma of the eyelid: a clinicopathologic comparison between isolated unilateral tumors and tumors demonstrating extrapalpebral involvement. Am J Dermatopathol. 2010;32(7):694–9.
57. Brun SC, Jakobiec FA. Kaposi's sarcoma of the ocular adnexa. Int Ophthalmol Clin. 1997;37(4):25–38.
58. Dammacco R, Lapenna L, Giancipoli G, et al. Solitary eyelid Kaposi sarcoma in an HIV-negative patient. Cornea. 2006;25(4):490–2.
59. Jhaj G, Ilyas G, Shinder R. Eyelid Kaposi's sarcoma in an immunocompetent woman. Ophthalmology. 2017;124(3):392.
60. Teixeira AI, Neno M, Badura R, et al. Kaposi sarcoma of the eyelid as an initial manifestation of AIDS. Dermatol Online J. 2016;22(7):13030.
61. Ulloa-Padilla JP, Ghassibi MP, Dubovy SR, Kerr DA. Clinicopathologic correlation of kaposi sarcoma involving the ocular adnexa: immunophenotyping of diagnostic and therapeutic targets. Ophthalmic Plast Reconstr Surg. 2020;36(2):185–90.
62. Brunetti AE, Guarini A, Lorusso V, et al. Complete response to second line Paclitaxel every 2 weeks of eyelid kaposi sarcoma: a case report. Ophthalmic Plast Reconstr Surg. 2013;29(5):e114–5.
63. Zhang ML, Suarez MJ, Bosley TM, Rodriguez FJ. Clinicopathological features of peripheral nerve sheath tumors involving the eye and ocular adnexa. Hum Pathol. 2017;63:70–8.
64. Butt Z, Ironside JW. Superficial epithelioid schwannoma presenting as a subcutaneous upper eyelid mass. Br J Ophthalmol. 1994;78(7):586–8.
65. Singh AD, Eagle RC Jr, Shields CL, Shields JA. Merkel cell carcinoma of the eyelids. Int Ophthalmol Clin. 1993;33(3):11–7.
66. Kivela T, Tarkkanen A. The Merkel cell and associated neoplasms in the eyelids and periocular region. Surv Ophthalmol. 1990;35(3):171–87.
67. Amber K, McLeod MP, Nouri K. The Merkel cell polyomavirus and its involvement in Merkel cell carcinoma. Dermatologic Surg. 2013;39(2):232–8.
68. Feng H, Shuda M, Chang Y, Moore PS. Clonal integration of a polyomavirus in human Merkel cell carcinoma. Science. 2008;319(5866):1096–100.
69. Hanafi H, Verdijk RM, Paridaens D. Eyelid Merkel cell carcinoma in a patient treated with golimumab. Orbit. 2018;37(1):21–5.
70. Sniegowski MC, Warneke CL, Morrison WH, et al. Correlation of American Joint Committee on Cancer T category for eyelid carcinoma with outcomes in patients with periocular Merkel cell carcinoma. Ophthalmic Plast Reconstr Surg. 2014;30(6):480–5.
71. Moll I, Kuhn C, Moll R. Cytokeratin 20 is a general marker of cutaneous Merkel cells while certain neuronal proteins are absent. J Invest Dermatol. 1995;104(6):910–5.
72. Walsh NM. Merkel cell carcinoma of the eyelid and periocular region: a review. Saudi J Ophthalmol. 2021;35(3):186–92.
73. Peters GB III, Meyer DR, Shields JA, et al. Management and prognosis of Merkel cell carcinoma of the eyelid. Ophthalmology. 2001;108(9):1575–9.
74. Tuskada A, Fujimura T, Hashimoto A, et al. Successful local control of cutaneous Merkel cell carcinoma on the eyelid with CyberKnife radiosurgery. Eur J Dermatol. 2013;23(5):725–6.
75. Pfeiffer ML, Savar A, Esmaeli B. Sentinel lymph node biopsy for eyelid and conjunctival tumors: what have we learned in the past decade? Ophthalmic Plast Reconstr Surg. 2013;29(1):57–62.
76. Nudelman NT, Ekhator N, Rothschild M, Wladis EJ. A SEER program study of survival trends in Merkel cell carcinoma of the eyelid: 2000-2019. Orbit. 2023;43(3):290–5.
77. Margo CE, Mulla ZD. Malignant tumors of the eyelid: a population-based study of non-basal cell and non-squamous cell malignant neoplasms. Arch Ophthalmol. 1998;116(2):195–8.
78. Graue GF, Finger PT, Maher E, et al. Ocular adnexal lymphoma staging and treatment: American Joint Committee on Cancer versus Ann Arbor. Eur J Ophthalmol. 2013;23(3):344–55.
79. Svendsen FH, Rasmussen PK, Coupland SE, et al. Lymphoma of the eyelid - an international multicenter retrospective study. Am J Ophthalmol. 2017;177:58–68.
80. Ahamed E, Samuel L, Tighe J. Extramedullary plasmacytoma of the eyelid. Br J Ophthalmol. 2003;87(2):244–5.
81. Yaghouti F, Nouri M, Mannor GE. Ocular adnexal granulocytic sarcoma as the first sign of acute myelogenous leukemia relapse. Am J Ophthalmol. 1999;127(3):361–3.
82. Rosai J, Dorfman RF. Sinus histiocytosis with massive lymphadenopathy. A newly recognized benign clinicopathological entity. Arch Pathol. 1969;87(1):63–70.
83. Hsu HY, Chen ZT, Tsai CY, et al. Atypical Rosai-Dorfman disease with lacrimal gland involvement. Semin Ophthalmol. 2013;28(4):253–5.
84. Jat KR, Panigrahi I, Srinivasan R, et al. Cutaneous Rosai-Dorfman disease: presenting as massive bilateral eyelid swelling. Pediatr Dermatol. 2009;26(5):633–5.
85. Levinger S, Pe'er J, Aker M, Okon E. Rosai-Dorfman disease involving four eyelids. Am J Ophthalmol. 1993;116(3):382–4.
86. Foucar E, Rosai J, Dorfman RF. The ophthalmologic manifestations of sinus histiocytosis with massive lymphadenopathy. Am J Ophthalmol. 1979;87(3):354–67.
87. Vemuganti GK, Naik MN, Honavar SG. Rosai dorfman disease of the orbit. J Hematol Oncol. 2008;1(1):7.
88. Wang G, Lin Y, Shen H, et al. Intracranial Rosai-Dorfman disease complicated by mucosa-associated lymphoid tissue: a case report. Oncol Lett. 2023;26(3):402.
89. McCulley TJ, Yip C-C, Kersten RC, Kulwin DR. An ectopic site of lacrimal gland secretion mimicking epiphora. Arch Ophthalmol. 2002;120(11):1586–7.
90. Gordon AJ, Patrinely JR, Knupp JA, Font RL. Complex choristoma of the eyelid containing ectopic cilia and lacrimal gland. Ophthalmology. 1991;98(10):1547–50.
91. Holbach LM, Naumann GO, Font RL. Neuroglial choristoma presenting as congenital lid tumor. Graefes Arch Clin Exp Ophthalmol. 1989;227(6):584–8.
92. Dithmar S, Schmack I, Volcker HE, Grossniklaus HE. Phakomatous choristoma of the eyelid. Graefes Arch Clin Exp Ophthalmol. 2004;242(1):40–3.
93. Ellis FJ, Eagle RC, Shields JA, et al. Phakomatous choristoma (Zimmerman's tumor). Immunohistochemical confirmation of lens-specific proteins. Ophthalmology. 1993;100(6):955–60.

Eyelid Tumors: Surgical Techniques

11

Jennifer I. Hui and David T. Tse

11.1 Introduction

The goals in the management of a malignant eyelid lesion are to establish an early accurate diagnosis, to achieve a permanent cure by total eradication of the tumor, and to preserve or restore both eyelid function and cosmesis.

11.2 General Principles

11.2.1 Diagnostic Biopsy

An eyelid lesion that exhibits clinical features suggestive of malignancy should first undergo biopsy to establish a definitive diagnosis. It is important to always photograph all lesions prior to any biopsy or excision being performed. Photographs must be obtained with the eyelid in normal position and the eyelid everted. If possible, a copy of the clinical photograph together with the markings of where the pathology specimen was obtained should be sent to the histopathologist. If the lesion is small, an excisional biopsy including at least a 2–3 mm margin of normal tissue should be considered. Following simple elliptical excision, the tissue margins of the specimen must be examined histologically to confirm tumor clearance. If the size of the anticipated excisional defect is such that closure might cause eyelid malposition, an incisional biopsy should first be considered to establish a pathologic diagnosis before proceeding with surgical excision and reconstruction. If a graft or flap is anticipated in the repair of the defect, the surgical margins must first be evaluated microscopically to confirm tumor eradication.

If sebaceous cell carcinoma is suspected, a full thickness excisional biopsy with 5 mm margins should be performed by removing a pentagonal wedge of the anterior and posterior lamella [1]. Given the tumor's propensity for pagetoid spread and skip lesions, multiple carefully mapped biopsies of the conjunctiva and tarsus should be considered for permanent section.

11.2.2 Definitive Treatment

Following histological confirmation of a malignant lesion, definitive excision is pursued. Mohs micrographic surgery and excision with frozen- or permanent-section control yield high cure rates [2]. The authors' treatment of choice for primary periocular malignant eyelid lesions is Mohs' micrographic surgery followed by immediate reconstruction. The Mohs' method allows for maximal tissue conservation with careful evaluation of surgical margins. First, the gross mass of the tumor plus a small peripheral margin of normal tissue is removed [2–6]. A thin layer of tissue (2 mm) is further excised from the base and edges of the wound. The specimen is divided and placed on glass slides and the edges are carefully marked with different-colored dyes to maintain orientation. Frozen sections are obtained from the undersurface and skin edges; the locations of residual tumor are mapped, and only those areas are subsequently re-excised (Fig. 11.1). Once tumor-free margins have been achieved, the oculoplastic surgeon reconstructs the eyelid defect on the same or the following day.

11.2.3 Sentinel Lymph Node Biopsy

In a patient with a biopsy-proven malignant eyelid lesion with demonstrated biological behavior for regional lymph

J. I. Hui
Orthopedic, Miller School of Medicine, University of Miami, Miami, FL, USA

D. T. Tse (✉)
Ophthalmology, Bascom Palmer Eye Institute, Miller School of Medicine, University of Miami, Miami, FL, USA
e-mail: dtse@med.miami.edu

B. C. K. Patel et al. (eds.), *Clinical Ophthalmic Oncology*, https://doi.org/10.1007/978-3-031-72328-5_11

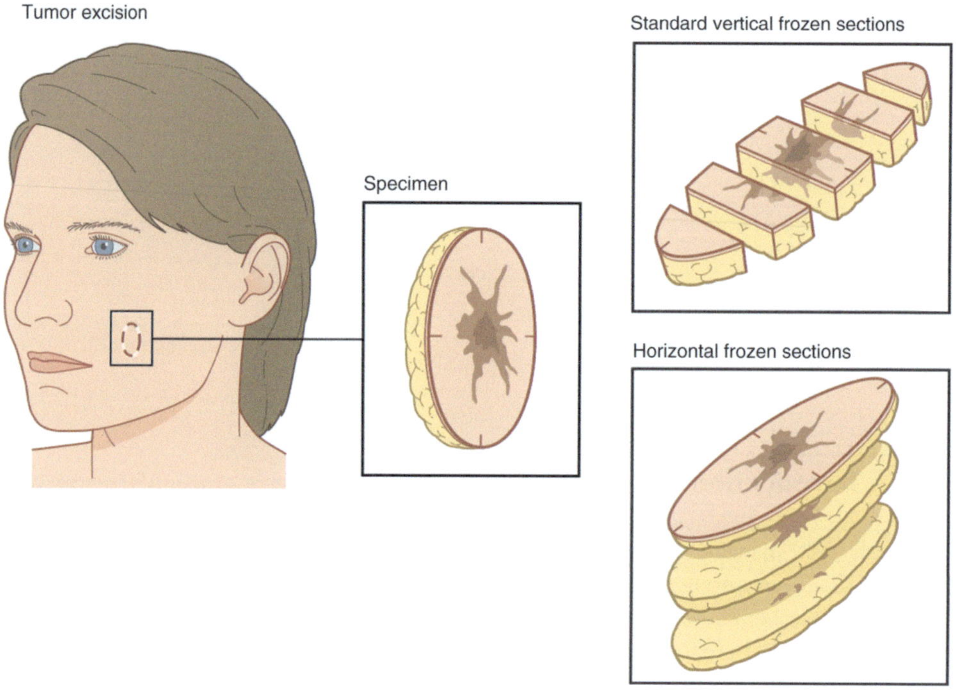

Fig. 11.1 Mohs' micrographic surgery. Frozen sections are obtained from the undersurface and skin edges of the excised lesion. Locations of residual tumor are marked on a map for subsequent second stage excision

node metastasis, careful evaluation of preauricular and submandibular lymph nodes is essential. An additional consideration is the use of lymphatic mapping and sentinel lymph node biopsy for early accurate staging of solid tumors exhibiting a propensity for regional nodal metastasis (Chap. 21) [7].

11.2.4 Eyelid Reconstruction

Optimum functional and cosmetic outcomes are possible if the following general principles of eyelid reconstruction are taken into consideration:

- The eyelid is a bilamellar structure; the anterior lamella consists of the skin and orbicularis oculi muscle, and the posterior lamella of the tarsal plate and conjunctiva.
- The anterior or posterior lamella must have its own inherent blood supply.
- Provision must be made for maximal horizontal stabilization with minimal vertical tension through proper canthal fixation, and an epithelialized internal surface to face the globe [8].
- Undermining should be sufficient to allow for tension-free closure.
- Identification of the transverse edge of the levator aponeurosis and a knowledge of facial nerve anatomy are essential in maintaining the opening and closing functions of the eyelid.

11.3 Lower Eyelid Defects (Fig. 11.2)

11.3.1 Anterior Lamellar Deficit, Lid Margin Intact

11.3.1.1 Primary Closure

In general, anterior lamellar defects without lid margin involvement may be closed primarily if this does not induce distortion. The wound is closed in two layers using deep, interrupted 5/0 or 6/0 Vicryl sutures and interrupted, superficial 6/0 or 7/0 nylon or silk sutures in the skin. If insufficient anterior lamella remains, a full-thickness pentagonal wedge, including the anterior lamellar defect, may be excised with Westcott scissors. The tarsal borders should be sharp and perpendicular to the lid margin. The resulting full-thickness defect may then be closed primarily as described below.

11.3.1.2 Skin Graft

For defects that are too large to close primarily, full-thickness skin grafts from hairless areas may be employed. Possible donor sites include the ipsilateral or contralateral upper eyelid, the preauricular or retroauricular skin, and less commonly the supraclavicular fossa and the upper inner arm. In general, split-thickness skin grafts are not recommended in eyelid reconstruction [2]. If a skin graft is obtained from the upper eyelid or retroauricular area, it must be thinned of subcutaneous fat and connective tissue. The graft is then trimmed to size and sutured to the edges of the defect with interrupted 7/0 nylon or silk sutures [9].

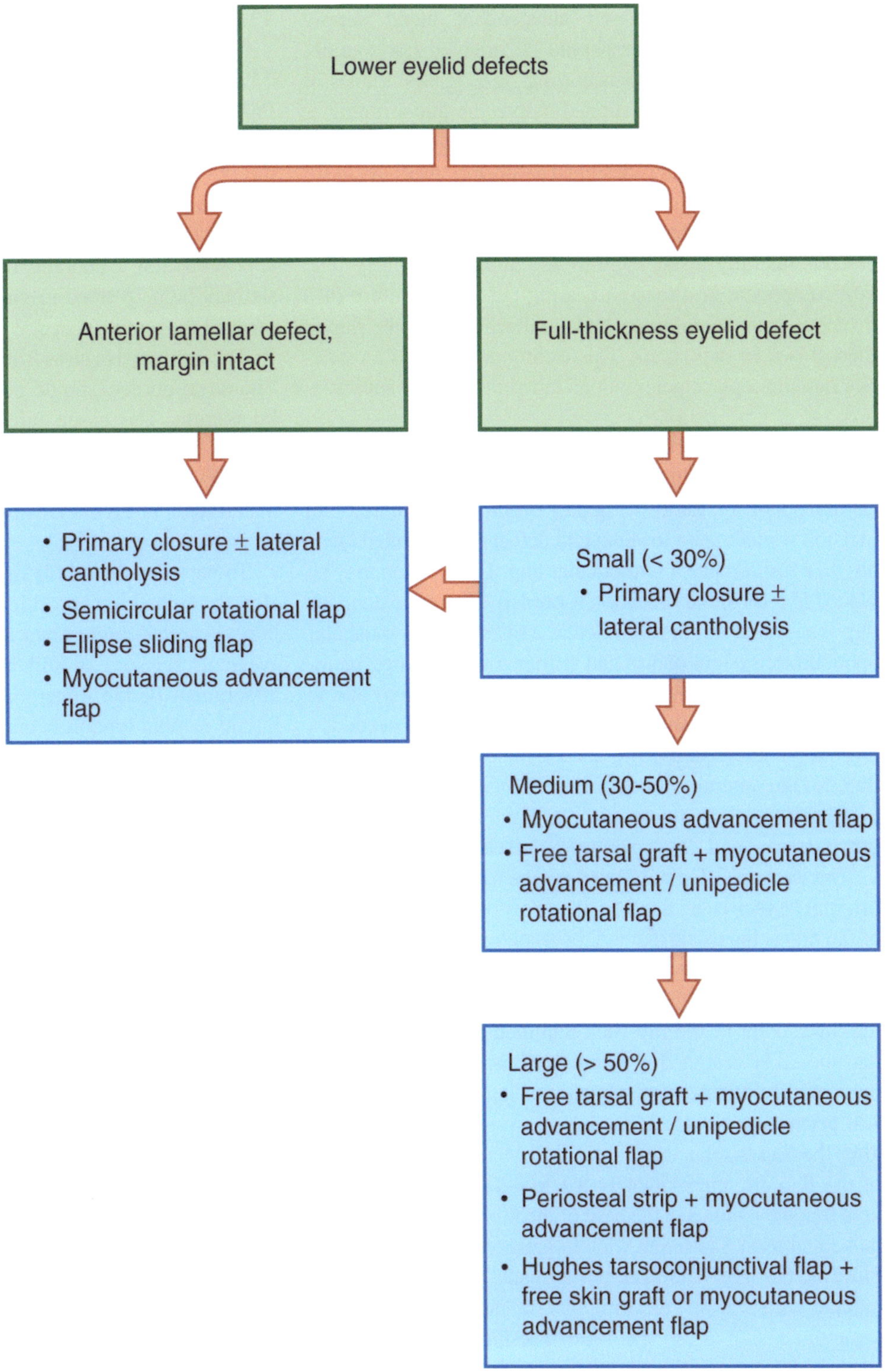

Fig. 11.2 Algorithm for the repair of lower eyelid defects

11.3.1.3 Ellipse Sliding Flap

An elliptical sliding flap may also be used to close some anterior lamellar defects [10]. This flap, however, should not be used to reconstruct anterior lamellar defects near the lid margin because ectropion or retraction may be induced by excessive perpendicular tension. The ellipse should be oriented parallel to the relaxed skin tension lines. The long axis should be four times longer than the short axis, with the ellipse angle at approximately 30°. The flap is secured in two layers.

11.3.1.4 Myocutaneous Advancement Flap

An ideal method to address a large anterior lamellar deficit is the myocutaneous advancement flap because it provides the best tissue match with an independent blood supply (Fig. 11.3). Incision lines should be oriented horizontally and blend within naturally occurring skin creases. Planes of dissection should be determined before the undermining is advanced past the lateral orbital rim [8, 9]. The flap consists of skin and muscle and is designed to advance medially to fill an anterior lamellar defect. The creation of a myocutaneous advancement flap begins with an infralash incision that extends laterally to the canthus and arches superiorly. The key component is a tension-bearing permanent suture (4/0 Prolene) at the zygoma or the lateral orbital rim; the flap is then closed in two layers. This technique provides an anterior lamella replacement with an inherent vascular supply.

11.3.1.5 Flip Back Technique (Fig. 11.4)

This technique is suited for moderate to large anterior lamellar defects of the lower (or upper) eyelid [11]. A horizontal incision is made for a lower eyelid defect and extended laterally in a fashion like a semicircular flap. The incision may be placed in a subsidiary location if needed. The myocutaneous flap is elevated in the suborbicular and superficial muscular aponeurotic system planes and redraped using a superotemporal vector. This overlaps the semicircular incision due to laxity in the cheek and lateral canthal regions. If needed, a 5-0 Vicryl suture is used to anchor the deep surface of the flap to the lateral orbital rim periosteum. This tension-bearing suspension suture supports the flap against gravitational descent and post-operative contracture.

The anchored flap now overlaps the superior edge of the original semicircular flap incision. This overlapping portion of the flap is the tissue that will be used for the flip-back flap. A marking pen is used to design a back-cut incision starting at the temporal apex of the semicircular flap and ending at the pivot point of the flip-back flap medially. The flip-back flap should be designed to ensure that it is wide enough to fill the vertical dimension of the anterior lamellar defect while still permitting closure of the lateral wound without tension after the flap is rotated and inset. In general, the dimensions of the flap are approximately 3:1 to 4:1. It is important to note that the isthmus at the base of the flip-back pedicle must be kept at least 5 to 6 mm wide to preserve the vascular viability of the flap. The back-cut is made in a full-thickness manner with scissors, ensuring that the muscle layer has the same dimension as the skin layer. The flip-back flap is then rotated 180° around the pivot point and inset into the recipient site. The flap is sutured into place medially with deep buried 5-0 Vicryl sutures, and the skin is closed with 7-0 Vicryl or nylon sutures.

When used to close an eyelid margin defect, the superior edge of the flip-back flap is sutured to the superior edge of the reconstructed posterior lamella with multiple 7-0 Vicryl mattress sutures. Lamellar passes are taken in the posterior lamella to avoid post-operative corneal abrasion.

11.3.2 Full-Thickness Eyelid Defect

11.3.2.1 Primary Closure

For small defects involving less than one-third of the lower eyelid margin, primary closure without lateral cantholysis is the best option. Primary layered closure provides the best tissue match, a smooth lid margin, and a continuous eyelash line. If tension is present and precludes proper lid margin approximation, a lateral canthotomy with inferior cantholysis may be performed to yield 5–6 mm of medial advancement of the temporal eyelid margin [9, 10].

The first step requires trimming of the eyelid defect edges. The tarsal borders should be sharp and perpendicular to the lid margin. The tissue inferior to the tarsus is cut into a wedge, forming a pentagonal-shaped defect. Direct closure may be utilized if the borders of this defect can be reapproximated without excess tension; otherwise, a lateral cantholysis is needed.

To perform a cantholysis, a 4- to 5-mm horizontal incision through skin and orbicularis muscle is made from the lateral canthal angle toward the orbital rim. The tip of the Westcott scissors should be used to identify the lateral attachment of the lower lid, and the inferior crus of the lateral canthal tendon is cut by making a vertical incision. If there is still need for further mobilization of the eyelid laterally, the scissors are used to release the lateral retinaculum and even the lateral inferior septum, both of which allow further mobilization of the eyelid so that the defect may be closed with minimal or no tension. The most important step in primary closure of the pentagonal lid margin defect is precise approximation of the tarsal edges. Accurate vertical alignment provides most of the tension-bearing support of the wound. Following lid margin reapproximation and repair of the tarsal defect as outlined in Fig. 11.5, the anterior lamella is closed in two layers. The site of the lateral canthotomy will require simple suture support to ensure that a reasonable lateral canthal angle is preserved.

11.3.2.2 Semicircular Rotational Flap

A lateral semicircular rotational flap may be used to reconstruct up to two-thirds of a central lower lid defect if there is a sufficient temporal tarsal remnant. The temporal tarsal remnant and a myocutaneous flap are moved as a unit [9]. The first step is to outline a semicircle, approximately 20 mm in diameter, starting at the lateral canthal angle. The outline should arc superiorly and temporally, but not pass the lateral extent of the brow. In addition, a lateral canthotomy of the inferior crus is performed with the scissors extending to the inside of the orbital rim. The lateral lower lid and flap are moved medially until the lid margin defect may be covered and closed without tension. Once the defect is closed, the lateral canthus is reformed. Fixation of the lateral edge of the

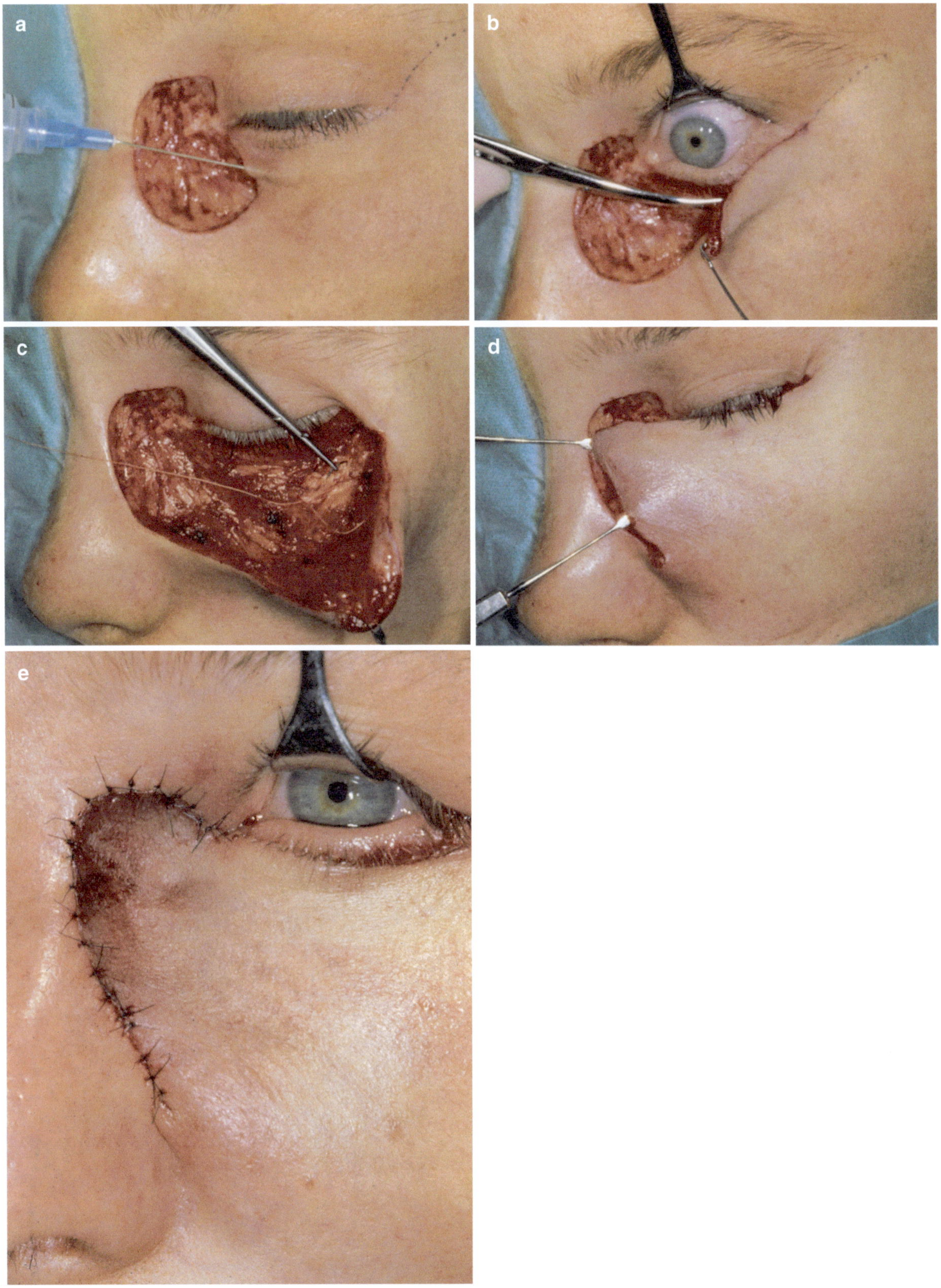

Fig. 11.3 Myocutaneous advancement flap. A large anterior lamella deficit may be repaired with a myocutaneous advancement flap because it provides the best tissue match with an independent blood supply (**a**). A flap of sufficient size that allows for tension-free closure is dissected from the underlying tissue (**b**). Proper placement of a tension-bearing permanent suture (4-0 Prolene) at the zygoma or the lateral orbital rim is important in securing the flap into position (**c**). Closure at the tip of the flap should be devoid of tension (**d**). The myocutaneous advancement flap with its inherent vascular supply now covers the anterior lamella defect (**e**)

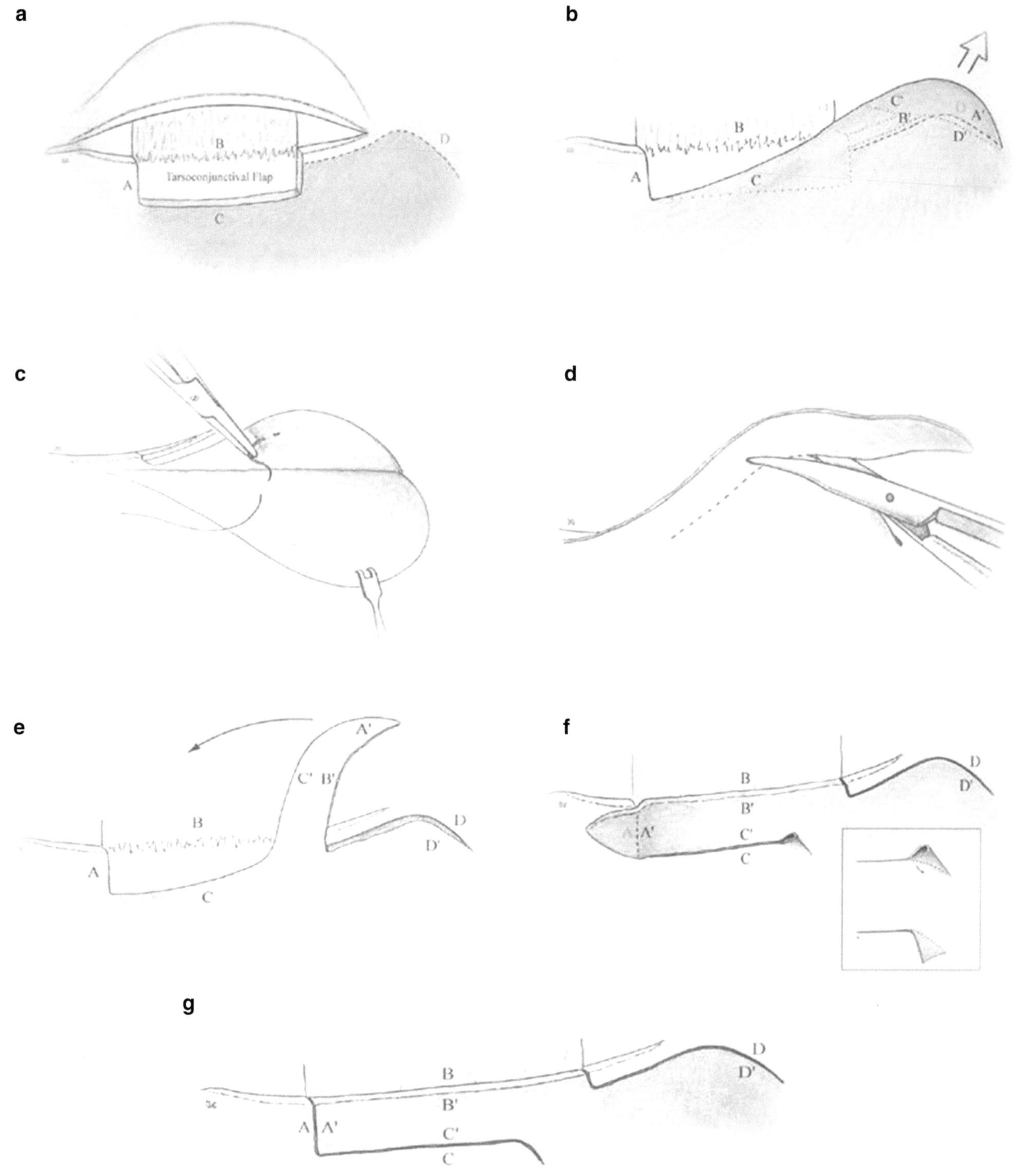

Fig. 11.4 Flip back flap: depicted here is a representative left lower eyelid defect with Hughes tarsoconjunctival flap inset. Letters correspond to the initial defect margins, while those with a prime symbol (e.g., A′) denote the flap edges that are rotated to meet them. The flap is started with a semicircular flap design as marked (**a**). The myocutaneous flap is then elevated in the suborbicularis and presuperficial muscular aponeurotic system planes, and redraped using a superotemporal vector (**b**). A 5-0 polygalactin suture is passed through the deep surface of the flap and anchored to the lateral orbital rim periosteum to support the flap (**c**). Flip-back flap creation with a back-cut starting at the temporal apex of the semicircular flap and ending at the pivot point of the flap (**d**). The flip-back flap should be designed to ensure that it is wide enough to fill the vertical dimension of the anterior lamellar defect, and the pedicle wide enough to ensure viability. The flip-back flap is then rotated 180° around the pivot point and inset into the recipient site. The tip of the flap is trimmed as needed (**e**). The dog-ear resulting from the rotation of the flap is excised inferiorly, taking care not to narrow the flap pedicle (**f**). The flap is then sutured into place medially with deep buried 5-0 polygalactin sutures, and the skin is closed with 7-0 polygalactin or permanent monofilament suture (**g**)

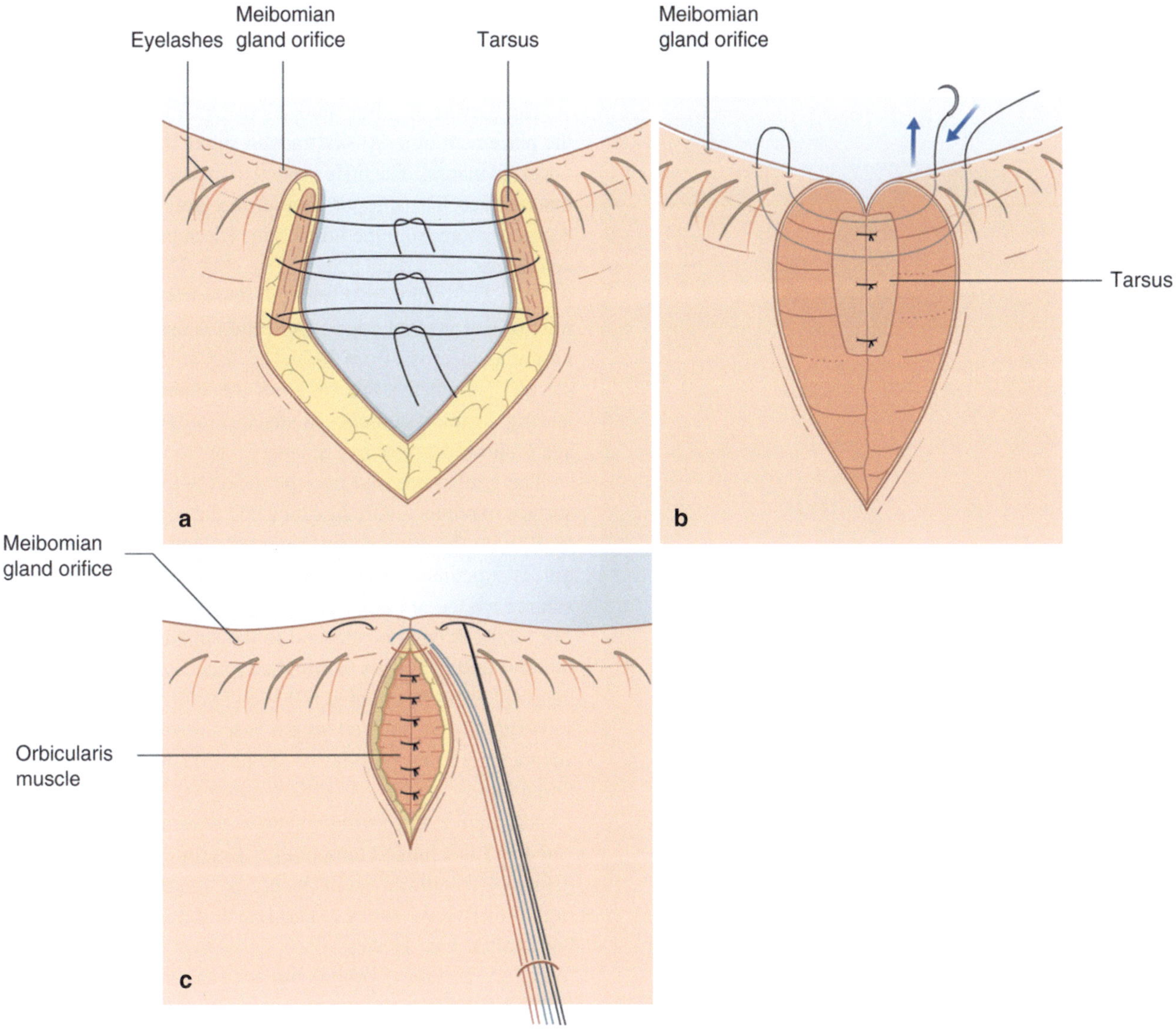

Fig. 11.5 Lid margin repair, full-thickness defect. The eyelid margin defect may be closed primarily if less than one-third of the margin is involved. An important step in primary closure of a full-thickness lid margin defect is precise approximation of the tarsal edges. Accurate vertical alignment provides the tension-bearing support of the wound. Three interrupted 5-0 Vicryl sutures are placed at partial thickness through the tarsal plate (**a**). The lid margin is closed with a vertical mattress suture using 6-0 silk suture which provides proper anteroposterior alignment. A vertical lid margin suture induces puckering of the wound edges to avoid notching after healing (**b**). Two additional sutures, one posterior and another inferior to the lashes, are placed to align the lid margin. The three 6-0 silk sutures should be left long and secured away from the wound onto the lower lid skin with a suture (**c**)

flap is needed to provide posterior and lateral vector forces so that the reconstructed lower eyelid lies in apposition with the globe. The deep edge of the flap is sutured to the inner aspect of the lateral orbital rim inferior to the superior crus using 4/0 Vicryl sutures. Finally, the conjunctival edge previously cut during the canthotomy is advanced superiorly and attached to the skin edge of the lateral lid margin with a running 7/0 Vicryl suture.

11.3.2.3 Free Tarsal Graft and Myocutaneous Advancement Flap

For larger defects where primary closure is not possible, a free tarsal graft from the ipsilateral or contralateral upper eyelid can be used for posterior lamella replacement [10]. The graft provides posterior lamellar support and a mucous membrane lining for the reconstructed lower lid. A myocutaneous advancement flap is then fashioned to provide blood supply to the free graft (Fig. 11.6). This option is most appro-

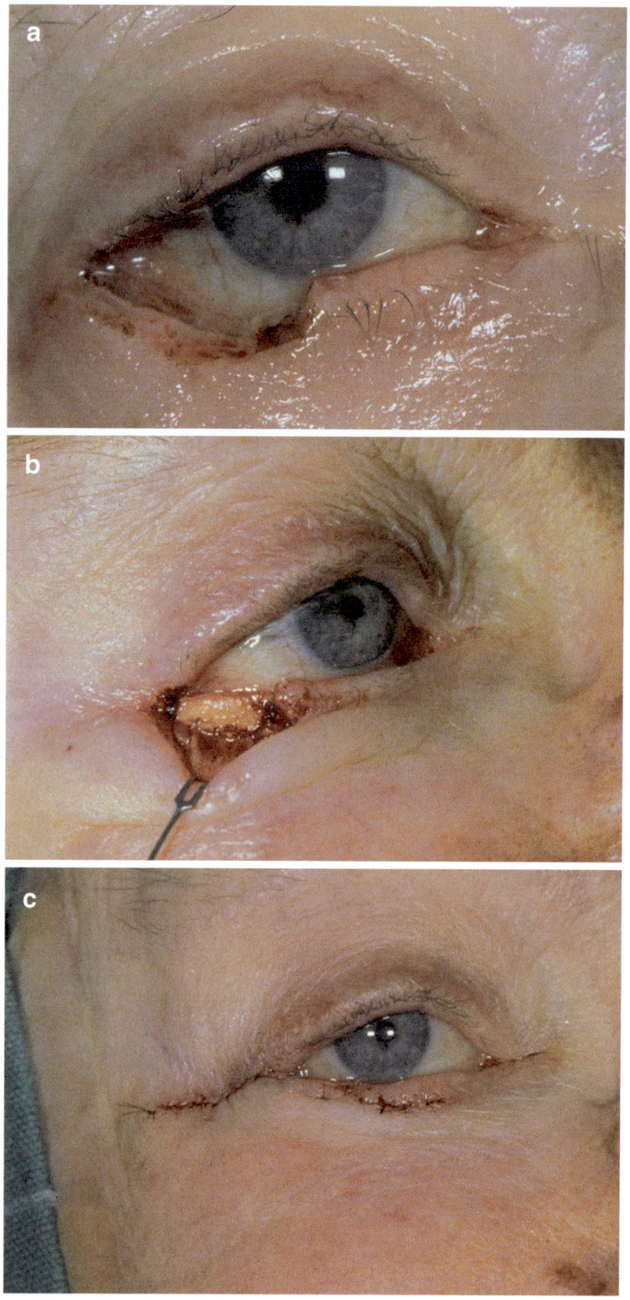

Fig. 11.6 Free tarsal graft plus myocutaneous advancement flap. A full-thickness lower eyelid defect may be repaired with a free tarsal graft for posterior lamella replacement and an overlying myocutaneous advancement flap to provide vascular support (**a**). The free tarsal graft harvested from either the ipsilateral or the contralateral upper eyelid provides posterior lamellar replacement (**b**). The myocutaneous advancement flap, fashioned in the manner of a lower eyelid blepharoplasty, provides an inherent blood supply to the underlying free tarsal graft. This figure demonstrates the key principle that either the reconstructed anterior or posterior lamella must have its own inherent vascular supply (pedicle flap), thus ensuring tissue survival and optimum surgical outcome for the patient (**c**)

priate for patients whose involved eyelid is on the side of the only seeing eye or who would not be able to tolerate closure of the eyelids with a Hughes flap (see below).

The harvest of a free autogenous tarsal graft first involves the placement of a 4/0 silk traction suture through the central upper lid margin. The lid is everted to expose the tarsoconjunctival surface. The inferior edge of the graft is parallel to and 4 mm or more from the lid margin. The superior tarsal border determines the vertical height of the graft. The incision is made through the conjunctiva and full-thickness tarsus along the inferior and vertical edges. Dissection is used to separate the levator aponeurosis from the underlying tarsus. Mueller's muscle and conjunctiva are cut from the superior tarsal border, leaving 2 mm of conjunctiva attached to the graft. The donor site is allowed to heal by secondary intention.

The graft is secured into the defect with the conjunctival surface in contact with the globe and the superior edge of the graft, with the conjunctival remnant along the new lid margin. The medial edges are secured with interrupted 5/0 Vicryl sutures passed at partial thickness to avoid ocular irritation. The superior edge is attached to the superior forniceal conjunctiva and the edges of Mueller's muscle and levator aponeurosis using interrupted 6/0 Vicryl sutures. The graft may subsequently be covered with a vascularized myocutaneous advancement flap (similar to the previously described rotational flap).

Alternatively, a swinging upper tarsal flap may be elevated and left hinged temporally. It is rotated down into the defect of the lower eyelid where it is sutured using interrupted 6-0 vicryl sutures. The lateral part of this swinging flap (called the "Hewes" flap) sometimes needs to be reinforced to the lateral orbital rim with interrupted 6-0 or 5-0 vicryl sutures to provide a firm support to the newly formed posterior lamella. The anterior lamella may then be repaired using a free skin graft or a myocutaneous flap or a bipedicled flap (bucket-handle flap or Tripier flap) or a mono-pedicled flap from the upper eyelid.

11.3.2.4 Periosteal Strip and Myocutaneous Advancement Flap

The periosteal strip with myocutaneous advancement flap is an alternative to the free tarsal graft [9]. This method may be used to reconstruct the lower lid when the lateral third of the tarsus is not present. The periosteal strip may also be used in combination with other procedures for larger defects. When fashioning the periosteal strip, the skin overlying the flap is first outlined with a marking pen in a semicircle or as a cheek flap extended 1–2 cm past the lateral commissure. Once the skin–muscle flap is mobilized and reflected, the lateral orbital rim is exposed. A rectangular strip of periosteum based at the inner aspect of the rim is then formed. The strip should be 1 cm wide, angled at 45° to follow the lower lid contour. The distance from the lateral edge of the tarsal defect to the orbital rim determines the length. The fascia is dissected from the temporalis muscle and separated from the bony rim with a periosteal elevator. The strip is reflected nasally to fill the tarsal defect. The anterior periosteum lies against the globe, and the distal end is secured to the lateral border of the remaining tarsus with partial-thickness 5/0 Vicryl sutures. The strip thus provides posterior lamellar support for the reconstructed lower eyelid. The myocutaneous advancement flap is then rotated and secured to fill the anterior lamellar defect.

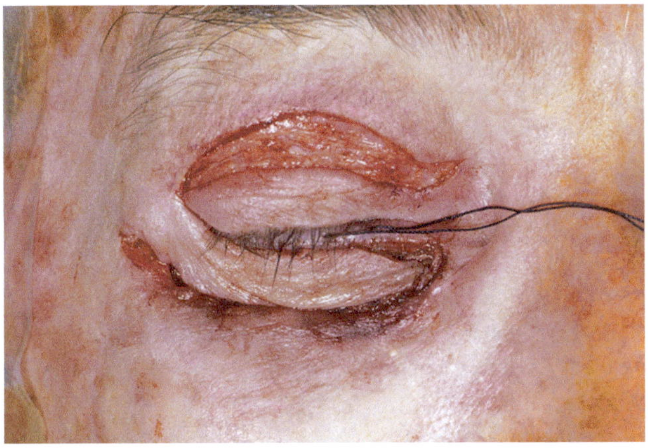

Fig. 11.7 Unipedicle flap. A unipedicle flap from the upper eyelid with an inherent vascular supply is used to replace an anterior lamella defect in the lower eyelid

11.3.2.5 Free Tarsal Graft and Unipedicle Flap from the Upper Eyelid

A free tarsal graft with a unipedicle flap from the upper eyelid is another method used to close full-thickness lower eyelid defects. The free tarsal graft is first harvested. Next, a flap is harvested from excess upper lid skin and subcutaneous tissue, based at the lateral canthus (Fig. 11.7), rotated inferiorly to fill the lower anterior lamellar defect, and then closed in two layers. The unipedicle flap may leave the patient with a lump of tissue at the lateral canthus. If necessary, a second procedure may be undertaken 6–8 weeks later to thin the base of the flap and remove this excess tissue.

11.3.2.6 Tarsoconjunctival (Hughes) Flap and Free Skin Graft or Myocutaneous Advancement Flap

For large defects involving more than 50% of the eyelid margin, a tarsoconjunctival flap (Hughes flap) with a free skin graft or myocutaneous advancement flap may be considered [9]. In this procedure (Fig. 11.8), a tarsoconjunctival flap from the upper eyelid is passed behind the upper eyelid mar-

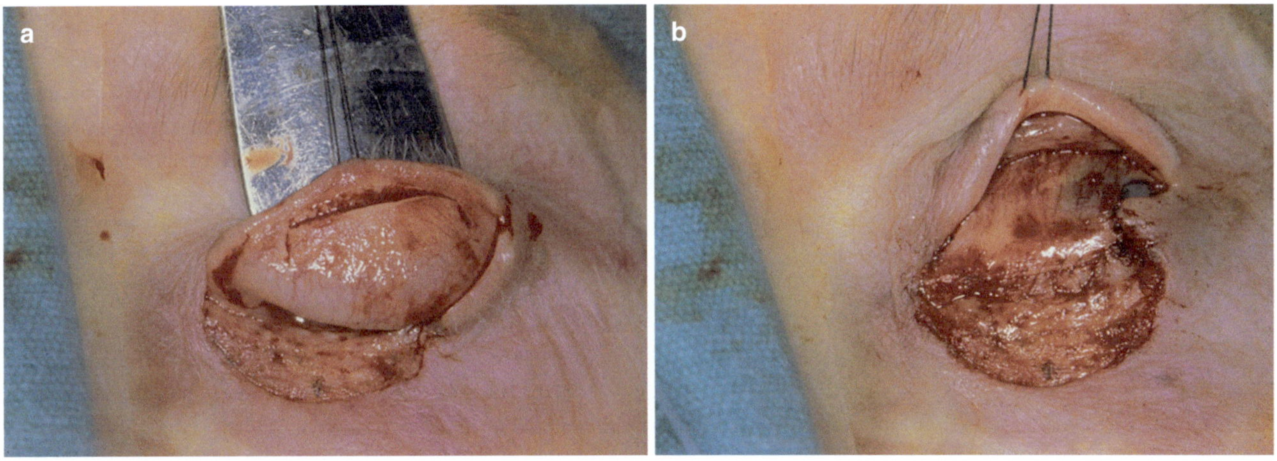

Fig. 11.8 Hughes tarsoconjunctival flap. With the upper eyelid everted over a retractor, a three-sided flap is created in the central tarsal conjunctiva of the upper eyelid. The horizontal incision should be at least 4 mm from the lid margin to avoid entropion, lid margin contour deformity, loss of lashes, and trichiasis. The vertical incisions course up toward the superior fornix perpendicular to the lid margin. All incisions are made through conjunctiva and tarsus. The Muller's muscle is dissected off the conjunctiva and remains in the upper eyelid proper (**a**). The tarsoconjunctival flap is mobilized into the lower lid defect to align the upper lid superior tarsal border with the lower lid margin remnant (**b**)

gin remnant and advanced into the posterior lamellar defect of the lower eyelid. The anterior lamella is then recreated with a skin advancement flap or a free skin graft from the preauricular or retroauricular area. The main disadvantage is that the pupil remains covered for 4–8 weeks by the tarsoconjunctival bridge. This vascularized pedicle is severed and released in a second procedure after the lower eyelid flap is revascularized. Although this is often called the "Hughes technique," it should rightfully be called the "Kollner technique" as Kollner described the use of a tarsoconjunctival flap and reconstruction of the anterior lamella with a skin graft in 1911. Hughes in 1937 simply used an advancement flap instead of a free conjunctival graft but termed his technique "A new method for rebuilding a lower eyelid." In reality, Hughes' technique should be called the modified Kollner technique.

We usually mobilize the orbicularis and cover the tarsus with the mobilized orbicularis as it gives the eyelid its more normal anatomical structure, and also allows for a skin graft to survive when the tarsoconjunctival flap is opened with a button hole or, indeed, taken down within a week which we frequently do. By creating the anatomical layer of orbicularis, the reconstructed eyelid has a very normal appearance.

11.4 Upper Eyelid Defects (Fig. 11.9)

11.4.1 Anterior Lamellar Deficit, Lid Margin Intact

11.4.1.1 Primary Closure

As in the case of the lower eyelid, small defects may be closed primarily if lid distortion will not be induced. If insufficient anterior lamella remains, a full-thickness pentagonal wedge may be used.

11.4.1.2 Skin Graft

For larger defects not involving the lid margin, a free full-thickness skin graft may be employed [8, 9].

11.4.1.3 Ellipse Sliding Flap

An elliptical sliding flap is a technique used to close some anterior lamellar defects, as described in the section on lower eyelid defects [9]. The main advantage of this flap is the ability to repair an anterior lamellar defect without sacrificing significant amounts of normal tissue.

11.4.1.4 Myocutaneous Advancement Flap

As with lower lid defects, a myocutaneous advancement flap may also be used. Flaps provide the best tissue match, the best cosmetic result, and an inherent vascular supply.

11.4.2 Full-Thickness Eyelid Defect

11.4.2.1 Primary Closure

Central upper lid defects—up to 30% in younger patients and 50% in older patients—may be closed using the same technique as in the lower lid. The main difference is that the vertical height of the tarsus is two to three times longer than that of the lower lid. Also, the levator aponeurotic attachments should not be disturbed, so as to avoid postoperative ptosis. If necessary, lateral cantholysis may provide 3–5 mm of medial mobilization of the remaining lateral eyelid margin.

11.4.2.2 Semicircular Rotational Flap

Up to half of the medial or central upper lid may be reconstructed with primary closure and a lateral semicircular or myocutaneous flap, similar to that described for the lower lid [9]. The first difference is an inferiorly, not superiorly, arching semicircle flap. The second is that the superior, not inferior, crus of the lateral canthal tendon should be lysed.

11.4.2.3 Free Tarsal Graft and Myocutaneous Advancement Flap

With larger defects, a free tarsal graft with a myocutaneous advancement flap may be needed [9]. A free tarsoconjunctival graft may be harvested from the contralateral upper eyelid. Once the flap is secured, the conjunctival remnant is advanced anteriorly and secured to the inferior flap skin edge with a running 7/0 Vicryl suture to reestablish the mucocutaneous junction. Finally, the superior eyelid must be immobilized and kept on stretch to minimize postoperative retraction. Some patients may require a formal recession of the levator aponeurosis as it is not uncommon to see secondary contracture of the upper eyelid retractors in such reconstructions. A temporary 4/0 silk suture is tied over bolsters and placed on inferior traction.

11.4.2.4 Tarsoconjunctival Flap (Cutler–Beard Flap) and Free Skin Graft or Myocutaneous Advancement Flap

The Cutler–Beard procedure is a less commonly used, two-stage method of closing large, full-thickness upper eyelid defects involving more than 50% of the lid margin. The procedure is similar to the Hughes flap. It involves the advancement of a lower eyelid flap, consisting of skin and muscle (anterior lamella) and conjunctiva, behind the lower eyelid margin remnant into the defect of the upper eyelid. The main disadvantage of the procedure is the creation of a thick, relatively immobile upper eyelid without tarsal support. Modifications to the Cutler–Beard approach include the use of a free tarsal graft to reconstruct the posterior lamella. This procedure, in combination with a myocutaneous advancement flap, is used when there are no alternative methods of closing the defect [8, 9].

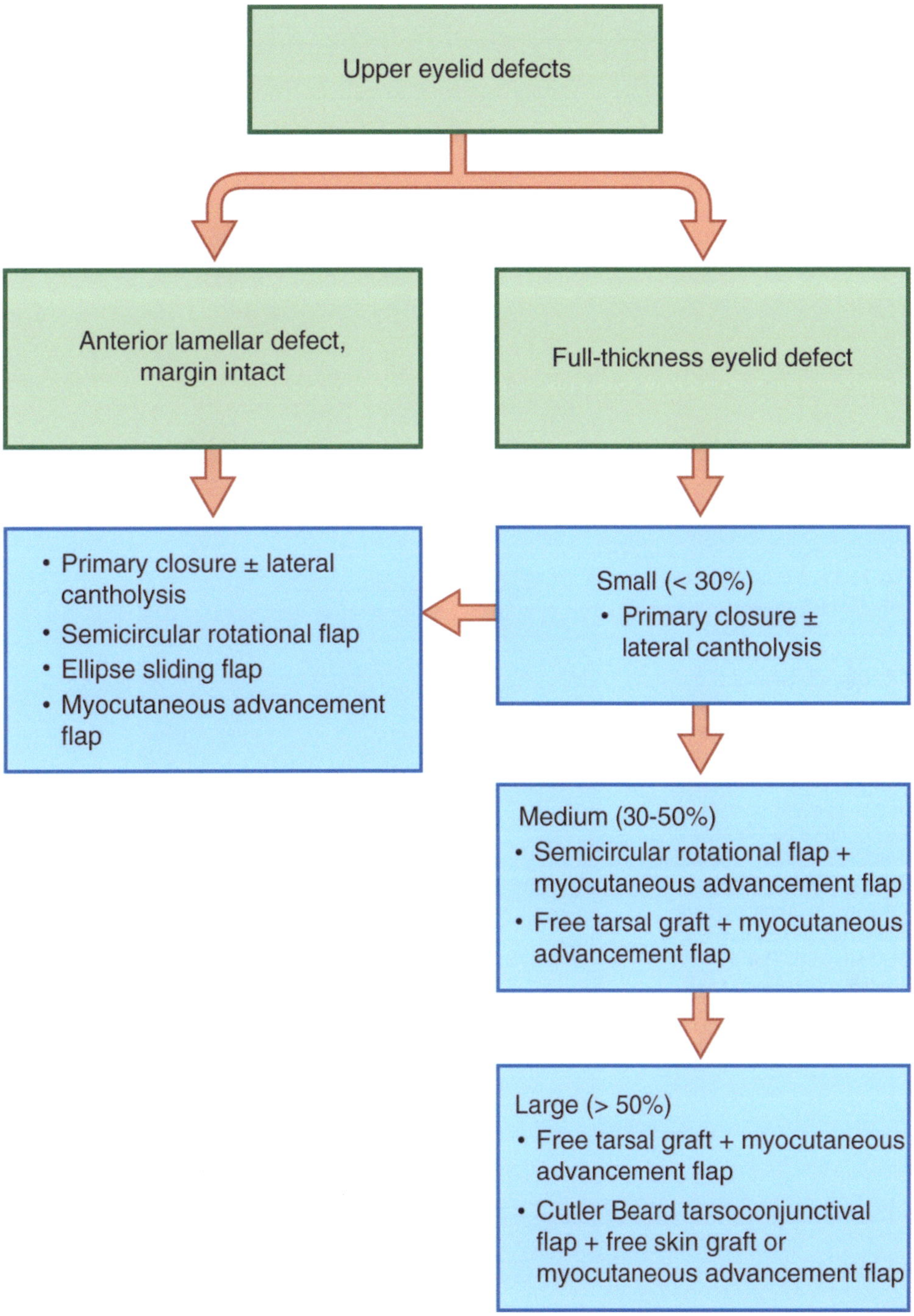

Fig. 11.9 Algorithm for the repair of upper eyelid defects

11.5 Special Circumstances (Fig. 11.10)

11.5.1 Medial Canthal Defect

11.5.1.1 Median Forehead Flap

The median forehead flap is a unipedicle flap used to close large anterior lamellar defects of the lower eyelid and medial canthus (Fig. 11.11) [8]. The flap is based on the axis of the contralateral supraorbital neurovascular bundle. Following 120–180° of rotation into the defect, the flap is secured with a two-layered closure. It may be combined with other rotational flaps for very large defects.

11.5.1.2 Glabellar Flap

Medial canthal defects may also be repaired with a glabellar flap, which is a modified V–Y rotation flap [8] in the shape of an inverted V, which begins at the midpoint of the glabella just above the brow, with an angle of less than 60°. Following

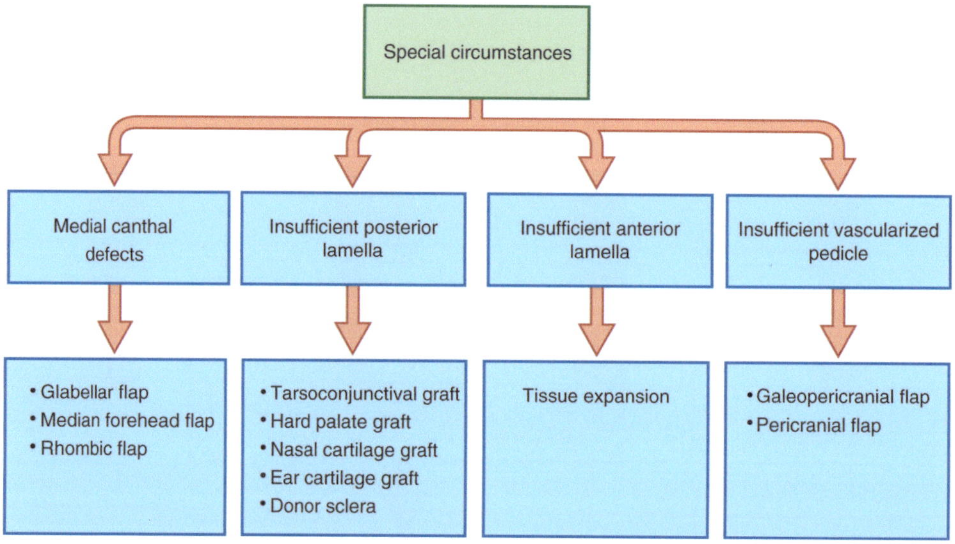

Fig. 11.10 Algorithm for surgical repair in special circumstances

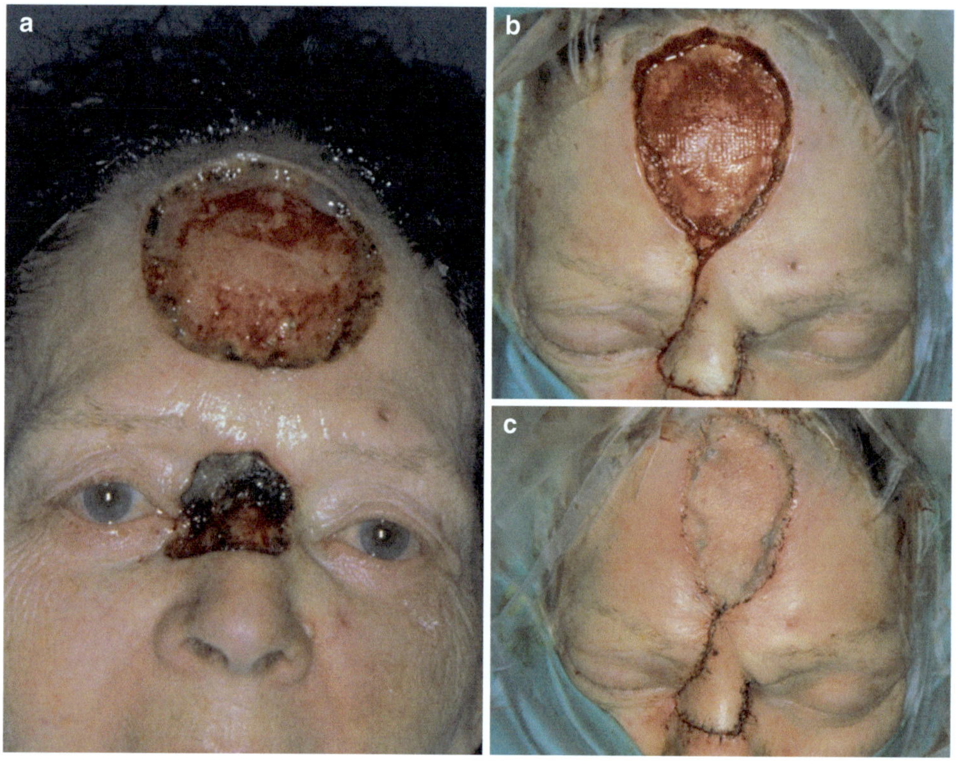

Fig. 11.11 Median forehead flap. This patient has a large forehead and right-sided medial canthal defects following excision of two lesions in these respective areas (**a**). The medial canthal defect is repaired by rotating a median forehead flap, with its own inherent vascular supply, down into the area of deficient tissue (**b**). The large forehead defect is not amenable to primary closure; thus it may be repaired with a free skin graft. This case illustrates the simultaneous use of two reconstructive options to correct two disparate defects (**c**)

rotation into the defect, the apex is placed at the lateral edge and the point at the inferior tip. Finally, the donor site is sutured in a V–Y closure which may induce a shortening of the interbrow distance. This flap may require secondary debulking.

11.5.1.3 Rhombic Flap

The rhombic flap (Limberg flap) is a non-transposition flap used in the closure of medial and lateral canthal defects [9]. With minimal sacrifice of normal tissue, most defects may be converted to a rhombic configuration with angles of 60° and 120° and all sides of equal length (Fig. 11.12). In practice, we often use the Dufourmentel flaps which are a modification of the Limberg rhombic flaps where angles other than 60° and 120° are used to reconstruct defects.

11.5.2 Insufficient Posterior Lamella

In defects with insufficient posterior lamella, tarsoconjunctival grafts are preferred because they provide a smooth surface over the cornea. If such a graft is not available, nasal or

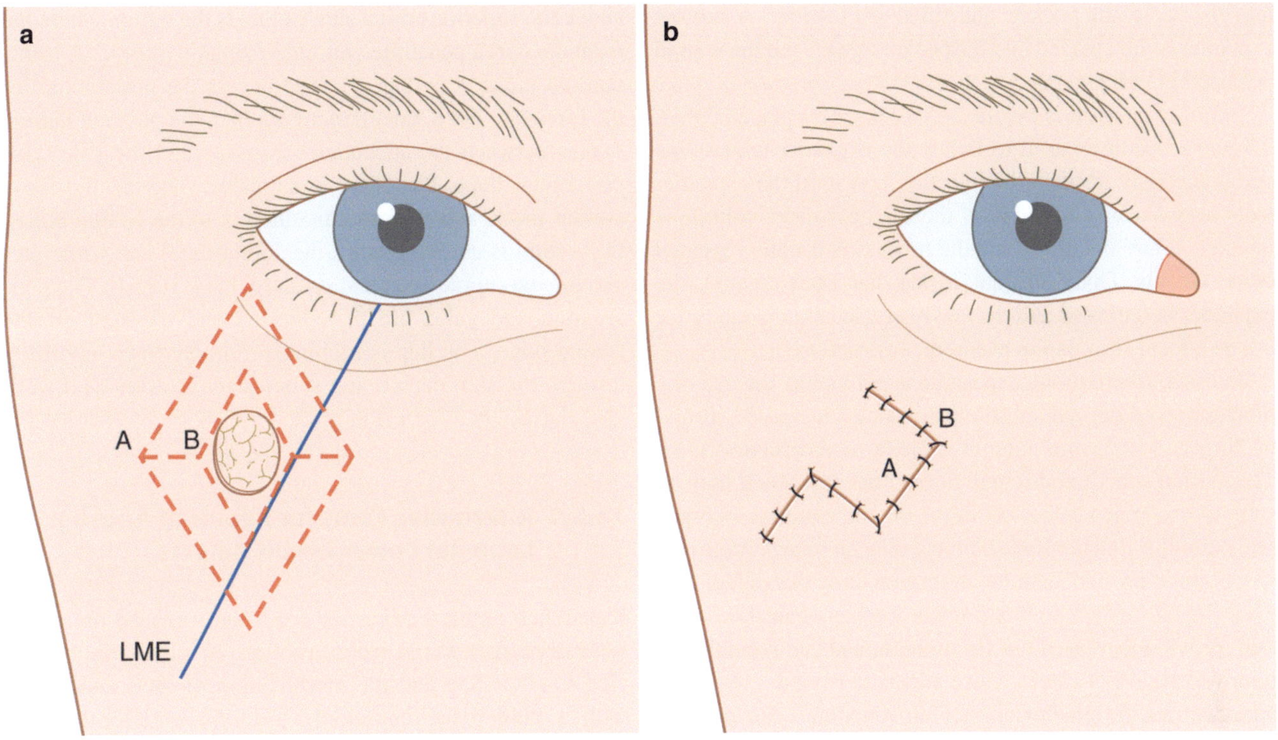

Fig. 11.12 Rhombic flap. First, the defect is made into a rhombus by marking two lines parallel to the lines of maximum extensibility (LME) (**a**). These LME are oriented perpendicular to the relaxed skin tension lines (RSTL). The first rhombic flap is made by placing two more parallel lines equal in length to and tangential to the defect at either 60° or 120° to the first set of lines while sacrificing the minimal amount of normal tissue possible. Next, a line is drawn from each end of the shorter diagonal that bisects the 120° angle. This line should be equal in length to the sides of the rhombus. Further lines are marked from the end of the previous mark at a 60° angle parallel to the sides of the rhombic defect. Of the four possible flaps that are designed, only one of the two flaps oriented to close the donor site along LME, which causes the least interference with surrounding structures, should be chosen. With medial rotation, this flap is advanced into the defect so that point B aligns with medial point of the defect, and point A is placed in the inferior apex (**b**)

ear cartilage grafts, donor sclera grafts, or dermis fat grafts may be used to reconstruct the deficiency. Hard palate grafts harvested from the gingival surface of the roof of the mouth have been used with greater frequency [12, 13]. The key points are the need to avoid the central palatine raphe, the anterior palatine rugae, and the area overlying the greater palatine foramen where the anterior palatine artery exits. Xenogenic spacer grafts made from a porcine collagen matrix have also become increasingly popular in cases of insufficient posterior lamella.

In patients who need more posterior lamellar augmentation or have concomitant volume deficiency, a dermis fat graft can be harvested from the postauricular area or abdomen. The graft should be oversized to account for postoperative contraction. The dermis is removed with a diamond burr or scalpel once a graft of sufficient thickness is harvested. The end point or dermabrasion is fine pinpoint bleeding of the graft. The graft is then placed into the eyelid defect with the dermis facing the globe. A frost suture or tarsorrhaphy should be used postoperatively to counteract contractile forces [14–16].

11.5.3 Insufficient Anterior Lamella

More extensive defects of the anterior lamella may require more involved methods of repair. The posterior lamella is first replaced with a graft, as described above. If a free graft is used, the anterior lamella must be reconstructed with a vascular flap. Tissue expanders allow for the use of vascularized skin that is similar in appearance, thickness, and texture to that adjacent to the defect without sacrificing normal tissue [17]. Most importantly, tissue expansion seems to enhance the vascularity of the skin flap. Other advantages include the non-hair-bearing nature and pliability of the created tissue. The main disadvantage is the creation of temporary disfigurement.

In tissue expansion, skin is recruited from the adjacent skin, such as the forehead, the temporalis and preauricular regions, and the lid proper. Adequate tissue area is created in a staged procedure. A skin incision is made along the hairline, brow, or a preexisting incision line, and a recipient pocket is dissected in the subcutaneous tissue. The expander is soaked in an antibiotic solution, tested for leaks, placed into the recipient pocket, and filled with saline. A remote expander is then placed into the pocket as well and the wound is closed in two layers.

Serial expansion is begun 2–3 weeks after placement. A 27-gauge needle is used to inflate the expander with saline percutaneously through the injection port until the expander feels taut. Usually 10–15% of the total expander volume is injected at any one time, and the process is usually repeated twice weekly. Once adequate tissue has been created, the expander is removed and the newly created skin is ready for use as a local skin flap in eyelid reconstruction.

In cases where tissue expansion is not viable, the use of a bioengineered dermal substitute allows for increased wound healing and adequate anterior lamella reconstruction [18]. The dermal substitute is cut to fit over the defect and may be sutured into place using 7/0 vicryl. As the material incorporates into the surrounding skin, its collagen matrix promotes vascularization and cellular migration into the defect. An overlying silicone membrane acts to protect against dessication, provide increased tensile strength, and can typically be removed after 2–4 weeks. Once adequate wound integration has occurred, the smaller anterior lamellar defect can undergo a secondary reconstructive procedure. In many cases, use of a dermal substitute can allow for complete closure of the defect without need for further reconstructive techniques.

11.5.4 Insufficient Vascularized Pedicle

For large defects with an insufficient vascularized pedicle, galeal and pericranial flaps may be used [19]. They provide an excellent vascular supply for the recipient site and any underlying free tarsoconjunctival or overlying skin grafts. The main difference from a median forehead flap is that skin is not transposed with a galeal or pericranial flap. The thinner nature of these flaps reduces the amount of bunching over the nasal bridge. Although both types of flap may be employed in upper eyelid reconstruction, the galeopericranial flap is thought to be superior to the pericranial flap because of its increased vascularity.

In the repair of large upper eyelid defects, the posterior lamella is first reconstructed using one of the previously described grafts. The galeopericranial or pericranial flap is then created to fill the soft tissue defect. A standard bicoronal incision is outlined over the skull vertex. It is important to avoid a transverse incision of the flap two fingerbreadths above the superior orbital rim, as this is the region where the frontalis nerve penetrates into the frontalis muscle. A transcoronal incision is then made to access the pericranium of the forehead. For a galeopericranial flap, the plane of dissection is between the subcutaneous tissue and the galea (for pericranial flaps, the plane is subgaleal, leaving the loose areolar tissue and periosteum adherent to the frontal bone). Dissection is carried toward the supraorbital rim while preserving the supraorbital and supratrochlear vessels. The pericranium and galea are then incised and elevated off the frontal bone. The flap is mobilized, turned down anteriorly through the skin defect, and subsequently serves as a well-vascularized bed for a skin graft.

11.5.5 Alternative Flaps for Repair of Anterior Lamellar Lower Eyelid Defects

Flaps such as the Fricke flap from the forehead are rarely used in modern facial reconstruction. However, the bipedicled Landolt flap and the modification of the Landolt flap with a uniflap are commonly used for anterior lamellar reconstruction. For larger defects, the Mustardé flap and inferiorly based rotation flaps provide a thick flap which can sometimes obivate the need for a posterior lamellar graft as long as the conjunctiva is mobilized to attach to the new eyelid margin. Various types of V-Y flaps with or without Z-plasty at the base are advancement-rotation flaps with one example shown.

11.6 Summary

The treatment of malignant eyelid lesions includes complete excision of the tumor as well as reconstruction to provide optimum function, globe protection, and esthetics. Mohs' micrographic surgery technique is the preferred method of excision of periocular malignancies, as it allows for clearance of the tumor margin while maximally conserving normal tissues. Repair of the eyelid depends on the size of the defect and whether the lid margin is involved. Most importantly, either the reconstructed anterior or the posterior lamella must have its own inherent blood supply (pedicle flap), as this will ensure tissue survival and optimal surgical outcome for the patient (Box 11.1).

Box 11.1

Anterior lamella defect lower eyelid, eyelid margin intact

1. Primary closure
   (a) With lateral cantholysis
   (b) Without lateral cantholysis
2. Skin graft (of non-hair-bearing skin)
   (a) Ipsilateral upper eyelid
   (b) Preauricular skin graft
   (c) Retroauricular skin graft
   (d) Supraclavicular skin graft
   (e) Upper inner arm skin graft
3. Ellipse sliding flap
4. Myocutaneous advancement flap

Full-thickness eyelid defect lower eyelid

1. Primary closure
   (a) With lateral cantholysis
   (b) Without lateral cantholysis
2. Semicircular rotational flap
   (a) Temporal tarsal remnant + myocutaneous advancement flap
   (b) Only feasible if sufficient temporal tarsal remnant
3. Free tarsal graft + myocutaneous advancement flap
4. Periosteal strip + myocutaneous advancement flap
5. Free tarsal graft + unipedicle rotational flap from the upper eyelid
6. Hughes tarsoconjunctival flap + free skin graft or myocutaneous advancement flap

Anterior lamella defect upper eyelid, eyelid margin intact

1. Primary closure
   (a) With lateral cantholysis
   (b) Without lateral cantholysis
2. Skin graft (of non-hair-bearing skin)
   (a) Contralateral upper eyelid
   (b) Preauricular skin graft
   (c) Retroauricular skin graft
   (d) Supraclavicular skin graft
   (e) Upper inner arm skin graft
3. Ellipse sliding flap
4. Myocutaneous advancement flap

Full-thickness eyelid defect upper eyelid

1. Primary closure
   (a) With lateral cantholysis
   (b) Without lateral cantholysis
2. Semicircular rotational flap
   (a) Temporal tarsal remnant + myocutaneous advancement flap
   (b) Only feasible if sufficient temporal tarsal remnant
3. Free tarsal graft + myocutaneous advancement flap
4. Cutler–Beard tarsoconjunctival flap + free skin graft or myocutaneous advancement flap

Medial canthal defect

1. Median forehead flap
2. Glabellar flap
3. Rhombic flap

Insufficient posterior lamella

1. Free autologous tarsal grafts
2. Tarsoconjunctival graft
3. Harvested irradiated tarsal plate
4. Hard palate graft
5. Nasal septal chondromucosa
6. Ear cartilage graft
7. Donor sclera
8. Harvested irradiated aorta
9. Human cadaveric dermis (Alloderm)
10. Porcine derived membrane from small intestine (TarSys)
11. Porcine acellular matrix (Enduragen)

Insufficient anterior lamella

1. Tissue expansion
2. Dermal substitute

Insufficient vascularized pedicle

1. Galeopericranial flap
2. Pericranial flap

References

1. Shields JA, Demirci H, Marr BP, Eagle RC, Shields CL. Sebaceous carcinoma of the ocular region: a review. Surv Ophthalmol. 2005;50(2):103–22.
2. Cook BE Jr, Bartley GB. Treatment options and future prospects for the management of eyelid malignancies: an evidence-based update. Ophthalmology. 2001;108:2088–98; quiz 2099–2100, 2121.
3. Tse DT, Gilberg SM. Malignant eyelid tumors. In: Krachmer JH, Mannis MJ, Holland EJ, editors. Cornea: surgery of the cornea and conjunctiva. 2nd ed. Philadelphia: Mosby; 2005.
4. Esmaeli B, Wang B, Deavers M, et al. Prognostic factors for survival in malignant melanoma of the eyelid skin. Ophthalmic Plast Reconstr Surg. 2000;16:250–7.
5. Coleman WP III, Davis RS, Reed RJ, Krementz ET. Treatment of lentigo maligna and lentigo maligna melanoma. J Dermatol Surg Oncol. 1980;6:476–9.
6. Zitelli JA, Mohs FE, Larson P, Snow S. Mohs micrographic surgery for melanoma. Dermatol Clin. 1989;7:833–43.
7. Esmaeli B. Sentinel lymph node mapping for patients with cutaneous and conjunctival malignant melanoma. Ophthalmic Plast Reconstr Surg. 2000;16:170–2.

8. Nerad JA. The requisites in ophthalmology oculoplastics surgery: eyelid reconstruction. In: Krachmer JH, editor. Requisites in ophthalmology: oculoplastic surgery. St. Louis: Mosby; 2001.
9. Kronish J. Eyelid reconstruction. In: Tse DT, editor. Color atlas of ophthalmic surgery: oculoplastic surgery. Philadelphia: JB Lippincott; 1992.
10. Kersten RC, Codére F, Dailet RA, et al. Basic and clinical science course: section 7, orbit, eyelids, and lacrimal system. San Francisco: American Academy of Ophthalmology; 2003.
11. Ko MJ, Erickson BP, Blessing NW, Tse DT. The flip-bck myocutaneous advancement flap for periocular reconstruction. Ophthalmic Plast Reconstr Surg. 2019;35(6):569–73.
12. Bartley GB, Kay PP. Posterior lamellar eyelid reconstruction with a hard palate mucosal graft. Am J Ophthalmol. 1989;107:609–12.
13. Beatty RL, Harris G, Bauman GR, Mills MP. Intraoral palatal mucosal graft harvest. Ophthalmic Plast Reconstr Surg. 1993;9:120–4.
14. Korn BS, Kikkawa DO, Cohen SR, Hartstein M, Annunziata CC. Treatment of lower eyelid malposition with dermis fat grafting. Ophthalmology. 2008;115:744–51.
15. Brock WD, Bearden W, Tann T 3rd, Long JA. Autogenous dermis skin grafts in lower eyelid reconstruction. Ophthalmic Plast Reconstr Surg. 2003;19:394–7.
16. Chang HS, Lee D, Taban M, Douglas RS, Goldberg RA. "En-glove" lysis of lower eyelid retractors with AlloDerm and dermis-fat grafts in lower eyelid retraction surgery. Ophthalmic Plast Reconstr Surg. 2011;27:137–41.
17. Tse DT, McCafferty LR. Controlled tissue expansion in periocular reconstructive surgery. Ophthalmology. 1993;100:260–8.
18. Chen TA, Ayala-Haedo JA, Blessing NW, Topping K, Alabiad CR, Erickson BP. Bioengineered dermal substitutes for the management of traumatic periocular tissue loss. Orbit. 2018;37(2):115–20.
19. Tse DT, Goodwin WJ, Johnson T, et al. Use of galeal or pericranial flaps for reconstruction or orbital and eyelid defects. Arch Ophthalmol. 1997;115:932–7.

Eyelid and Conjunctival Tumors: Sentinel Lymph Node Biopsy

12

Tracy J. Lu and Bita Esmaeli

12.1 Introduction

In the 1990s, the technique of sentinel lymph node (SLN) biopsy was developed as a less morbid alternative to complete lymphadenectomy (CLND) [1–3]. SLN biopsy is based on the principle that the disease status of the first node in the lymphatic chain to which the tumor drains is representative of the disease status of the rest of the nodes in the chain. If pathologic analysis demonstrates that the SLN is negative, then there is no need for CLND.

Various approaches have been used to identify SLNs. In 1992, Morton et al. described identifying SLNs through the use of intraoperative lymphatic mapping with vital dyes [3]. A year later, Alex and Krag introduced injection of radioactive tracer followed by use of a handheld gamma probe passed over the skin to allow dissection of SLNs through a small incision [4]. In 1996, Glass et al. investigated the combination of dye and radiotracer; they concluded that using dye plus radiotracer had the potential to increase the rate of successful SLN localization compared to the rate with blue dye alone [5].

SLN biopsy has been used for many years for patients with melanoma and breast cancer. The first reports of SLN biopsy in patients with eyelid and conjunctival neoplasms (e.g., melanoma, squamous cell carcinoma, sebaceous carcinoma, Merkel cell carcinoma) appeared around the year 2000 [6]. In this chapter, we will describe the clinical principles underlying SLN biopsy for periocular malignancies and then discuss various aspects of the application of this technique in clinical practice.

T. J. Lu · B. Esmaeli (✉)
Department of Plastic Surgery, Orbital Oncology and Ophthalmic Plastic Surgery, The University of Texas MD Anderson Cancer Center, Houston, TX, USA

12.2 Lymphatic Drainage of the Eyelid and Periocular Region

The human eyelid has two distinct lymphatic systems: a superficial system between the skin and orbicularis muscle and a deeper system between the orbicularis muscle and tarsus [7]. The lymphatic drainage pattern for the periocular area was historically believed to be preauricular for the lateral aspect and submandibular for the medial aspect. However, in 2002, Cook et al. published a report demonstrating that the drainage pattern was more complex [8]. Using lymphoscintigraphy in a monkey model, these investigators confirmed that the lateral canthus drained to the preauricular nodes, but they found that the central upper eyelid drained to both preauricular and submandibular-anterior cervical nodes [8]. Furthermore, these investigators demonstrated that the medial upper eyelid and medial canthus drained to the preauricular region, whereas the medial and central lower eyelid drained to the submandibular-anterior cervical region.

Nijhawan et al. demonstrated the variable drainage patterns in the normal human eyelid. Their study included 28 patients who underwent injection of radioactive tracer followed by lymphatic mapping using a gamma camera. Sites of injection of radiotracer included the lateral and medial upper eyelid, medial canthus, and medial and lateral lower eyelid [9]. In the 25 patients with identifiable nodes, the preauricular area was the most common site of SLNs irrespective of the radiotracer injection site. Conversely, for each of the radiotracer injection sites, drainage could be to the preauricular area or the submandibular and deep cervical chains.

12.3 Fundamentals of Lymphoscintigraphy

Lymphoscintigraphy is mapping of the lymphatic system through administration of a radioactive tracer followed by sequential or dynamic imaging (Fig. 12.1).

One key factor in optimal lymphoscintigraphy is the imaging method. A cobalt 57 source behind the patient is

B. C. K. Patel et al. (eds.), *Clinical Ophthalmic Oncology*, https://doi.org/10.1007/978-3-031-72328-5_12

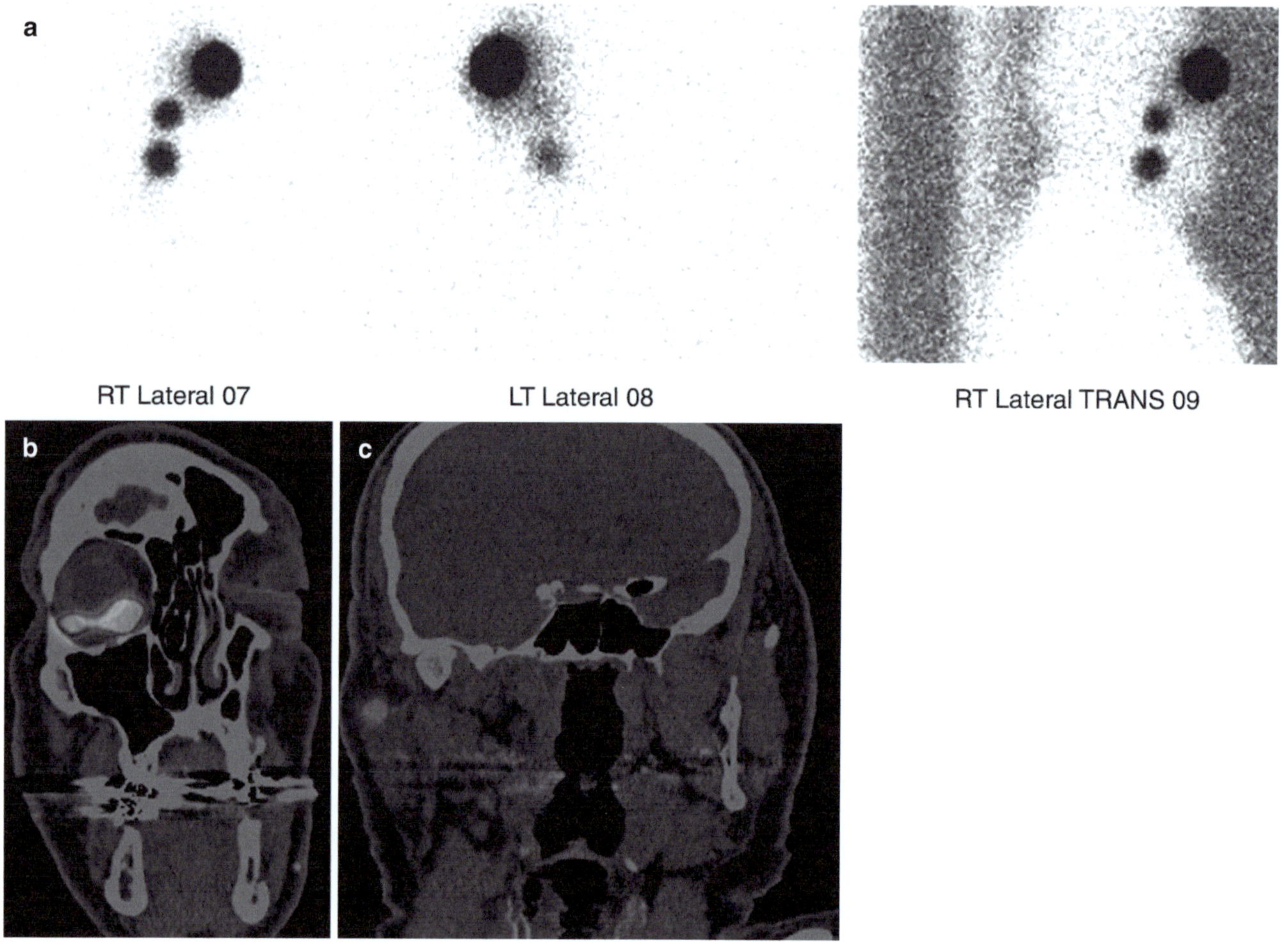

Fig. 12.1 Preoperative lymphoscintigraphy in a patient with a lower eyelid melanoma (**a**). The area of injection and the draining nodes are seen. SPECT/CT scan in the same patient (**b**). The area of injection of technetium (in blue) in the lower eyelid is seen (**c**). The draining sentinel lymph node (in blue) in the right parotid area is seen with much higher anatomic resolution compared with the standard lymphoscintigraphy image

useful for anatomical delineation of drainage along with lateral views [10]. The use of single photon emission computed tomography/computed tomography (SPECT/CT) in addition to traditional lymphoscintigraphy has been advocated to help identify additional SLNs and drainage locations (Fig. 12.1b) [11, 12]. SPECT/CT is a system with a dual-head gamma camera and CT scanner. This system allows high-resolution anatomical images to be fused with functional images from the radioactive tracer.

The other key factor in optimal lymphoscintigraphy is tracer characteristics. The smaller the tracer, the faster its drainage. Tracer smaller than 5 nm can penetrate the capillary membrane and enter the bloodstream, whereas tracer larger than 500 μm may be unable to migrate from the injection site [10]. The types of radioactive compounds used can be categorized as radiocolloids, radiolabeled molecules, and radiolabeled macromolecules. Colloids are phagocytosed by macrophages in lymph nodes and thus have a longer resident time in the lymph nodes than noncolloidal macromolecules such as human serum albumin. Antimony sulfide colloid is the most widely used colloid because of its ideal size, 3–25 nm, and its clearance rate of 40% over 4 h [13]. Colloids can be filtered to select for smaller particles, which will have shorter transit times. An example of a filtered colloid is filtered technetium ^{99m}Tc sulfur colloid.

Many different technetium ^{99m}Tc-labeled compounds have been tried for lymphoscintigraphy in cutaneous melanoma, including sulfur colloid, tin colloid, phytate, and human serum albumin. ^{99m}Tc-labeled human serum albumin has also been used commonly in melanoma involving the trunk. When ^{99m}Tc-labeled human serum albumin is injected intradermally, it drains rapidly; some would argue that this radiotracer is associated with better definition of the lymphatic system and better reproducibility of results than sulfur colloid [14].

12.4 Technical Considerations in SLN Biopsy for Eyelid and Conjunctival Tumors

12.4.1 Preoperative Lymphoscintigraphy

Preoperative identification of the SLN through lymphoscintigraphy aids in surgical planning and preoperative patient counseling. For SLN biopsy of the eyelid or conjunctival tumors, most authors to date have performed preoperative lymphoscintigraphy using filtered ^{99m}Tc-labeled sulfur colloid. The lymphoscintigraphy procedure is usually done 1–2 days before the SLN biopsy procedure as described in the following paragraphs.

The filtered ^{99m}Tc-labeled sulfur colloid is injected intradermally 1–2 mm around the eyelid tumor or, in the case of conjunctival tumors, in the subconjunctival space at two to four spots around the tumor. The dose of ^{99m}Tc-labeled sulfur colloid used is from 0.3 to 0.4 mCi in a volume of 0.2 mL [15, 16]. It is important to ensure that the injection is in the area immediately surrounding the tumor of interest so that the lymphatic drainage mapped reflects the pattern of lymphatic drainage from the tumor site.

At 15 min after radiotracer injection and every 5 min thereafter, a gamma camera is used to take dynamic photos at 30 s/frame (Fig. 12.1a). Transmission images are also taken with a low-activity cobalt 57 sheet source every 3 min. It is important to obtain lateral images with and without transmission images. Anatomical markers with cobalt 57 disks are also taped at the thyroid cartilage and suprasternal notch for reference [15, 16].

To allow more precise anatomical delineation, SPECT/CT has been utilized in conjunction with preoperative lymphoscintigraphy [17]. In this approach, SPECT images are acquired with a matrix size of 128 × 128 pixels, at 22 s/view over 180°. Axial CT images are used for classification of lymph node level, but the parameters for CT acquisition depend on the CT scanner used and site-specific protocols. Figure 12.1b, c shows the specific identification of an SLN in a patient with conjunctival melanoma using SPECT/CT and traditional lymphoscintigraphy.

A study of 403 patients with cutaneous melanoma in which 149 (37%) patients had preoperative SPECT/CT found that lymphoscintigraphy plus SPECT/CT identified more SLNs per patient than lymphoscintigraphy alone: a median of 0.34 SLNs versus 0.32 SLNs [12]. The increase in the number of SLNs per patient with SPECT/CT compared to lymphoscintigraphy alone was particularly pronounced in patients who were obese (body mass index of 30 kg/m^2 or higher): 25% of such patients had SLNs detected with SPECT/CT, and only 9.1% had SLNs detected with lymphoscintigraphy alone. Furthermore, univariate and multivariate analysis showed the use of SPECT/CT to be significantly correlated with better disease-free survival.

12.4.2 Intraoperative SLN Detection

In the preoperative holding area, approximately 1–1.5 h prior to planned surgery, ^{99m}Tc-labeled unfiltered sulfur colloid (0.3 mCi in 0.2 mL) can be injected in the same fashion as described above for preoperative lymphoscintigraphy. Alternatively if the preoperative lymphoscintigraphy or SPECT/CT scan is scheduled 1 day prior to surgery, there is usually no need for reinjection of sulfur colloid. Intraoperatively, the surgeon passes a handheld gamma probe (Fig. 12.2a) over the skin in the area where SLNs were identified on preoperative lymphoscintigraphy, using the lymphoscintigram as a guide. Once the area of high radioactivity is identified, an incision is made directly over this area (Fig. 12.2b). The SLN is then carefully dissected and sent for histopathologic evaluation (Fig. 12.2c).

Some authors have injected isosulfan blue dye (Fig. 12.2d) in addition to technetium ^{99m}Tc sulfur colloid to facilitate visual identification of SLNs in patients with eyelid and conjunctival tumors, but this technique has proven to be of no additional value. One possible reason for the lack of benefit is the fast transition in the head and neck region. Another possible reason is that in the case of conjunctival melanoma, the volume of blue dye injected is smaller (0.2 cc) than for tumors at other anatomic sites in order to avoid diffuse infiltration of the blue dye in all conjunctival quadrants and thus inaccurate and nonspecific drainage [15]. This small volume of blue dye used for conjunctival tumors is probably not large enough to make the SLN blue.

12.4.3 Histopathologic Processing

The histologic evaluation of SLNs is one of the most important aspects of SLN biopsy and can significantly impact the rate of detection of micrometastases. In the past, lymph nodes dissected during elective lymph node dissection were bisected through the hilum, which contains a number of lymphatic vessels, and then cut into 5- to 7-μm-thick sections. However, this method can be inconsistent when the nodes are small and can leave areas of the capsule unexamined. Pathologic evaluation of the SLN entails making very thin slices perpendicular to the long axis from one end of the node to the other to yield 1- to 2-mm-thick slices, a technique sometimes referred to as "bread loafing the SLN." Each slice is then cut into 5- to 7-μm-thick sections, which are stained with hematoxylin–eosin in the usual fashion. The bread-loafing technique allows for better evaluation of the

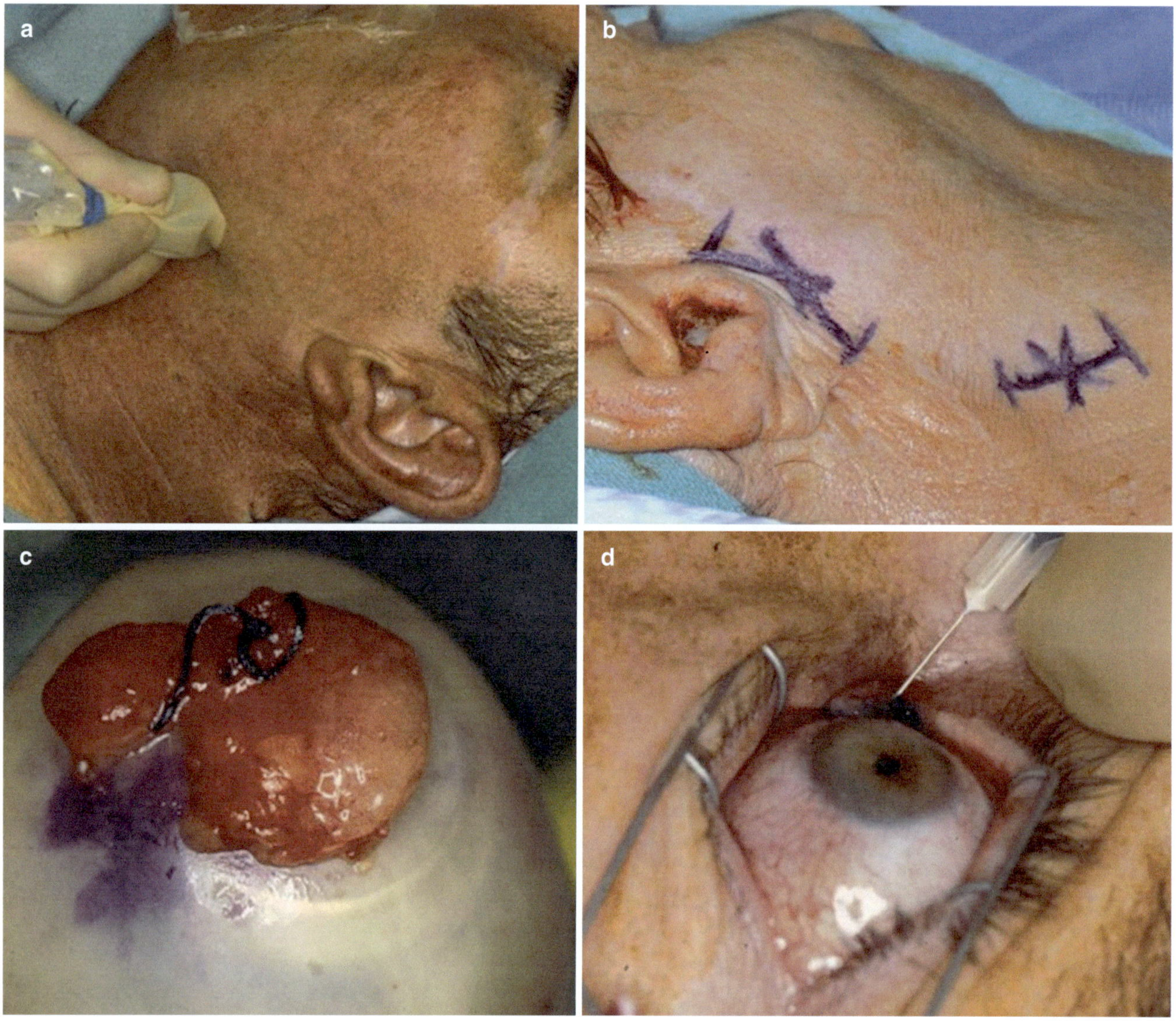

Fig. 12.2 Steps involved in sentinel lymph node biopsy for a conjunctival melanoma are outlined. (**a**) Intraoperative photograph of the gamma probe which detects the area of increased radioactive uptake (of technetium) corresponding to the draining sentinel lymph nodes based on the preoperative lymphoscintigraphy or preoperative SPECT/CT scan. (**b**) This photograph shows small skin incisions that are made directly overlying the areas of increased uptake in the draining lymphatic basins to facilitate biopsy of the sentinel lymph nodes. (**c**) The photograph shows a sentinel lymph node that has been removed from its lymphatic basin. The amount of radioactivity in the sentinel node is checked compared with the background to ensure it represents the draining lymph node from the primary eyelid or conjunctival lesion. (**d**) Subconjunctival injection of blue dye can be done using a 30-G needle, but given the very small volume that would be required to avoid nonspecific spread of the blue dye in the subconjunctival space, the yield of "blue nodes" was so low in our early experience that the use of the blue dye was abandoned after the first 16 patients who had SLN biopsy for conjunctival tumors as part of the prospective clinical trial at MD Anderson. We now use technetium only as the tracer for sentinel lymph node biopsy for conjunctival and eyelid tumors and find excellent identification rate of the sentinel lymph nodes using technetium alone. (Reprinted from Esmaeli [18]. With permission from Wolters Kluwer Health, Inc.)

capsule but may miss the hilum. If the initial section is negative, deeper sections of the block are cut [19]. Using careful serial sectioning of the sentinel lymph nodes can lead to the detection of very small foci of microscopic metastasis that are well below the resolution of even the most sophisticated imaging studies (Fig. 12.3).

Immunohistochemical staining is done if hematoxylin–eosin staining of the bread-loafed sections is negative for metastasis or when there are areas of suspicious morphology. Immunohistochemical stains used to evaluate SLNs include anti-S100, HMB-45, anti-MART1, and anti-tyrosinase for melanoma [19]; cytokeratin 20, chromogranin, and antibodies to Cam5.2 for Merkel cell carcinoma and sebaceous carcinoma [21]; and anti-adipophilin and anti-perilipin antibodies for sebaceous carcinoma [22].

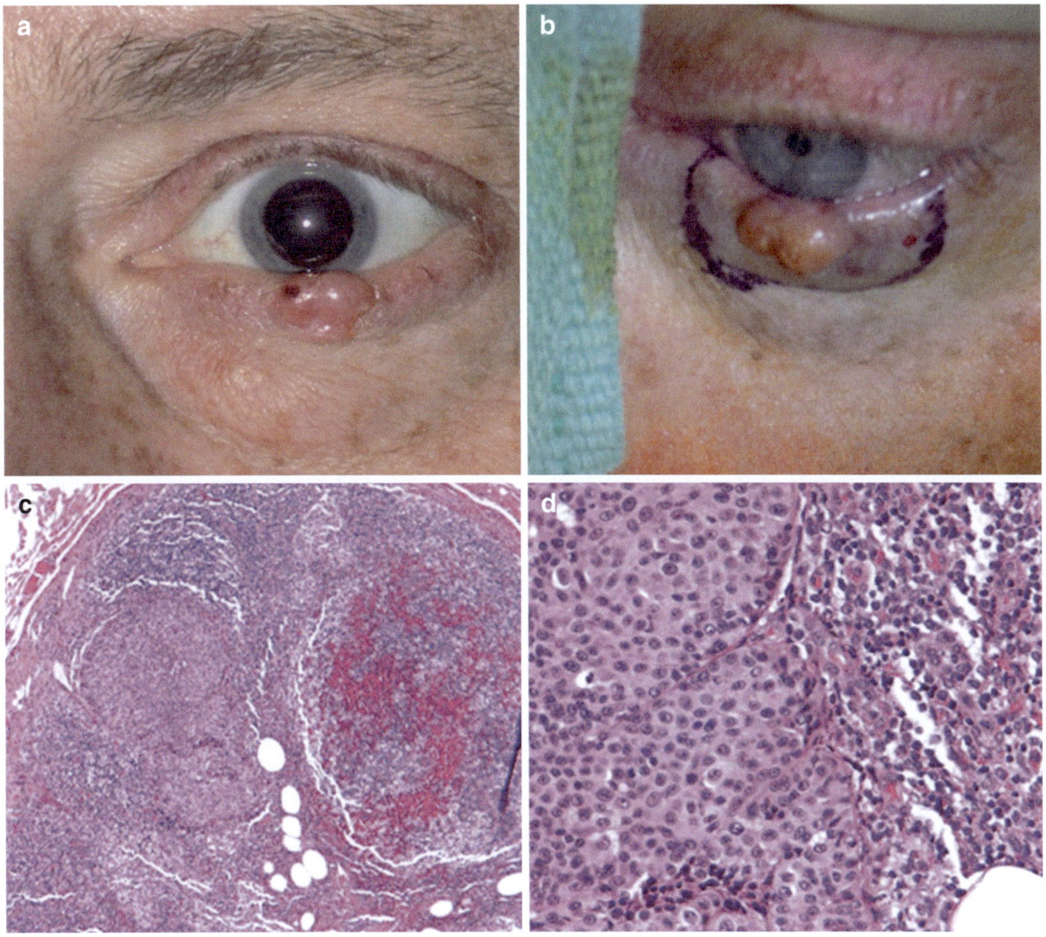

Fig. 12.3 (**a**) External photograph of a lower eyelid amelanotic melanoma (Breslow thickness 3.8 mm Clark level IV). The patient had a negative systemic work-up including a negative MRI of head and neck and a negative ultrasound of the parotid area prior to undergoing sentinel lymph node biopsy. (**b**) Wide surgical excision of the lesion was carried out along with sentinel lymph node biopsy. One positive lymph node was detected in the parotid tail. (**c**) Histologic section through the parotid sentinel lymph node shows a very small focus of metastatic melanoma that measures 0.8 × 0.5 mm with no extracapsular extension. (**d**) High-power magnification of the microscopic melanoma metastasis in the sentinel lymph node. This patient subsequently underwent completion neck dissection and parotidectomy which did not reveal any additional positive lymph nodes. (Reprinted from Sanchez et al. [20]. With permission from Wolters Kluwer Health, Inc.)

12.5 Indications for SLN Biopsy for Eyelid and Conjunctival Tumors

Accurate determination of regional lymph node status in patients with eyelid and conjunctival neoplasms not only is important for staging disease and estimating prognosis but also may increase survival through early detection of microscopic metastasis. This begins with the clinical examination on palpation of the lymph nodes in the preauricular, submandibular, or cervical areas. If no enlarged lymph node is palpated, we routinely request an ultrasonographic examination of the head and neck by an experienced radiologist to detect suspicious lymph nodes which can then undergo a fine needle aspiration biopsy. Large areas of lymph node metastasis could sometimes be detected on standard computed tomography or positron–emission tomography/computed tomography (PET/CT) prior to surgery, but smaller metastases may be detected on ultrasonography and otherwise missed on CT or PET/CT. If any of the above examinations show a suspicious lymph node, a fine needle aspiration (FNA) is done to assess for malignant cells in the lymph node. Sentinel lymph node biopsy is only appropriate after the above tests are done and are negative. Here, we discuss the rationale for and indications for SLN biopsy for the major types of eyelid and conjunctival neoplasm.

12.5.1 Melanoma

Experience with SLN biopsy for cutaneous malignancy started with melanoma, and most of the research to date on SLN biopsy for cutaneous malignancy has been done in patients with this disease. A study of 670 consecutive patients with melanoma found that patients who had SLN biopsy had a significantly better recurrence-free survival, distant metastasis-free survival, and overall survival compared with patients with similar characteristics who did not have SLN biopsy. Five-year melanoma-specific survival rate with Kaplan–Meier analysis was 84.8% in patients with SLN biopsies versus 80.3% without [23]. The international Multicenter Selective Lymphadenectomy Trial (MSLT-I) randomly assigned 1661 patients with primary cutaneous melanoma to undergo wide excision and nodal observation with lymphadenectomy for nodal relapse (observation group), or wide excision and SLN biopsy with immediate lymphadenectomy for nodal metastases detected on biopsy (biopsy group). The 10-year results of this important study found that the 10-year disease-free survival rates were significantly improved in the biopsy group as compared with the observation group, among patients with intermediate-thickness melanomas (defined as 1.20–3.50 mm; 71.3% vs. 64.7%, $p = 0.01$) and those with thick melanomas (defined as >3.50 mm; 50.7% vs. 40.5%, $p = 0.03$). They found that biopsy-based management improved the 10-year rate of distant disease-free survival and the 10-year rate of melanoma-specific survival for patients with intermediate-thickness melanoma with a positive SLN compared with those who had nodal metastasis discovered during the observation period. The authors concluded that biopsy-based staging of melanomas thicker than 1.2 mm provides important prognostic information and early identification of patients with nodal metastases leads to better survival outcomes for the subset of patients with melanoma who harbor nodal metastasis [24]. The subsequent MSLT-II study found that immediate CLND was not associated with increased melanoma-specific survival among 1934 patients with sentinel node metastases, underscoring the potential therapeutic effect of SLN biopsy [25].

Based on a study of 44 patients with eyelid skin melanoma, the Collaborative Eyelid Skin Melanoma Group concluded that melanoma of the eyelid has a regional nodal metastasis rate of 11% and a distant metastasis rate of 7%, with a mean follow-up of 34 months [26]. A larger single-center study of 64 well-documented cases of eyelid melanomas reported 10% of patients diagnosed with lymph node metastasis at presentation (8% via SLN biopsy and 2% via ultrasound-guided FNA) [27]. In this series, 5 of 14 patients (36%) who had SLN biopsy had a positive SLN detected, and all 5 patients had a T category greater than T2b (AJCC 7th edition) Breslow thickness greater than 1.5 mm and more than one mitotic figure per mm^2. Six of 17 patients (35%) who presented with greater than T2b tumor (AJCC 7th edition) had nodal metastasis at presentation, compared with none of 46 patients who presented with the T category of T2b or less ($p = 0.0026$). Another study, of 29 patients with eyelid skin melanoma from Australia, found that 17% of patients experienced local recurrence and 7% (2 of 29 patients) of patients died of metastatic melanoma [28]. Several studies have demonstrated that the risk of nodal metastasis increases with increasing tumor thickness [26, 29].

The first report of an SLN biopsy for conjunctival melanoma came from our institution in 2001 and served as a proof of concept that preoperative lymphoscintigraphy and SLN biopsy can be performed safely in patients with conjunctival melanoma [15]. Since then we have published our experience with SLN biopsy of melanoma of the eyelid or conjunctiva in several reports [30–32]. In the largest series to date of SLN biopsy for ocular adnexal melanomas, 51 patients with conjunctival and/or eyelid melanoma had SLN biopsy [29]. The report was a mix of eyelid melanoma and conjunctival melanoma, since eight patients (16%) had melanoma involving both structures. When comparing patients with and without nodal metastases, histologic features associated with a positive SLN included greater tumor thickness (median thickness 3.5 mm vs. 2.2 mm, $p = 0.04$), greater number of mitotic figures (median count/10 hpf of 6 vs. 2, $p = 0.03$), and presence of ulceration (80% vs. 26%, $p = 0.003$) (Fig. 12.4) [29]. Cohen et al. conducted a prospective study in which they performed SLN biopsy on patients with conjunctival melanoma who met the following selection criteria: tumor thickness ≥2 mm, were in an unfavorable (e.g., nonbulbar) location, or recurrent conjunctival melanoma associated with the "florid phase" of primary acquired melanosis [33]. These features were determined based on previous reports that found thickness greater than 1–2 mm to carry a higher risk for metastases [34, 35]. Only 26 patients met the selection criteria, of 70 patients who presented with conjunctival melanoma to that center over the 4 years of the study, and 22 patients eventually consented to undergo SLN biopsy. Their SLN identification rate using ^{99m}Tc injection was 82%, which the authors term "injection failure" and attribute to previous local surgeries that led to scarring and disruption of the normal lymphatic drainage. Two of 18 patients (11%) had an SLN which was positive for metastases, and no false-negative cases were identified over a median follow-up of 20 months (range 6–36). A recently published review of the literature by Aziz et al. confirmed that high-risk features for nodal involvement associated with conjunctival melanoma included clinical features of nonlimbal location and thickness >2 mm and histologic features of ulceration and mitotic rate >1/mm^2 [36].

12.5.2 Squamous Cell Carcinoma

Although it accounts for only 9% of eyelid tumors, squamous cell carcinoma is the second most common eyelid malignancy after basal cell carcinoma [37]. Squamous cell

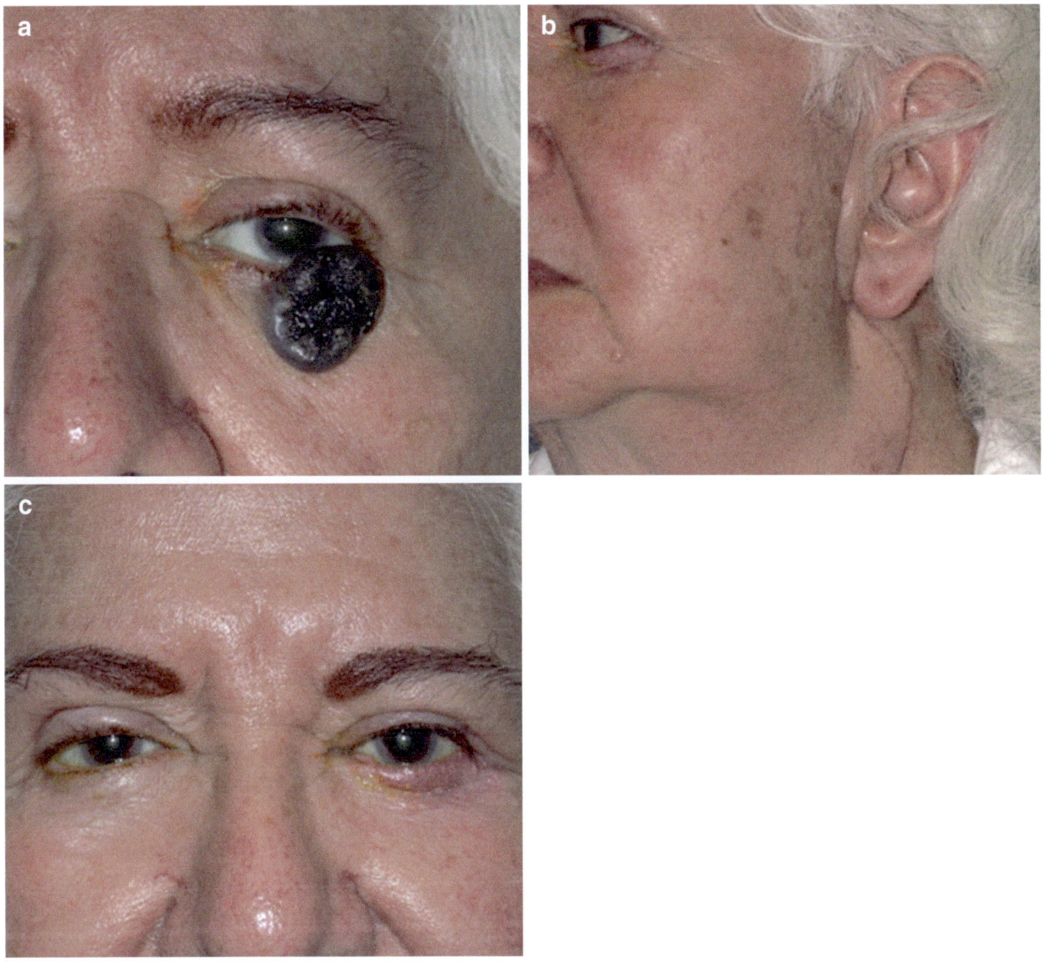

Fig. 12.4 (**a**) Left lower eyelid melanoma (Breslow thickness 7.2 mm with histologic ulceration Clark level II) with no palpable lymph nodes with a negative ultrasound and MRI of the regional lymph nodes. The patient underwent surgical removal of the melanoma simultaneous with sentinel lymph node biopsy which demonstrated one positive sentinel lymph node in the parotid gland. (**b**) The patient subsequently had completion neck dissection and parotidectomy which showed two additional positive nodes (in addition to the previous positive sentinel lymph node). The photograph shows the incision for the parotidectomy/neck dissection which is much larger than the incisions needed for the sentinel lymph node biopsy; parotidectomy and completion lymph node dissection only become necessary in patients who have a positive sentinel lymph node. (**c**) This patient was doing well without evidence of disease at last follow-up 3 years after removal of her eyelid melanoma and additional treatments for her positive sentinel lymph node. (Reprinted from Savar et al. [32]. With permission from Elsevier Inc.)

carcinoma has a higher rate of local recurrence than basal cell carcinoma, and squamous cell carcinoma, unlike basal cell carcinoma, has the potential for regional nodal metastasis. In a series of 111 patients with advanced eyelid squamous cell carcinoma treated at our center, local recurrence occurred in 41 patients (36.9%), and regional nodal metastasis occurred in 27 patients (24.3%) [38]. Distant metastasis occurred in only seven patients, but five of them died of the metastatic disease. In another series from our center with less advanced cases, we found that local recurrence occurred in 7 of 65 patients (11%) with a median time of 30 months from presentation to local recurrence, and no patient was found to have distant metastases at last follow-up (median, 27 months; range, 1–150 months) [39]. These had routine screening for LN metastases prior to surgery (see paragraph 21.5) but did not undergo SLN biopsy. Four patients (6%) had regional LN metastasis at the time of diagnosis (with T-stage tumors of T2b, T3b, and T4), and two patients with a T3a and T4 disease (AJCC 7th edition) were found with LN metastases on follow-up 2 weeks and 8 months after surgery, respectively. In a more recent review that validated the updated AJCC 8th edition staging system for eyelid and periorbital SCC, 4 of 109 patients (3.7%) had nodal metastasis at presentation and 7 of 109 (6.4%) developed nodal metastasis during follow-up, with a median time to nodal metastasis of 5.2 months (range 0.7–57.9). This study found a significant association between T category and nodal metastasis, with clinical stage of T2c or worse (AJCC 8th edition) portending a higher risk of nodal metastasis and death of disease, suggesting a potential role for SLN biopsy or at least strict nodal surveillance in such patients [40].

A review of the literature found 14 retrospective studies and case series that reported an SLN biopsy positivity rate of 0–44% in patients with SCC (in various locations in the body) and high-risk features [41]. The definition of high-risk features was variable between studies but mostly included size >2 cm, depth of invasion >4–5 mm, perineural invasion, and anatomic location. Some of these retrospective studies suggest that positive SLN biopsy was associated with worse prognosis [42–45], but this was not consistent in all studies [46].

Experience with SLN for periocular SCC has been reported in small case-series. Maalouf et al. reported their experience with SLN biopsy in nine patients with squamous cell carcinoma of the eyelid and conjunctiva with a median follow-up of 22 months. SLNs were successfully identified in all nine patients, and one of the nine patients had a positive SLN [47]. There were no local recurrences or deaths in their series. In another small case series, Chak et al. described five patients with a large (2.0–4.3 cm) primary poorly differentiated periocular squamous cell carcinoma who underwent SLN biopsy using preoperative ^{99m}Tc injection and intraoperative isosulfan blue injection after imaging failed to show metastatic disease. All patients were found to have a positive SLN and therefore had adjuvant radiation or systemic treatment [48].

With advances in medical treatments for metastatic cutaneous carcinomas, for example, the efficacy of immune checkpoint inhibitors (ICIs) and EGFR inhibitors for metastatic squamous carcinomas, identification of early metastasis associated with squamous cell carcinoma of the periocular region is crucial and could lead to consideration of systemic treatments that would be expected to have high efficacy for patients with cutaneous SCC [49, 50].

12.5.3 Sebaceous Carcinoma

Sebaceous carcinoma is often associated with a delay in diagnosis because it can mimic benign lesions such as chalazion and blepharoconjunctivitis. In a series of 60 patients with sebaceous carcinoma of the eyelid, 11 patients (18%) had local recurrence, and 5 patients (8%) had clinical nodal metastasis. Of the patients with clinically palpable nodal metastasis, 4 patients (80%) died of metastatic disease [51]. Another study of 50 patients demonstrated that lymph node metastasis was correlated with American Joint Committee on Cancer (AJCC) T category for eyelid carcinoma (7th edition) in patients with eyelid sebaceous carcinoma [31, 52]. This study further demonstrated that the T category of T2b is significantly associated with worse prognosis and that patients with the T category of T3b or worse (AJCC 7th edition) at presentation had poorer disease-specific survival. In a series of 100 patients with eyelid sebaceous carcinoma, 10 patients (10%) had LN metastases and none had distant metastases at presentation [53]. During a median follow-up of 32 months (range, 1–192), 12 additional patients (12%) developed LN metastasis for a total of 22% lymph node metastasis during the study period.

At the University of Texas MD Anderson Cancer Center, we have performed SLN biopsy for sebaceous carcinoma of the eyelid as part of a prospective clinical trial for the past 22 years. In an early report of ten patients with sebaceous carcinoma of the eyelid, one patient had a positive SLN [31]. In a later report, we described a patient with a T3 tumor (AJCC 7th edition) in the upper eyelid who had a positive SLN identified at the time of tumor excision. The patient underwent complete neck dissection and parotidectomy and adjuvant radiation therapy and was without recurrence at 20 months of follow-up [54]. These early reports suggested that SLN biopsy can be successfully carried out for sebaceous carcinoma of the eyelid, can identify microscopic metastasis, and may be most appropriate for tumors with the T category greater than T2b (AJCC 7th edition) [52]. In our most recent data of 140 patients with eyelid sebaceous carcinoma, 38 patients (27%) underwent SLN biopsy, and 5 of them (13%) with T2c tumor (1 patient, AJCC 8th edition), T3c tumor (2 patients), T4a (1 patient), and T4b (1 patient) were found to have positive lymph nodes (unpublished data, personal communication, B Esmaeli).

12.5.4 Merkel Cell Carcinoma

Merkel cell carcinoma is a rare and aggressive malignancy. Twenty percent of all cases of Merkel cell carcinoma occur in the periocular and eyelid area [55]. Historically, the 5-year overall survival rate for patients with Merkel cell carcinoma is reported to be 40–45% and as low as 25% in patients with distant metastasis [34]. The incidence of positive SLNs in patients with Merkel cell carcinoma who present with localized disease has been reported to be as high as 20–30% [56]. An analysis of the National Cancer Data Base that included more than 5800 patients with Merkel cell carcinoma found that the 5-year survival rate was 76% in patients with pathologically proven negative nodal status but only 42% in patients with positive nodes [57]. A recent report of 150 patients with MCC (in various body locations) who underwent SLN biopsy found that 26% had a positive SLN, and patients with a positive SLN had a higher risk for in-transit recurrence [58]. This study, however, failed to find a difference in overall survival or disease-specific survival between patients with a positive or negative SLN [58]. The importance of nodal status in Merkel cell carcinoma is reflected in the 2018 American Joint Committee on Cancer staging system 8th edition, in which disease associated with positive lymph nodes, or micrometastasis, is classified as stage III irrespective of tumor size. The National Comprehensive Cancer Network (NCCN) guidelines for MCC also include SLN biopsy for patients with clinical N0 disease as part of the management algorithm (NCCN guidelines for Merkel cell carcinoma, version 1.2018).

There are a few recent reports on periocular MCC. In a study of 14 patients with periocular MCC, lymph node metastasis occurred in 3 patients (21.4%), all of whom had negative margins at surgery [59]. Two of these patients had metastasis to the parotid nodes and one to the submandibular nodes. The time from diagnosis to nodal metastasis ranged from 11 months to 30 months. Only one patient died of metastatic disease, and this patient was one of the patients with nodal involvement. As a proof of concept, in 2002 we described a 61-year-old man with Merkel cell carcinoma of the eyelid who had a positive SLN in the parotid area and subsequent underwent parotidectomy and neck dissection, which revealed Merkel cell carcinoma in an additional lymph node and the deep parotid gland [60]. This report provided proof of the principle that SLN biopsy can be successfully carried out for Merkel cell carcinoma of the eyelid. Since then SLN biopsy has become part of the management algorithm recommended by NCCN. In a more recent study of 18 patients with periocular MCC from MD Anderson Cancer Center, 22% of patient had LN involvement at presentation with the T category of T3a in three patients and Tx in one patient (AJCC 7th edition) [61]. Of these four patients, two had clinically positive LN verified by biopsy, and two of three other patients who underwent SLN biopsy were found with a positive LN. In a series of 21 patients with MCC of the eyelid from five different centers from Australia and the United Kingdom, the authors reported regional nodal metastatic rate of 10% and distant metastatic rate of 19% and with the lowest T-category tumor of T2a (AJCC 7th edition for eyelid carcinoma) measuring 8 mm to develop either [62]. However, the methodology of systemic work-up in this study was inconsistent between centers, and only one patient underwent SLN biopsy, and only eight patient had head/neck imaging.

In recent years, SLN biopsy for all patients with MCC without clinical nodal disease has become more the standard of care due to its proven prognostic value [63, 64]. This shift is partly spurred by recent advances in medical therapy for MCC, such as the use of ICIs, that make a more compelling argument to support the use of SLN biopsy for staging purposes [65–68]. PD-L1 and PD1 inhibitors avelumab and pembrolizumab, respectively, were approved by the Food and Drug Administration (FDA) in 2017 and 2018, respectively, for the treatment of both locally advanced and metastatic MCC, with reported response rates from 33 to 58% that have been durable [67, 69–71]. Immunotherapy is now the standard of care for MCC, and there are ongoing studies for nivolumab, another PD-1 inhibitor, as well as other forms of immunotherapy utilizing adoptive T cells and natural killer cells for the treatment of MCC [72, 73].

12.6 Adverse Effects of SLN Biopsy in the Head and Neck and Periocular Region

SLN biopsy is a relatively noninvasive procedure associated with much less morbidity than elective neck dissection. A meta-analysis of the morbidity of SLN biopsy in patients with melanoma found that SLN biopsy is associated with lymphedema in 0.66–6% of patients, hematoma or seroma in 1.12–2.31%, and wound infection in 1.08–4% [74]. In the same study, pain was reported by only 0.75% of patients.

Analyses of SLN biopsy specifically in the head and neck region also indicate that complications are rare. In a study by Wasserberg et al. of 35 patients who had SLN biopsy in the head and neck region, one patient had seroma, and one patient had sensory disturbance [75]. Furthermore, a large series of SLN biopsy in the periocular region showed that complications were rare and insignificant [29, 31]. An infrequent (6%) reported side effect is the temporary weakness of the marginal mandibular branch of the facial nerve that resolved spontaneously after a few weeks [29].

The SLN biopsy procedure typically adds 30–90 min of additional surgery time and probably is best done at the same time as the definitive surgery for the eyelid tumor. In our prospective trials at MD Anderson of SLN biopsy for more than 90 patients with sebaceous carcinoma and melanoma of the ocular adnexa, we used the blue dye in only the first 16 patients and then stopped using it and now use technetium as a tracer only. This is due to the fact that the addition of blue dye did not improve the rate of detection of SLNs. Furthermore for conjunctival tumors, in particular, the volume of blue dye needed to expect a draining blue lymph node which is typically 1 cc would be too large to inject in the subconjunctival space and would lead to nonspecific drainage from the wide area of the ocular surface. In the 16 patients who had blue dye injection in our early experience with SLN biopsy for conjunctival melanomas, we used only 0.2 cc volume of blue dye. In these 16 patients, there were no blue SLNs although among these patients some had microscopically positive SLNs found using technetium as the tracer. Furthermore, there were no cases of permanent blue discoloration of the ocular surface, and there were no cases of anaphylactic shock secondary to the blue dye [31].

12.7 Salient Diagnostic Findings

12.7.1 Lymph Node Identification Rate

The SLN identification rate for ocular tumors (eyelid and conjunctival tumors) is high and reported to be more than 95% in most series. Of the three largest series published to date on SLN biopsy for ocular tumors, two are from MD Anderson and describe patients enrolled in prospective trials of SLN biopsy for melanoma and sebaceous carcinoma; the third report is from France.

In the earlier report from MD Anderson, published in 2007, Ho et al. reported successful identification of SLNs in 24 of 25 patients with sebaceous carcinoma of eyelid (10 patients) and melanoma (15 patients) [31]. One patient had an SLN identified on preoperative lymphoscintigraphy, but no SLN was identified intraoperatively with use of a gamma probe. In a follow-up report from MD Anderson on SLN biopsy in conjunctival and eyelid melanomas, Savar et al. reported successful SLN identification in 29 of 30 patients (96.7%) on preoperative lymphoscintigraphy and in all 30 patients on intraoperative mapping using a gamma probe [32], yet an updated report with a larger cohort of patients with longer follow-up from MD Anderson reported an overall intraoperative identification rate of 98% [29]. We have observed that in the rare patient who has poor drainage on preoperative lymphoscintigraphy, often a slight modification of the injection technique leads to successful drainage on the day of surgery. We have also observed that in patients with sebaceous carcinoma, who often have had multiple eyelid procedures prior to correct diagnosis and appropriate referral for definitive oncologic surgery, lymphatic drainage may be altered, and as a consequence, there may be no drainage during lymphoscintigraphy or surgery.

Maalouf et al. reported on results of SLN biopsy in 17 patients with a variety of types of eyelid tumors, including melanoma (4 patients), Merkel cell carcinoma (4 patients), squamous cell carcinoma (8 patients), and sebaceous carcinoma (1 patient) [47]. SLNs were identified in all patients; however, the authors did not specify whether SLNs were identified on lymphoscintigraphy, SLN biopsy, or both.

Although both preoperative lymphoscintigraphy and intraoperative use of a gamma probe are associated with high rates of SLN identification, it is important to use the two techniques in combination. Savar et al. in one of the published reports from MD Anderson found a poor correlation between findings on preoperative lymphoscintigraphy and findings on intraoperative use of a gamma probe [32]. Only 7 of 30 patients (23%) had correlation between preoperative and intraoperative findings in all basins, and 16 patients (53%) had correlation in at least one basin. More recently, the use of intraoperative indocyanine green angiography has been reported for sentinel lymph node biopsy for breast carcinomas [76–78].

12.7.2 False-Negative Rate

Findings on SLN biopsy are deemed false-negative if a patient in whom SLN biopsy is negative (meaning no microscopic metastasis found) is later diagnosed with clinical nodal metastasis. In an early report from MD Anderson, Ho et al. found that with a median follow-up time of 25 months, one of ten patients with sebaceous carcinoma who had a negative SLN biopsy result developed nodal metastasis after SLN biopsy [31]. In this patient, rereview of the pathology slides of the SLN demonstrated the presence of a microscopic focus that had been missed during the initial pathologic review.

In a more recent updated report from MD Anderson in a larger cohort of patients and with longer follow-up time, Pfeiffer et al. reported on 51 patients with ocular adnexal melanoma, of whom 41 patients had a negative SLN. Three of these 41 patients later developed a nodal recurrence, making the false-negative rate to be 7% (95%CI, 1.5–9.9) [29]. The authors pointed out that all three patients with false-negative findings on SLN biopsy were among the first patients who had SLN biopsy at MD Anderson; there were no false-negative events in any of the subsequent patients after the year 2004 suggesting the presence of a learning curve and importance of experience with sentinel lymph node biopsy in the head and neck region and for ocular adnexal cancers in particular.

Maalouf et al. reported no false-negative events—none of their patients with negative findings on SLN biopsy had had a nodal recurrence at median follow-up times of 18.7 months for the 4 patients with Merkel cell carcinoma, 22 months for the 8 patients with squamous cell carcinoma, 27.2 months for the 4 patients with melanoma, and 30 months for the 1 patient with carcinoma [47].

12.8 Care of Patients with a Positive SLN

Once micrometastasis is discovered on SLN biopsy, historically completion lymph node dissection is recommended according to the 2018 National Comprehensive Cancer Network Melanoma Practice Guideline (version 2.2018). In a series of 90 patients with cutaneous melanoma and positive SLNs, 15–29% of patients with positive SLNs had metastasis in non-SLNs based on findings on completion lymphadenectomy [79–81].

Adjuvant high-dose radiation therapy, with or without concurrent chemotherapy, has been shown to be effective in obtaining local–regional control for patients with melanoma [82], squamous cell carcinoma [83], sebaceous carcinoma [84], and Merkel cell carcinoma with positive lymph nodes [85]; however, a long-term survival benefit from radiation with or without concurrent chemotherapy has not been established. Systemic chemotherapy alone has also been used as postoperative adjuvant therapy for patients with lymph node metastasis. Historically, adjuvant systemic chemotherapy with single agents, with multiple agents, or in combination with interferon had not demonstrated benefit over observation [86]; similar negative results were found in patients with melanoma treated with immune stimulants or vaccination [87]. Some benefit had been observed from adjuvant use of interferon as demonstrated in the Eastern Cooperative Oncology Group trial E1694, of 774 patients with melanoma, high-dose interferon-alpha-2b resulted in longer relapse-free and overall survival than GMK vaccine at a median follow-up time of 16 months [88].

However, the management of melanoma patients with positive SLN biopsies has changed over the past few decades. Two large randomized trials, MSLT-II and DeCOG-SLT, comparing CLND versus observation in patients with a positive SLN biopsy, both showed no survival benefit for CLND over observation [25, 89]. These results, along with the morbidity associated with CLND, have led to reductions in its use. Furthermore, the discovery of effective systemic treatments for melanoma and for Merkel cell carcinoma has significantly changed the management of patients with a positive SLN. Strong consideration is given to use of ICIs, specifically PD-1 inhibitors, instead of CLND.

Despite not so great historical data for patients with metastatic melanoma, we have seen a remarkable improvement in disease-free and overall survival in patients with metastatic melanoma in large part due to the advent of ICIs for the treatment of metastatic or recurrent melanoma [90, 91]. These promising results provide an even stronger argument for identifying patients with microscopically positive early metastasis in the sentinel lymph nodes so that we can offer early adjuvant treatments with ICIs. And although ICI therapies were evaluated in clinical trials as adjuvant therapy after CLND was completed, there is growing evidence for the use of ICI instead of CLND for melanoma patients with a positive SLN biopsy [92]. Torphy et al. retrospectively evaluated patients who received ICI without CLND compared to observation alone [93]. The authors reported that among 56 patients who received adjuvant therapy and 34 who underwent observation alone, disease recurrence was 35% and 20% in the adjuvant therapy versus observation groups, respectively. Furthermore, adjuvant therapy was associated with a significantly improved 24 month distant metastasis-free survival among patients with stage 3b/c disease (86% vs. 59%, $p=0.04$).

Although no standard treatment protocols have been established for metastatic conjunctival melanoma, its molecular and pathophysiological similarities to cutaneous melanoma suggest that ICIs could also be beneficial, and this is supported by several cases in the literature [94]. We have reported a positive response to ICI therapy in several patients with locally advanced or metastatic conjunctival melanoma, and with melanoma metastatic to the orbit [95–97]. ICI therapy also has efficacy for other periocular cutanous malignancies such as SCC and MCC as mentioned previously [65, 98–102].

12.9 Future Research

The studies to date on SLN biopsy for eyelid and conjunctival tumors have proven the feasibility of SLN biopsy for this anatomic location; demonstrated excellent rates of success in identification of SLNs; and demonstrated positive SLNs in patients with eyelid melanoma, conjunctival melanoma, sebaceous carcinoma of the eyelid, squamous cell carcinoma of the eyelid, and Merkel cell carcinoma of the eyelid [103, 104]. These findings support continued use and further study of SLN biopsy for ocular tumors. A positive SLN indicates a more advanced cancer stage and should prompt additional treatments. A negative SLN, on the other hand, augurs a better prognosis.

Given the steep learning curve for SLN biopsy studies in the head and neck region and for ocular tumors in particular and given the risk, albeit low, of false-negative events, we recommend continued surveillance of the regional lymph nodes in all patients with high-risk tumors with negative SLNs. There is no question that early detection of microscopic metastasis in the regional lymph nodes leads to earlier interventions for nodal metastasis and potential eligibility of patients for additional systemic treatments. This is particularly true given the recent drug discoveries for metastatic melanoma and the very real possibility that early microscopic detection of metastasis would allow for earlier treatments with ICIs, or multi-drug targeted therapy, all recent strategies that have proven effective and associated with prolonged survival for patients with metastatic melanoma [97].

Whether there is a survival benefit from the addition of SLN biopsy to the treatment regimen for patients with eyelid or conjunctival tumors specifically is more difficult to address. Determining whether such a benefit exists would require much larger studies and longer follow-up times than are reflected in the currently available literature on SLN biopsy for ocular tumors. However, the MSLT I, in which 1347 patients with intermediate-thickness (1.2–3.5 mm) cutaneous melanoma were randomly assigned to SLN biopsy or observation, showed a significantly better 5-year disease-free survival rate for patients with nodal metastasis found early via SLN biopsy than for patients with nodal metastasis detected when the nodes became palpable on clinical examination: 72.3% versus 52.4% [105].

Future research should focus on identifying primary tumor characteristics that correlate with a positive SLN for each diagnosis category. Some recent strides have been made in this direction. For example, several studies on patients with conjunctival melanoma have suggested that tumor thickness of at least 2 mm, presence of histologic ulceration, presence of mitotic figures, and for conjunctival melanoma, palpebral location are correlated with a higher risk of nodal metastasis [29, 106, 107]. In a series of 150 patients with conjunctival melanoma, Shields et al. found on multivariate analysis that lateral tumor margin involvement and melanoma not involving the limbus were also associated with a higher risk of nodal metastasis [108]. For SCC we found that T category at presentation was associated with nodal metastasis at any time, and that patients with T2c or worse tumors had a higher risk of nodal metastasis (AJCC 8th edition) [40]. For sebaceous carcinoma, we also found a significant correlation between T2c or worse category and lymph node metastasis and distant metastasis (AJCC 8th edition) [53]. For Merkel cell carcinoma, we found that in our series of 18 patients, all patients with a positive nodal metastasis had a T3a disease (AJCC 7th edition eyelid carcinoma criteria) except for 1 patient who had a Tx disease [61].

Future research should focus on management of patients with a positive SLN using ICI therapy or other targeted therapy with overall goal to decrease surgical morbidity associated with other traditional approaches such as CLND and to potentially decrease the likelihood of distant metastasis.

Acknowledgement the authors thank Dr Yin and Dr Sagiv for previous contributions to this chapter.

References

1. Bennett LR, Lago G. Cutaneous lymphoscintigraphy in malignant melanoma. Semin Nucl Med. 1983;13(1):61–9.
2. Wanebo HJ, Harpole D, Teates CD. Radionuclide lymphoscintigraphy with technetium 99m antimony sulfide colloid to identify lymphatic drainage of cutaneous melanoma at ambiguous sites in the head and neck and trunk. Cancer. 1985;55(6):1403–13.
3. Morton DL, Wen DR, Wong JH. Technical details of intraoperative lymphatic mapping for early stage melanoma. Arch Surg. 1992;127(4):392–9.
4. Alex JC, Krag DN. Gamma-probe guided localization of lymph nodes. Surg Oncol. 1993;2(3):137–43.
5. Glass LF, Messina JL, Cruse W. The use of intraoperative radiolymphoscintigraphy for sentinel node biopsy in patients with malignant melanoma. Dermatologic Surg. 1996;22(8):715–20.
6. Esmaeli B. Sentinel lymph node mapping for patients with cutaneous and conjunctival malignant melanoma. Ophthalmic Plast Reconstr Surg. 2000;16(3):170–2.
7. Cook BE, Lucarelli MJ, Lemke BN. Eyelid lymphatics I: histochemical comparisons between the monkey and human. Ophthalmic Plast Reconstr Surg. 2002;18(1):18–23.
8. Cook BE, Lucarelli MJ, Lemke BN. Eyelid lymphatics II: a search for drainage patterns in the monkey and correlations with human lymphatics. Ophthalmic Plast Reconstr Surg. 2002;18(2):99–106.
9. Nijhawan N, Marriott C, Harvey JT. Lymphatic drainage patterns of the human eyelid: assessed by lymphoscintigraphy. Ophthalmic Plast Reconstr Surg. 2010;26(4):281–5.
10. Valdes Olmos RA, Hoefnagel CA, Nieweg OE. Lymphoscintigraphy in oncology: a rediscovered challenge. Eur J Nucl Med. 1999;26(4):S2–S10.
11. Veenstra HJ, Vermeeren L, Olmos RA. The additional value of lymphatic mapping with routine SPECT/CT in unselected patients with clinically localized melanoma. Ann Surg Oncol. 2012;19:1018–23.
12. Stoffels I, Boy C, Poppel T, Kuhn J. Association between sentinel lymph node excision with or without preoperative SPECT/CT and metastatic node detection and disease-free survival in melanoma. JAMA. 2012;308:1007–14.
13. Kramer EL. Lymphoscintigraphy: radiopharmaceutical selection and methods. Nucl Med Biol. 1990;17:57–63.
14. Tonakie A, Sondak V, Yahanda A. Reproducibility of lymphoscintigraphic drainage patterns in sequential 99mTc human serum albumin and 99mTc sulfur colloid studies: implication for sentinel node identification in melanoma. Surgery. 2000;127:955–62.
15. Esmaeli B, Eicher S, Popp J. Sentinel lymph node biopsy for conjunctival melanoma. Ophthalmic Plast Reconstr Surg. 2001;17:436–42.
16. Amato M, Esmaeli B, Ahmadi MA. Feasibility of preoperative lymphoscintigraphy for identification of sentinel lymph nodes in patients with conjunctival and periocular skin malignancies. Ophthalmic Plast Reconstr Surg. 2003;19:102–6.
17. Mar MV, Miller SA, Kim E. Evaluation and localization of lymphatic drainage and sentinel lymph nodes in patients with head and neck melanomas by hybrid SPECT/CT lymphoscintigraphic imaging. J Nucl Med Technol. 2007;35:10–6.
18. Esmaeli B. Advances in the management of malignant tumors of the eyelid and conjunctiva: the role of sentinel lymph node biopsy. Int Ophthalmol Clin. 2002;42(2):151–62.
19. Prieto CG, Clark SH. Processing of sentinel lymph nodes for detection of metastatic melanoma. Ann Diagn Pathol. 2002;6:257–64.
20. Sanchez R, Ivan D, Esmaeli B. Eyelid and periorbital cutaneous malignant melanoma. Int Ophthalmol Clin. 2009;49(4):25–43.
21. Allen PJ, Busam K, Hill AD. Immunohistochemical analysis of sentinel nodes from patients with Merkel cell carcinoma. Cancer. 2001;92:1650–5.
22. Ansai S, Takeichi H, Arase S, et al. Sebaceous carcinoma: an immunohistochemical reappraisal. Am J Dermatopathol. 2011;33:579–87.
23. Satzger I, Meier A, Hoy L. Sentinel node dissection delays recurrence and prolongs melanoma-related survival: an analysis of 673 patients from a single center with long-term follow-up. Ann Surg Oncol. 2011;18:514–20.
24. Morton DL, Thompson JF, Cochran AJ. Final trial report of sentinel-node biopsy versus nodal observation in melanoma. N Engl J Med. 2014;370(7):599–609.
25. Faries MB, Thompson JF, Cochran AJ. Completion dissection or observation for sentinel-node metastasis in melanoma. N Engl J Med. 2017;376(23):2211–22.
26. Esmaeli B, Youssef A, Naderi A. Margins of excision for cutaneous melanoma of the eyelid skin: the Collaborative Eyelid

Skin Melanoma Group Report. Ophthalmic Plast Reconstr Surg. 2003;19(2):96–101.
27. Yin VT, Warneke CL, Merritt HA, Esmaeli B. Number of excisions required to obtain clear surgical margins and prognostic value of AJCC T category for patients with eyelid melanoma. Br J Ophthalmol. 2014;98(12):1681–5.
28. Chan FM, O'Donnell BA, Whitehead K. Treatment and outcomes of malignant melanoma of the eyelid: a review of 29 cases in Australia. Ophthalmology. 2007;114(1):187–92.
29. Pfeiffer ML, Ozgur OK, Myers JN. Sentinel lymph node biopsy for ocular adnexal melanoma. Acta Ophthalmol. 2017;95(4):e323–8.
30. Nijhawan N, Ross MI, Diba R. Experience with sentinel lymph node biopsy for eyelid and conjunctival malignancies at a cancer center. Ophthalmic Plast Reconstr Surg. 2004;20(4):291–5.
31. Ho VH, Ross MI, Prieto VG. Sentinel lymph node biopsy for sebaceous cell carcinoma and melanoma of the ocular adnexa. Arch Otolaryngol. 2007;133(8):820–6.
32. Savar A, Ross MI, Preito VG. Sentinel lymph node biopsy for ocular adnexal melanoma: experience in 30 patients. Ophthalmology. 2009;116:2217–23.
33. Cohen VM, Tsimpida M, Hungerford JL. Prospective study of sentinel lymph node biopsy for conjunctival melanoma. Br J Ophthalmol. 2013;97(12):1525–9.
34. Shields CL. Conjunctival melanoma: risk factors for recurrence, exenteration, metastasis, and death in 150 consecutive patients. Trans Am Ophthalmol Soc. 2000;98:471–92.
35. Missotten GS, Keijser S, Keizer De RJ, De Wolff-Rouendaal D. Conjunctival melanoma in the Netherlands: a nationwide study. Invest Ophthalmol Vis Sci. 2005;46(1):75–82.
36. Aziz HA, Gastman BR, Singh AD. Management of conjunctival melanoma: critical assessment of sentinel lymph node biopsy. Ocul Oncol Pathol. 2015;1(4):266–73.
37. Francis IC, Benecke PS, Kappagoda MB. A ten-year hospital survey of eyelid cancer. Aust J Ophthalmol. 1984;12:121–7.
38. Faustina M, Diba R, Ahmadi A. Pattern of regional and distant metastasis in patients with eyelid and periocular squamous cell carcinoma. Ophthalmology. 2004;111:1930–2.
39. Nasser QJ, Roth KG, Warneke CL. Impact of AJCC 'T' designation on risk of regional lymph node metastasis in patients with squamous carcinoma of the eyelid. Br J Ophthalmol. 2014;98(4):498–501.
40. ShiqiongX,OdedS,LauraRM,Ho-SeokS,TetzlaffMT,Priyadharsini N, Jing N, Bita E. JAMA Ophthalmol. 2019;137(5):537. https://doi.org/10.1001/jamaophthalmol.2019.0238.
41. Ahadiat O, Higgins S, Sutton A. SLNB in cutaneous SCC: a review of the current state of literature and the direction for the future. J Surg Oncol. 2017;116(3):344–50.
42. Reschly MJ, Messina JL, Zaulyanov LL. Utility of sentinel lymphadenectomy in the management of patients with high-risk cutaneous squamous cell carcinoma. Dermatologic Surg. 2003;29(2):135–40.
43. Ross AS, Schmults CD. Sentinel lymph node biopsy in cutaneous squamous cell carcinoma: a systematic review of the English literature. Dermatologic Surg. 2006;32(11):1309–21.
44. Renzi C, Caggiati A, Mannooranparampil TJ. Sentinel lymph node biopsy for high risk cutaneous squamous cell carcinoma: case series and review of the literature. Eur J Surg Oncol. 2007;33(3):364–9.
45. Takahashi A, Imafuku S, Nakayama J. Sentinel node biopsy for high-risk cutaneous squamous cell carcinoma. Eur J Surg Oncol. 2014;40(10):1256–62.
46. Durham AB, Lowe L, Malloy KM. Sentinel lymph node biopsy for cutaneous squamous cell carcinoma on the head and neck. JAMA Otolaryngol. 2016;142(12):1171–6.
47. Maalouf TJ, Dolivet G, Angioi KS. Sentinel lymph node biopsy in patients with conjunctival and eyelid cancers: experience in 17 patients. Ophthalmic Plast Reconstr Surg. 2012;28:30–4.
48. Chak G, Morgan PV, Joseph JM, Tao JP. A positive sentinel lymph node in periocular invasive squamous cell carcinoma: a case series. Ophthalmic Plast Reconstr Surg. 2013;29(1): 6–10.
49. Morena F, Della CCM, Di LR, Giuseppe V, Francesca S, Lucia IM, Fernando P, Antonio P, Stefania N, Giulia M, Floriana M, Salvatore C, Fortunato C. Immunotherapy for head and neck cancer: present and future. Critical Reviews. Oncology. 2022;174:103679. https://doi.org/10.1016/j.critrevonc.2022.103679.
50. Renata F, William N, Tseng JE, Shanthi M, Shin DM, Barbara M, Cohen Ezra EW, Thomas CY, Richard W, Jan C, Nusrat H, Jack LJ, Wistuba IW, Haddad RI, Glisson BS. Randomized phase II trial of cixutumumab alone or with cetuximab for refractory recurrent/metastatic head and neck squamous cell carcinoma. Oral Oncol. 2018;82:83–90. https://doi.org/10.1016/j.oraloncology.2018.05.014.
51. Shields JA, Demirci H, Marr BP. Sebaceous carcinoma of the eyelids: personal experience with 60 cases. Ophthalmology. 2004;111:2151–7.
52. Esmaeli B, Nasser QJ, Cruz H. American Joint Committee on Cancer T category for eyelid sebaceous carcinoma correlates with nodal metastasis and survival. Ophthalmology. 2012;119(5):1078–82.
53. Ho-Seok S, Laura RM, Shiqiong X, Jing N, Michael T, Oded S, Kandl Thomas J, Bita E. Prognostic factors for local recurrence, metastasis and survival for sebaceous carcinoma of the eyelid: observations in 100 patients. Br J Ophthalmol. 2019;103(7):980–4. https://doi.org/10.1136/bjophthalmol-2018-312635.
54. Connor M, Droll L, Ivan D. Management of perineural invasion in sebaceous carcinoma of the eyelid. Ophthalmic Plast Reconstr Surg. 2011;27:356–9.
55. Agelli M, Clegg LX. Epidemiology of primary Merkel cell carcinoma in the United States. J Am Acad Dermatol. 2003;49:832–41.
56. Donepudi S, DeConti RC, Samlowski WE. Recent advances in the understanding of the genetics, etiology, and treatment of Merkel cell carcinoma. Semin Oncol. 2012;39:163–72.
57. Lemos BD, Storer BE, Iyer JG. Pathologic nodal evaluation improves prognostic accuracy in Merkel cell carcinoma: analysis of 5823 cases as basis of the first consensus staging system. J Am Acad Dermatol. 2010;63:751–61.
58. Sims JR, Grotz TE, Pockaj BA. Sentinel lymph node biopsy in Merkel cell carcinoma: The Mayo Clinic experience of 150 patients. Surg Oncol. 2018;27(1):11–7.
59. Peters GB, Meyer DR, Shields JA. Management and prognosis of Merkel cell carcinoma of the eyelid. Ophthalmology. 2001;108:1575–9.
60. Esmaeli B, Naderi A, Hidaji L. Merkel cell carcinoma of the eyelid with a positive sentinel node. Arch Ophthalmol. 2002;120:646–8.
61. Sniegowski MC, Warneke CL, Morrison WH. Correlation of American Joint Committee on Cancer T category for eyelid carcinoma with outcomes in patients with periocular Merkel cell carcinoma. Ophthalmic Plast Reconstr Surg. 2014;30(6): 480–5.
62. Herbert HM, Sun MT, Selva D. Merkel cell carcinoma of the eyelid: management and prognosis. JAMA Ophthalmol. 2014;132(2):197–204.
63. Marie-Léa G, Cynthia A, Becker JC, Astrid B, Veronique B, Brigitte D, Veronique DM, Forsea AM, Fargnoli MC, Jean-Jacques G, Fabio G, Axel H, Christoph H, Catherine H, Nicole K-S, Roland K, Aimilios L, Josep M, David M-R, Ketty P, Giovanni P, Philippe S, Stratigos AJ, Ricardo V, Iris Z, van Akkooi Alexander CJ, Paul L, Claus G, Céleste L. Diagnosis and treatment of Merkel cell carcinoma: European consensus-based interdisciplinary guideline – Update. Eur J Cancer. 2022;171:203–31. https://doi.org/10.1016/j.ejca.2022.03.043.

64. Melika M, Raghav T, Scott JF. Utilization of sentinel lymph node biopsy for Merkel cell carcinoma. J Am Acad Dermatol. 2022;87(6):1404–6. https://doi.org/10.1016/j.jaad.2022.09.002.
65. Nghiem PT, Bhatia S, Lipson EJ. PD-1 blockade with pembrolizumab in advanced Merkel-cell carcinoma. N Engl J Med. 2016;374(26):2542–52.
66. Kaufman HL, Russell J, Hamid O. Avelumab in patients with chemotherapy-refractory metastatic Merkel cell carcinoma: a multicentre, single-group, open-label, phase 2 trial. Lancet Oncol. 2016;17(10):1374–85.
67. D'Angelo SP, Jeffery R, Céleste L, Bartosz C, Thilo G, Jean-Jacques G, Felix K, Guilherme R, Patrick T, Isabella Z, Marcis B, Meliessa H, Kaufman HL. Efficacy and safety of first-line avelumab treatment in patients with stage IV metastatic merkel cell carcinoma. JAMA Oncol. 2018;4(9):e180077. https://doi.org/10.1001/jamaoncol.2018.0077.
68. Walker John W, Celeste L, Giovanni G, Paul N, Luc D, Eyal F, Antonio AP, Shahneen S, Rodrigo M, Elena B, Sarah F, Josh R, Arne E, Subramanian H, Vijay K. Efficacy and safety of avelumab treatment in patients with metastatic Merkel cell carcinoma: experience from a global expanded access program. J Immunother Cancer. 2019;8(1):e000313. https://doi.org/10.1136/jitc-2019-000313.
69. D'Angelo Sandra P, Shailender B, Brohl Andrew S, Omid H, Mehnert Janice M, Patrick T, Shih Kent C, Isaac B, Celeste L, Lewis Karl D, Linette Gerald P, Michele M, Sara G, Parantu S, Barbara E-L, Marcis B, Gülseren G, Nghiem PT. Avelumab in patients with previously treated metastatic Merkel cell carcinoma: long-term data and biomarker analyses from the single-arm phase 2 JAVELIN Merkel 200 trial. J Immunother Cancer. 2019;8(1):e000674. https://doi.org/10.1136/jitc-2020-000674.
70. Paul N, Shailender B, Lipson EJ, Sharfman WH, Kudchadkar RR, Brohl AS, Friedlander PA, Adil D, Kluger HM, Reddy SA, Boulmay BC, Riker AI, Burgess MA, Hanks BA, Thomas O, Kim M, Lundgren LM, Abha S, Nirasha R, Candice C, Park SY, Shinohara MM, Bob S, Taube JM, Bird SR, Nageatte I, Fling SP, Blanca HM, Elad S, Cheever MA, Topalian SL. Durable tumor regression and overall survival in patients with advanced merkel cell carcinoma receiving pembrolizumab as first-line therapy. J Clin Oncol. 2019;37(9):693–702. https://doi.org/10.1200/JCO.18.01896.
71. Paul N, Shailender B, Lipson Evan J, Sharfman William H, Kudchadkar Ragini R, Brohl Andrew S, Friedlander Philip A, Adil D, Kluger Harriet M, Reddy Sunil A, Boulmay Brian C, Adam R, Burgess Melissa A, Hanks Brent A, Thomas O, Kari K, Candice C, Tomoko A, Nirasha R, Shinohara Michi M, Bob S, Taube Janis M, Erin J, Mizuho K, Fling Steven P, Blanca HM, Elad S, Cheever Martin A, Topalian SL. Three-year survival, correlates and salvage therapies in patients receiving first-line pembrolizumab for advanced Merkel cell carcinoma. J Immunother Cancer. 2021;9(4):e002478. https://doi.org/10.1136/jitc-2021-002478.
72. Wendel NR, Antoine H, Tim M, Michael-John D, Ana O, Joseph K, López-Picazo JM, Jean-Pascal M, Jean-Pierre D, Evans Thomas RJ, Valentina B, Emiliano C, Topalian SL, Tian C, Ibrahima S, Li Bin G, Junchen ZR, Moore KN. Safety and efficacy of nivolumab monotherapy in recurrent or metastatic cervical, vaginal, or vulvar carcinoma: results from the phase I/II CheckMate 358 trial. J Clin Oncol. 2022;37(31):2825–34. https://doi.org/10.1200/JCO.19.00739.
73. Hernandez LE, Noreen M, Marita Y, Stefano FF, Isabella D, Keyvan N. Merkel cell carcinoma: an updated review of pathogenesis, diagnosis, and treatment options. Dermatol Ther. 2022;35(3):15292. https://doi.org/10.1111/dth.15292.
74. Cigna E, Gradilone A, Ribuffo D. Morbidity of selective lymph node biopsy for melanoma: meta-analysis of complications. Tumori. 2012;98:94–8.
75. Wasserberg N, Tulchinsky H, Schachter J. Sentinel-lymph-node biopsy for melanoma is not complication-free. Eur Oncol. 2004;30:851–6.
76. Troyan SL, Kianzad V, Gibbs-Strauss SL. The F intraoperative near-infrared fluorescence imaging system: a first-in-human clinical trial in breast cancer sentinel lymph node mapping. Ann Surg Oncol. 2009;16:2943–52.
77. Sugie T, Sawada T, Tagaya N. Comparison of the indocyanine green fluorescence and blue dye methods in detection of sentinel lymph nodes in early-stage breast cancer. Ann Surg Oncol. 2013;20:2213–8.
78. Rubinstein TJ, Perry JD, Korn JM. Indocyanine green-guided sentinel lymph node biopsy for periocular tumors. Ophthalmic Plast Reconstr Surg. 2014;30(4):301–4.
79. McMasters K, Swetter SM. Current management of melanoma: benefits of surgical staging and adjuvant therapy. J Surg Oncol. 2003;82:209–16.
80. Elias N, Tanabe KK, Sober AJ. Is completion lymphadenectomy after a positive sentinel lymph node biopsy for cutaneous melanoma always necessary? Arch Surg. 2004;139:400–5.
81. Yasuhiro F, Otsuka F. The benefit of a sentinel lymph node biopsy and adjuvant therapy in thick 4 mm melanoma multicenter retrospective study of 291 Japanese patients. Melanoma Res. 2012;22:362–7.
82. Mendenhall WM, Amdur RJ, Grobmyer SR. Adjuvant radiotherapy for cutaneous melanoma. Cancer. 2008;112:1189–96.
83. D'Souza J, Clark J. Management of neck in metastatic cutaneous squamous cell carcinoma of the head and neck. Curr Opin Otolaryngol Head Neck Surg. 2011;19:99–105.
84. Yen MT, Tse DT, Wu X. Radiation therapy for local control of eyelid sebaceous cell carcinoma: report of two cases and review of literature. Ophthalmic Plast Reconstr Surg. 2000;16:211–5.
85. Hedina-Franco H, Urist MM. Multimodality treatment of Merkel cell carcinoma: case series and literature review of 1024 cases. Ann Surg Oncol. 2001;8:204–8.
86. Sondak VK, Wolfe JA. Adjuvant therapy for melanoma. Curr Opin Oncol. 1997;9:189–204.
87. Eggermont AMM, Gore M. Randomized adjuvant therapy trials in melanoma: surgical and systemic. Semin Oncol. 2007;34:509–15.
88. Kirkwood JM, Ibrahim JG, Sosman JA. High-dose interferon alfa-2b significantly prolongs relapse-free and overall survival compared with the GM2-KLH/QS-21 vaccine in patients with resected stage IIb-III melanoma: results of intergroup trial E1694/S9512/C509801. J Clin Oncol. 2001;19:2370–80.
89. Ulrike L, Rudolf S, Cornelia M, Werner H, Norbert B, Carola B, Cord S, Martin K, Klaus-Werner S, Percy L, Thomas V, Jens U, Rudolf H, Wolfgang G, Jan-Christoph S, Ulrike K, Peter M, Claus G. Complete lymph node dissection versus no dissection in patients with sentinel lymph node biopsy positive melanoma (DeCOG-SLT): a multicentre, randomised, phase 3 trial. Lancet Oncol. 2016;17(6):757–67. https://doi.org/10.1016/S1470-2045(16)00141-8.
90. Hodi FS, O'Day SJ, McDermott DF. Improved survival with ipilimumab in patients with metastatic melanoma. N Engl J Med. 2010;363(8):711–23.
91. Larkin J, Chiarion-Sileni V, Gonzalez R. Combined nivolumab and ipilimumab or monotherapy in untreated melanoma. N Engl J Med. 2015;373(1):23–34.
92. Masoud SJ, Perone JA, Farrow NE, Mosca PJ, Tyler DS, Beasley GM. Sentinel lymph node biopsy and completion lymph node dissection for melanoma. Curr Treat Options in Oncol. 2018;19:11. https://doi.org/10.1007/s11864-018-0575-4.

93. Torphy RJ, Chloe F, Felix H, Leonard LD, Daniel T, Lewis KD, Medina TM, Robinson WA, Gonzalez RC, Stewart CL, Nicole K, McCarter MD, Ana G. Adjuvant therapy for stage III melanoma without immediate completion lymph node dissection. Ann Surg Oncol. 2016;29(2):806–15. https://doi.org/10.1245/s10434-021-10775-8.
94. Grimes JM, Shah NV, Samie FH, Carvajal RD, Marr BP. Conjunctival melanoma: current treatments and future options. Am J Clin Dermatol. 2020;21(3):371–81. https://doi.org/10.1007/s40257-019-00500-3.
95. Ford J, Thuro BA, Thakar S. Immune checkpoint inhibitors for treatment of metastatic melanoma of the orbit and ocular adnexa. Ophthalmic Plast Reconstr Surg. 2017;33(4):e82–5.
96. Oded S, Thakar SD, Kandl TJ, Joshua F, Sniegowski MC, Wen-Jen H, Bita E. Immunotherapy with programmed cell death 1 inhibitors for 5 patients with conjunctival melanoma. JAMA Ophthalmol. 2018;136(11):1236. https://doi.org/10.1001/jamaophthalmol.2018.3488.
97. Yau-Bun HB, Ford JR, Glitza IC, Torres Cabala Carlos A, Michael T, Prieto VG, Richard P, Claire D, Bita E. Immune checkpoint inhibitor therapy as an eye-preserving treatment for locally advanced conjunctival melanoma. Ophthalmic Plast Reconstr Surg. 2021;37(1):e9–e13. https://doi.org/10.1097/IOP.0000000000001700.
98. Hamid O, Robert C, Daud A. Safety and tumor responses with lambrolizumab (anti–PD-1) in melanoma. N Engl J Med. 2013;369(2):134–44.
99. Taube JM, Galon J, Sholl LM. Implications of the tumor immune microenvironment for staging and therapeutics. Mod Pathol. 2018;31(2):214–34.
100. Renata F, Moran A, Priyadharsini N, Laura RM, Ying Y, Diana B, El-Naggar AK, Johnson JM, Morrison WH, Rosenthal DI, Glisson BS, Johnson FM, Charles L, Mott FE, Bita E, Diaz EM, Gidley PW, Goepfert RP, Lewis CM, Weber RS, Wargo JA, Sreyashi B, Fei D, Yadav SS, Padmanee S, Allison JP, Myers JN, Gross ND. Correction: pilot phase II trial of neoadjuvant immunotherapy in locoregionally advanced, resectable cutaneous squamous cell carcinoma of the head and neck. Clin Cancer Res. 2022;28(8):1735. https://doi.org/10.1158/1078-0432.CCR-22-0468.
101. Allan GJ, Renata F, Neil G, Ryan G, Matthew DJ, Brandon G, Priyadharsini N, Bita E. Immune checkpoint inhibitors for treatment of periorbital squamous cell carcinoma. Br J Ophthalmol. 2023;107(3):320–3. https://doi.org/10.1136/bjophthalmol-2021-319417.
102. Fan J, Goldberg H, Torres-Cabala C, Nagarajan P, Debnam M, Crouse E, Lu T, Ferrarotto R, Esmaeli B. Complete response to immunotherapy using pembrolizumab in a patient with conjunctival squamous cell carcinoma with nodal metastasis. OPRS. 2024;40(5):e171–4.
103. Freitag SK, Aakalu VK, Tao JP, Wladis EJ, Foster JA, Sobel RK, Yen MT. Sentinel lymph node biopsy for eyelid and conjunctival malignancy. Ophthalmology. 2020;127(12):1757–65. https://doi.org/10.1016/j.ophtha.2020.07.031.
104. Bita E, Freitag R, et al. Ophthalmic technology assessment: sentinel lymph node biopsy for eyelid and conjunctival malignancy: a report by the American Academy of Ophthalmology. Ophthalmology. 2020;127:1757–65. https://doi.org/10.1016/j.ophtha.2021.01.012.
105. Morton DL, Thompson JF, Cochran AJ. Sentinel-node biopsy or nodal observation in melanoma. N Engl J Med. 2006;355(13):1307–17.
106. Esmaeli B, Roberts D, Ross M. Histologic features of conjunctival melanoma predictive of metastasis and death. Trans Am Ophthalmol Soc. 2012;110:64–73.
107. Tuomaala S, Kivela T. Metastatic pattern and survival in disseminated conjunctival melanoma: implications for sentinel lymph node biopsy. Ophthalmology. 2004;111:816–21.
108. Shields CL, Shields JA, Gunduz K. Conjunctival melanoma: risk factors for recurrence, exenteration, metastasis, and death in 150 consecutive patients. Arch Ophthalmol. 2000;118:1497–507.

Eyelid Tumors: Emerging Medical Therapy

13

Almila Sarigul Sezenoz and Hakan Demirci

Malignant tumors of the eyelid account for between 5% and 10% of all skin cancers, with an incidence of 15.7 cases per 100,000 individuals per year in the United States [1]. The most common eyelid malignancy is basal cell carcinoma (BCC) representing 86% of the cases, followed by squamous cell carcinoma (SCC) (7%), sebaceous cell carcinoma (Seb Ca) (3%), and Merkel cell carcinoma and melanoma (<1%) [2, 3]. The standard primary treatment for all eyelid cancers involves surgical excision with negative margins, though there still remains debate over the appropriate margin recommendations for each type of malignancy [4]. Alternative treatments are needed to preserve ocular and periorbital tissues in patients with locally advanced or recurring tumors, especially after several prior operations, or in patients with metastasis.

Molecular targeted therapy and immunotherapy are the main emerging medical treatment options for these patients. Significant advances in the recent years have been made in the development of both molecular targeted therapy and immunotherapy drugs for BCC, SCC, and melanomas, which has revolutionized the treatment of these patients [5]. Molecular targeted therapy aims to hinder molecular pathways that play a crucial role in malignancies, while immunotherapy stimulates the host's immune system to attack and destruct the tumor cells.

A. S. Sezenoz
Department of Ophthalmology and Visual Sciences, Kellogg Eye Center, University of Michigan, Ann Arbor, MI, USA

Faculty of Medicine, Department of Ophthalmology, Baskent University, Ankara, Turkey

H. Demirci (✉)
Department of Ophthalmology and Visual Sciences, Kellogg Eye Center, University of Michigan, Ann Arbor, MI, USA
e-mail: hdemirci@med.umich.edu

13.1 Targeted Drug Therapies

The traditional chemotherapeutics act by suppressing the rapid cell division and DNA synthesis [6]. However, they can also cause cytotoxicity to other rapidly dividing non-cancerous cells like bone marrow and epithelial cells. In contrast to the traditional chemotherapeutics that cause non-selective cell death throughout the body, targeted therapy interferes specific pathways and molecules responsible for tumor growth and proliferation. The National Cancer Institute defines targeted therapy as "A type of treatment that uses drugs or other substances to identify and attack specific types of cancer cells with less harm to normal cells" [7].

13.1.1 Hedgehog Pathway Inhibitors for Basal Cell Carcinoma

The 5-year recurrence incidence of primary excised BCC with margin control is reported to be 10% with traditional wide surgical excision and 1–3% with Mohs micrographic surgery [8]. Periocular locally advanced BCC, which is defined by involvement of the orbit or extensive periocular structures, can often lead to severe disfigurement and unfavorable outcomes after surgical removal [9]. For recurrent and locally advanced cases of BCC, wide margin excision of the eyelid, adjuvant radiotherapy, or exenteration are possible treatment options which lead to significant ocular morbidity [9, 10]. Targeted therapy and immunotherapy have gained importance in the recent years as alternative tissue sparing treatment methods for locally advanced and metastatic periocular BCC cases [10].

The Hedgehog (HH) signaling cascade is a pathway for signal transmission from the cell membrane to the nucleus and plays a crucial role in normal cell growth and development [11]. In a normal cell, this pathway is mostly inactive but aberrant activation of this pathway can be involved in tumor development processes [12]. Three proteins are involved in the HH pathway stimulation: HH ligand,

B. C. K. Patel et al. (eds.), *Clinical Ophthalmic Oncology*, https://doi.org/10.1007/978-3-031-72328-5_13

Patched (PTCH), and Smoothened (SMO) transmembrane proteins. SMO signals cells to divide while the PTCH prevents SMO signaling. The HH ligand binds to PTCH-1 receptor, preventing the inhibition of SMO [13]. Approximately 90% of periocular BCCs display a deactivating mutation in the PTCH-1 gene, causing reversal of the inhibition of SMO resulting in overactivation of the HH signaling cascade, uncontrolled cellular proliferation and tumor development [3, 9].

The inhibition of HH pathway through the SMO receptor protein is an established targeted therapy for BCC patients. Vismodegib (Erivedge, Genentech; 150 mg daily orally) and sonidegib (Odomzo, Sun Pharmaceutical Industries; 200 mg daily or 200 mg every other day orally) are the two SMO blocking therapies authorized by the Food and Drug Administration (FDA) in 2012 and 2015, respectively [5]. FDA-approved indications for these drugs are treatment of locally advanced BCC that has recurred after primary surgical excision, and patients who are not eligible for surgery or radiation [14, 15]. Only vismodegib was approved for metastatic BCC as the objective response rate of sonidegib for metastatic disease was only reported to be 7.7%, while that for vismodegib was found to be as high as 48.5% [14, 16]. HH inhibitors can be used as primary or neoadjuvant treatment methods for periocular BCC patients (Fig. 13.1) [17].

As a primary treatment, the drug is administered until maximal clinical response is achieved without further improvement over 2 consecutive months, disease progression

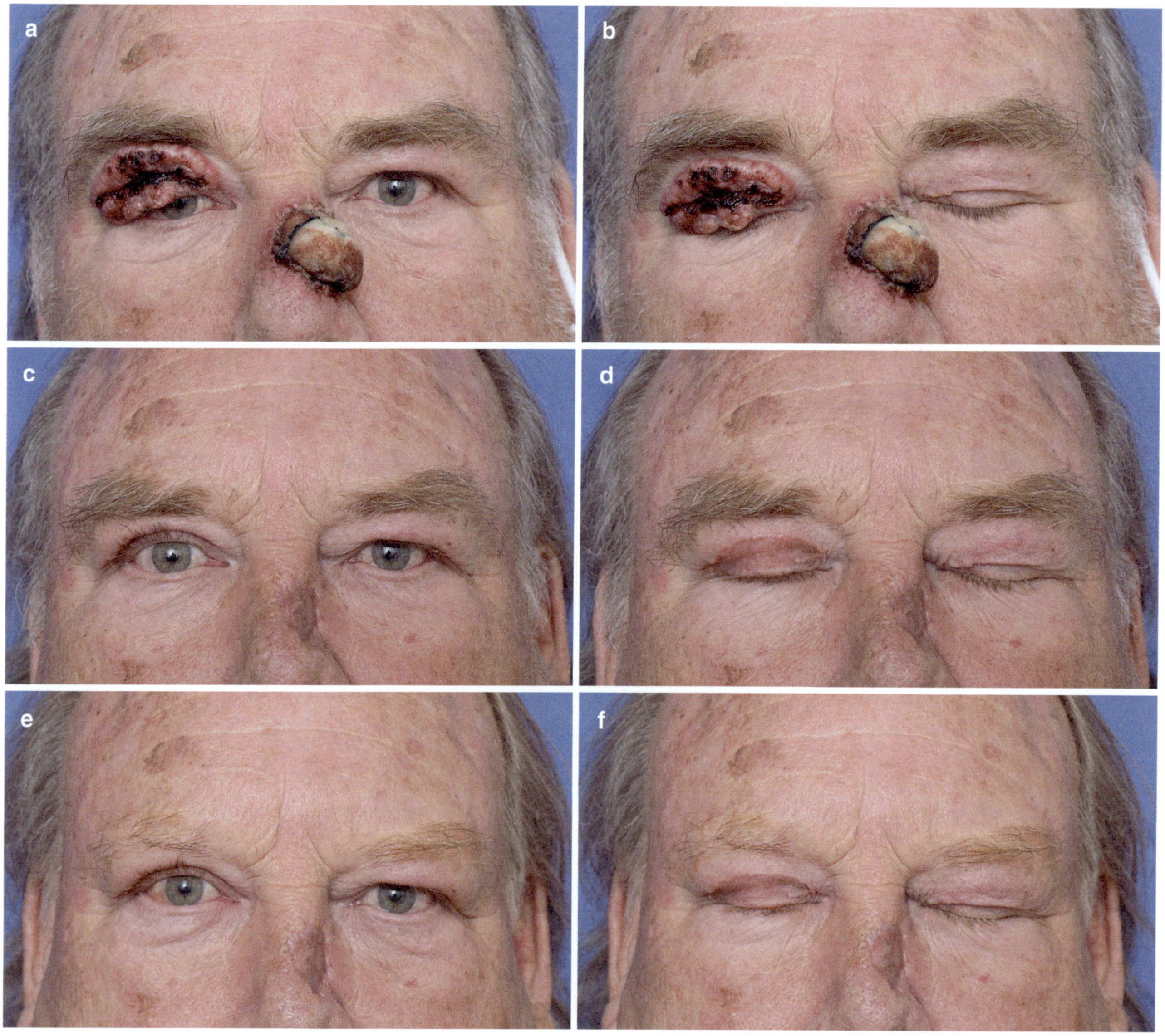

Fig. 13.1 A 60-year-old male patient presented with locally advanced basal cell carcinoma (BCC) involving the entire right upper eyelid, with overlying ulceration and a BCC located on the nasal dorsum (**a**, **b**); regressed lesions after five cycles of vismodegib treatment (**c**, **d**); the regressed lesions with skin irregularities after eight cycles of vismodegib treatment (**e**, **f**)

is observed under treatment, or unacceptable toxicity of the drug is experienced by the patient [18]. The median duration of primary treatment is 9 months (range: 7–19 months). The median time to treatment response is 2.5 months for sonidegib and 4.7 months for vismodegib [14, 15]. After primary treatment, 43% of patients require surgery for the excision of residual tumors. In neoadjuvant treatment, a 3–6 months interval is suggested to be the best time range providing maximal tumor reduction enabling globe preservation with minimal drug toxicity and side effects, as in most cases the side effects become more prominent after 5 months [19, 20]. As the response to treatment starts earlier and adverse effects appear later with sonidegib, providing a suitable time for the neoadjuvant treatment, sonidegib is proposed as a better option for neoadjuvant therapy [21]. In assesment of the patients' eligibility to treatment, the prediction model of Tiosano et al. [22] can be helpful. According to this model, if a patient responds to treatment with at least 20% reduction in tumor size at 3 months and 68% reduction at 6 months, the chances of achieving a complete response with vismodegib treatment are higher (83% and 95% respectively) [22]. In a recent paper, authors suggest a new regimen for neoadjuvant therapy [21]. Accordingly, they suggest that periocular BCCs that are not surgical candidates have four cycles of neoadjuvant sonidegib at 200 mg daily (one cycle meaning 30 days of 200 mg/day sonidegib), which is the period required to achieve steady state. If this treatment results in a full response, a pulsed therapy (sonidegib 200 mg daily for one week on and three weeks off) can be used until intolerable side effects arise. If the neoadjuvant method produces a partial response and the lesion is resectable, the patient may have surgery followed by pulsed therapy. If there is a partial response but the BCC cannot be excised, the patient may be started on the recommended sonidegib dose of 200 mg every other day for 3 cycles before being reviewed for resectability.

According to a recent review, the overall response rate to vismodegib treatment is 75%, complete response rate is 36% and partial response rate is 39% [10]. In patients with orbital involvement, the complete response rate to vismodegib is reported to be 51%, partial response as 45% and the rate of patients undergoing exenteration eventually was reported to be 11% [10]. The rate of orbital exenteration was significantly decreased from 46% with the use of vismodegib treatment [23]. On the other hand, according to a recent panel of European experts, at the 21-month follow-up, the overall response rate for vismodegib was 48%, with 22% complete and 25% partial response rate, while at the 18-month follow-up, the overall response rate of sonidegib was 61% with 21% complete and 39% partial response [24].

After completion of initial vismodegib treatment, the median recurrence rate was found to be 8% (range: 0–23%), with a 20 months (range: 8–38 months) median time of onset after cessation of treatment [10]. Therefore, after discontiuation of the drug, patients should be closely monitored, and some authors also advice a maintenance dose of 150 mg/week vismodegib for 1 year after complete remission, which was shown to reduce the rate of recurrence [25].

13.1.1.1 Adverse Effects of Hedgehod Inhibitors

Almost all of the patients experience mild to moderate side effects when using vismodegib treatment [10]. The most commonly faced adverse effects are alopecia, muscle spasms, dysgeusia, and weight loss [26]. Sonidegib has the advantage of having an alternate dose profile in patients who cannot tolerate the drug, as 200 mg every other day instead of daily 200 mg [21]. Also, another advantage of sonidegib is that the adverse effects appear slightly later, the incidence of most side effects is 10% lower and the severity is less than vismodegib [24].

Although very rarely, life threatening side effects can also occur. A 0.8% death rate was reported in the literature caused by myocardial infarction as an adverse effect of vismodegib treatment [26]. Another important issue is that HH inhibitors are teratogenic, so men and women of childbearing age must use effective contraception during treatment with these drugs [5]. Also, it should be kept in mind that especially in conditions of basal cell nevus syndrome, as the treatment does not treat the underlying genetic mutation, after discontinuation of the drug, new BCC lesions may occur so the patients should be closely monitored [27].

13.1.2 Epidermal Growth Factor Inhibitors for Squamous Cell Carcinoma

SCC is the second most common eyelid malignancy. In most cases, the treatment is wide surgical excision, either with or without adjuvant radiation therapy [9]. To avoid orbital exenteration in these patients, alternative therapies are widely being investigated.

The epidermal growth factor receptor (EGFR) (or ERB1/HER1) is a transmembrane receptor protein that belongs to the tyrosine kinase family. When the ligands (epidermal growth factor (EGF), epiregulin, and transforming growth factor-alpha) bind to the receptor's extracellular domain, this initiates EGFR dimerization. This, in turn, activates receptor tyrosine kinase activity and leads to EGFR autophosphorylation on specific tyrosine residues [28]. These phosphorylated tyrosines recruit signal transducers or adaptors that initiate various intracellular signaling pathways, including Ras/Raf/MEK/MAPS which regulate cellular proliferation, migration, and differentiation [28]. Overexpression of EGFR is a characteristic of SCC, present in 78% of cutaneous SCC cells and 62% of actinic keratoses [29, 30]. The activation of EGFR within keratinocytes has anti-apoptotic effects, leading to increased cellular proliferation and migration, and hindering cellular differentiation, resulting in severe epidermal disorganization and invasion [31, 32].

Small molecule tyrosine kinase inhibitors (gefitinib and erlotinib) and monoclonal antibodies of EGFR (cetuximab), which have better specificity but require intravenous delivery, are the two forms of EGFR inhibitors [31]. Periocular SCC treatment with surgical excision and radiotherapy is challenging, resulting in unfavorable cosmesis and function. The emerging systemic treatment methods including EGFR inhibitors are therefore gaining popularity in the recent years.

Cetuximab (Erbitux, Lilly) is a mouse-human chimeric monoclonal antibody that prevents binding of EGF to EGFR and inhibits downstream kinase activation. It is approved by FDA for use in locally advanced SCC of head and neck in conjunction with radiotherapy or recurrent or metastatic SCC progressing after platinum-based chemotherapy [5]. Although there is no definitive consensus on the treatment with cetuximab of the periocular region carcinomas, studies report promising results [33]. The cetuximab treatment can be given as an adjuvant therapy with combined radiotherapy in periocular locally advanced SCC patients. As an adjuvant therapy, the dosage can be administered as 400 mg/m^2 loading dose after excision of the lesion, followed by 6 weekly infusions of 250 mg/m^2 [33]. Significantly improved overall survival and disease free survival rates were reported with radiotherapy and cetuximab combination compared to radiotherapy alone in patients with locally advanced cutaneous SCC [34]. The most common adverse effect of cetuximab is known to be acne-like rash [35].

Erlotinib (Tarceva, Genentech) is an orally administered tyrosine kinase inhibitor EGFR antagonist that has been explored as an off-label potential therapy for locally advanced head and neck SCC [36]. Limited data show favourable outcomes with erlotinib for the treatment of orbital SCC recurring from previously excised eyelid SCC located at the lateral canthus in order to avoid orbital exenteration and the treatment of metastatic disease. Although there are no randomized clinical trials, in a case report of orbital SCC, the dosage of erlotinib was administered as 150–200 mg and the patient was followed up for 11 months on treatment without any significant adverse reactions [37].

13.1.2.1 Adverse Effects of EGFR Inhibitors

Acneiform rash, itching, changes in nails, diarrhea, and secondary infections are the most commonly reported adverse effects associated with EGFR inhibitors. Studies suggest that patients with a more severe rash experience a significantly better response to EGFR inhibitor treatment and better overall survival rates for cancer [38]. Additionally, EGFR inhibitors have been linked to superficial keratopathy, trichomegaly, and rarely uveitis [39].

13.1.3 Targeted Therapies for Other Eyelid Tumors

Approximately half of all cutaneous and conjunctival melanomas have been revealed to express BRAF mutations, the majority of which are V600E mutations, and confirming the BRAF mutational status is now a standard of care in eyelid melanoma [5, 9, 40]. Combination of anti-BRAF and anti-MEK targeted treatments has revolutionized the treatment of BRAF-mutated cutaneous melanoma [41]. Although there are no randomized clinical trials on eyelid melanomas, BRAF and MEK inhibitors are used in treatment of metastatic and unresectable mutation positive cutaneous melanomas and individual case reports indicate their potential effectiveness in eyelid melanomas [5, 42]. We previously reported a case of a 70-year-old female patient with extensive conjunctival melanoma involving upper and lower eyelids. After incisional biopsy, the tumor was tested positive for BRAF V600E mutation and neoadjuvant systemic BRAF inhibitor (dabrafenib) and MEK inhibitor (trametinib) treatments were administered to the patient. After 3 months of treatment, the tumor was regressed and local excision of the lesion was successfully performed. During follow-up, the patient did not develop any local recurrence, but she developed metastasis after 1 year [42].

The most common adverse effects of BRAF inhibitor therapy include adverse skin events such as rashes, photosensitivity, hyperkeratosis, papillomas, keratoacanthomas, and SCC development [43].

To date, no randomized controlled clinical study has reported the use of targeted therapies in eyelid sebaceous carcinoma and Merkel cell carcinoma. However, recently it was shown that HH pathway was upregulated in sebaceous carcinoma so these tumors may also favor SMO inhibitor treatments like BCC [44].

13.2 Immunotherapy for Eyelid Tumors

Immunotherapies aim to stimulate the host's own immune system to attack and eliminate the hidden tumor cells. Immune checkpoint inhibitor therapy is a special type of immunotherapy. The immune checkpoint proteins, known as programmed cell death-1 (PD-1), programmed cell death ligand-1(PDL-1) and cytotoxic T-lymphocyte antigen-4 (CTLA-4), are normal parts of the immune system. They are found on cell surfaces, and are responsible for keeping the T-cells inactive until they are needed to avoid autoimmune reactions. However, some tumor cells can also present these immune checkpoint proteins on their surface and take advantage of these to inactivate T-cells and gain immuntolerance. Immune checkpoint inhibitor drugs block these checkpoint proteins from binding with their partner proteins expressed on tumor cells, and activate the T-cells to destroy the tumors [45].

The first FDA approved checkpoint inhibitor was a CTLA-4 inhibitor, ipilimumab (Yervoy, Bristol-Myers Squibb), used against metastatic melanoma in 2011 [46]. CTLA-4 is a receptor expressed on T-cells and compete with another T-cell surface receptor, CD28, to bind with the CD80 and CD86 ligands present on the surface of antigen presenting cells [47, 48]. When binded with its ligand, CTLA-4 inactivates the cytotoxic T-cell. Ipilimumab is still the only FDA approved CTLA-4 inhibitor, used in the treatment of cutaneous melanoma [49]. Ipilimumab is licensed by the FDA for the treatment of metastatic or unresectable cutaneous melanoma, as well as an adjuvant therapy for patients with melanoma following complete lymphadenectomy, who had lymph node metastases of more than 1 mm [5].

PD-1 is a receptor present on both the T-cells, and the antigen presenting cells. Different from the CTLA-4, instead of inactivation of the T-cell, PD-1 is only presented after T-cell activation and it limits the action of T-cells. When interacted with its ligand, PD-1 induces apoptosis in antigen recognizing T-cells and inhibits apoptosis in T-regulatory cells [50]. There are currently three FDA approved PD-1 inhibitors (pembrolizumab (Keytruda, Merck), nivolumab (Opdivo, Bristol-Myers Squibb), and cemiplimab (Libtayo, Regeneron)), and they are indicated in metastatic or unresectable melanoma and metastatic or recurrent cutaneous SCC [46]. PDL-1 can be expressed on tumor cells inducing resistance to T-cells [51]. When the interaction of the PD-1 and PDL-1 is inhibited, T-cell expansion and activation occur at the tumor site without an increase in systemic immune system activity [52]. Currently available PDL-1 inhibitors are atezolizumab, avelumab (BAVENCIO, EMD Serono), and durvalumab [46]. Table 13.1 shows the properties of the immuncheckpoint inhibitor drugs, currently used in treatment of eyelid tumors.

13.2.1 Immunotherapy for Eyelid Malignant Melanoma

There are no randomized clinical studies on treatment of eyelid tumors with immuncheckpoint inhibitors but there are case reports with favorable outcomes. Case reports show that ipilimumab (1 mg/kg) and nivolumab (3 mg/kg) combination intravenously given every 3–4 weeks is an effective treatment for recurrent eyelid melanoma [53, 54]. Although long time follow-up is needed, authors reported a case of eyelid melanoma that had no recurrence after 3 years of follow-up [53]. We reported a neoadjuvant immune checkpoint therapy in a 60-year-old woman with recurrent conjunctival melanoma who developed locally advanced BRAF-negative melanoma in her nasal cavity and lymphadenopathy in thorax. She received four cycles of combined ipilimumab and nivolimab therapy, followed by maintanance nivolumab. Her melanoma in the nasal cavity experienced a dramatic response and underwent complete resection with a melanoma free 1-year follow-up [55]. In treatment of melanoma patients, combining anti-CTLA-4 with anti-PD-1/PD-L1 therapies has been shown to be more effective than either therapy alone [46]. To maximize its effects, immune checkpoint inhibitors can be coupled with regular chemotherapy, targeted drugs, and/or radiation [56].

13.2.2 Immunotherapy for Eyelid Squamous Cell Carcinoma

Immuncheckpoint inhibitors cemiplimab and pembrolizumab can be used as initial treatment for locally advanced or metastatic eyelid SCC as well as secondary treatment in recurrent cases after surgical excision. Although no randomized clinical trials are available for eyelid tumors, case reports of periocular SCC treated with pembrolizumab and cemiplimab show favorable outcomes [57, 58]. There is no

Table 13.1 The immuncheckpoint inhibitor drugs used in eyelid tumors and their properties

Generic name	Brand name	Target	Type of tumor	Regimen
Ipilimumab	Yervoy	CTLA-4	Metastatic and unresectable cutaneous melanoma, adjuvant therapy in patients with lymph node metastasis>1 mm	1 mg/kg, IV, q3 weeks
Nivolumab	Opdivo	PD-1	Metastatic or unresectable melanoma; metastatic and recurrent squamous cell carcinoma of head and neck	3 mg/kg, IV, q3 weeks
Pembrolizumab	Keytruda	PD-1	Metastatic melanoma, metastatic and recurrent squamous cell carcinoma of head and neck	2 mg/kg, IV, q3 weeks
Avelumab	Bavencio	PDL-1	Metastatic Merkel cell carcinoma	10 mg/kg, IV, q2 weeks
Cemiplimab	Libtayo	PD-1	Unresectable and metastatic cutaneous squamous cell carcinoma	350 mg, IV, q3 weeks

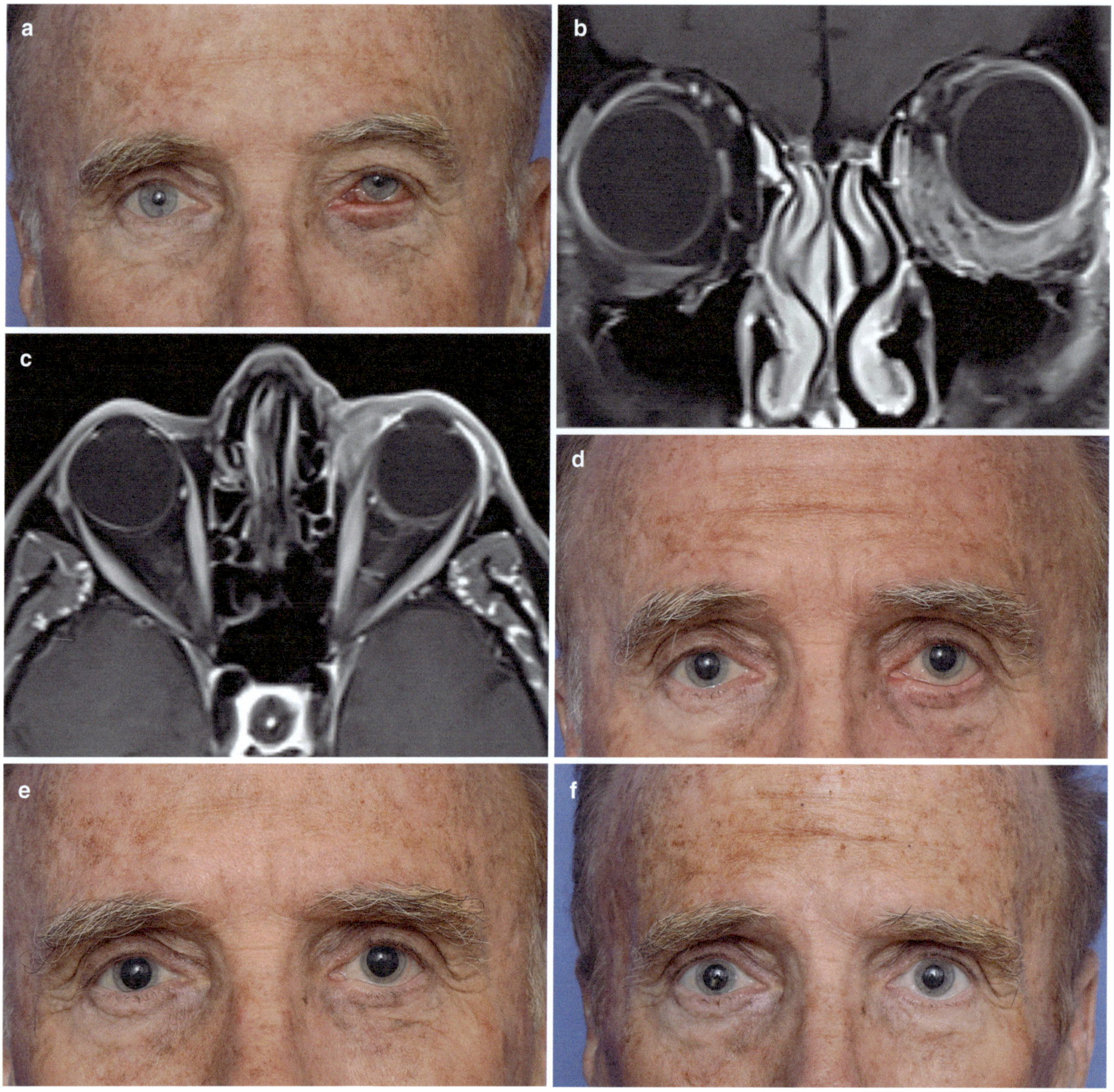

Fig. 13.2 A 72-year-old male patient presented with locally advanced squamous cell carcinoma (SCC) involving the inferior left lower eyelid, with eyelid swelling (**a**), and inferior and medial anterior orbital involvement (**b**, **c**); regression after 4th and 7th cycles of cemiplimab treatment (**d**, **e**); the regressed SCC 14 months after last cycle of cemiplimab treatment with skin irregularities after 8 cycles of vismodegib treatment (**f**)

consensus on the treatment regimen yet, and therefore treatments can be modified according to the patient's response and side effect profile. In a recent report, a large periocular SCC was unable to undergo surgical resection. However, pembrolizumab was utilized, resulting in a significant decrease in tumor size [58]. Dihillon et al. reported a case of recovery in a metastatic eyelid SCC treated with 6 cycles of cemiplimab given at a dose of 350 mg intravenously every 3 weeks. The authors intended to give cemiplimab as a neoadjuvant therapy first but the tumors were sufficiently regressed and no additional therapies other than eyelid reconstruction surgery was needed for the patient [57]. In a case series from our institution, we reported the management of locally advanced conjunctival SCC patients with eyelid and orbital involvement with either cemiplimab (350 mg every 3 weeks) in 3 patients and pembrolizumab (200 mg every 3 weeks) in 2 patients (Figs. 13.2 and 13.3). Complete response was obtained in four out of five patients without any recurrence after a mean follow-up of 6 months [59].

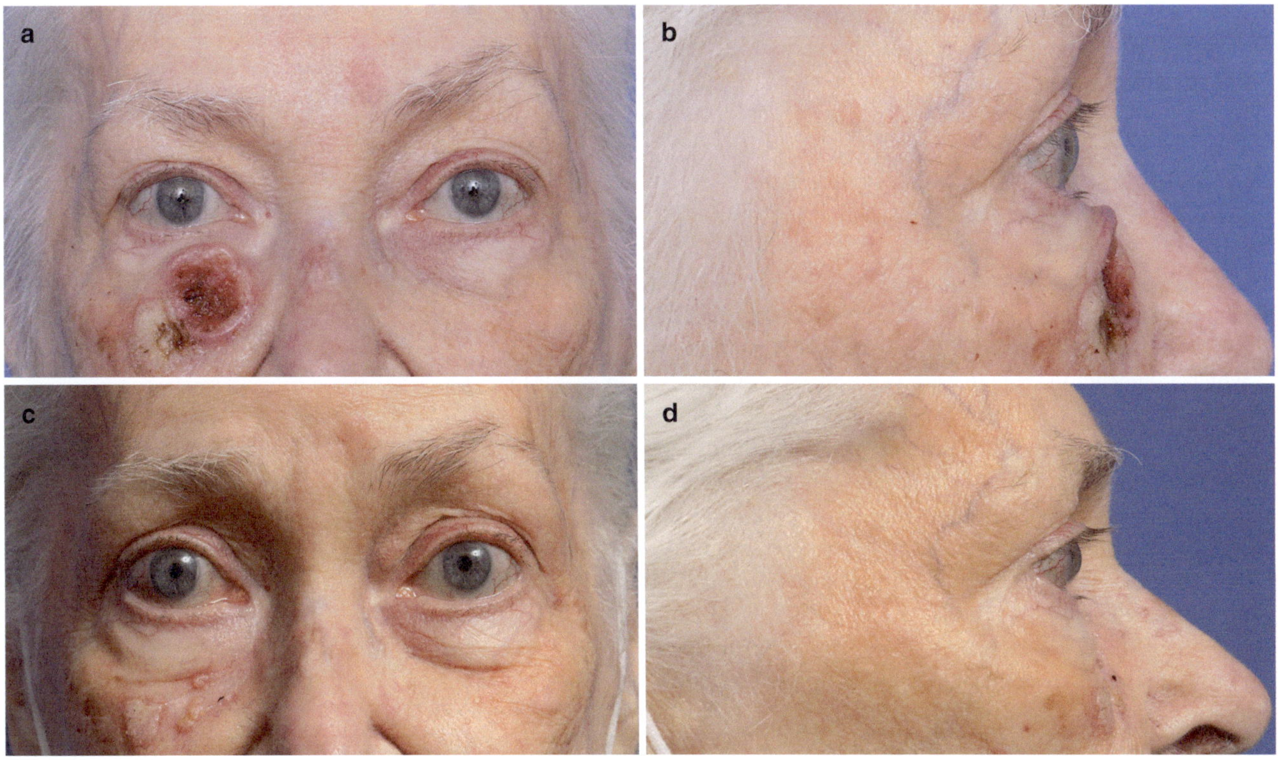

Fig. 13.3 A 95-year-old female patient presented with a biopsy proven squamous cell carcinoma (SCC) involving the right lower eyelid and cheek area, (**a**, **b**); regressed lesion after seven cycles of pembrolizumab treatment (**c**, **d**)

13.2.3 Immunotherapy for Eyelid Basal Cell Carcinoma

Although rare, BCCs can be metastatic and there has been a reported high mutational burden in these tumors, along with PD-1 amplification. Therefore, immuncheckpoint inhibitors can also be effective in treatment of BCC lesions [60]. An incidental reduction in size of a BCC lesion was observed in a patient under ipilimumab therapy for metastatic melanoma and a remission with pembrolizumab was reported in a patient with metastatic BCC [61, 62]. Mohan et al. reported a case of a male patient with metastatic cutaneous melanoma and BCC. The patient was started on ipilimumab and after 6 weeks of treatment, although the melanoma continued to progress his BCC lesion was noted to be regressed, showing significant response to ipilimumab [61]. Fischer et al. reported the case of an 81-year-old male patient with pulmonary metastases of a BCC that was progressing despite treatment with HH pathway inhibitors commenced treatment with pembrolizumab. Following treatment, the patient had a rapid clinical improvement with computed tomography exhibiting near-complete remission after five cycles [62].

13.2.4 Immunotherapy for Eyelid Sebaceous Cell Carcinoma

Recently, evidence of high expression of the PD-1/PDL-1 interaction was discovered in periocular Seb Ca, implying that PD-1 inhibitors may play a role in the treatment of such patients with unresectable or metastatic tumors [63, 64]. Periocular Seb Ca is shown to demonstrate a high expression of PD-1, PD-L1 and PD-L2 [63, 65]. Tumor mutational burden and PD-L1 expression can be indicators of treatment response of these patients [66].

Seb Ca can occur as a component of Muir-Torre Syndrome, which is caused by the germline mutation of DNA mismatch repair proteins leading to microsatellite instability [67]. Seb Ca lesions linked with Muir-Torre Syndrome demonstrate an elevated tumor mutational burden and higher expression of PD-L1 [66]. As a result, Muir-Torre Syndrome and microsatellite instability can serve as beneficial indicators for improved treatment response in Seb Ca patients [66]. A recent case report showed the regression of an eyelid Seb Ca with neoadjuvant pembrolizumab treatment [68]. Woods et al. reported a 58-year-old male patient with bilateral Seb Ca of the eyelids associated with Muir-Torre

Syndrome. The patient showed a good response to neoadjuvant pembrolizumab treatment with tumors shrinking to less than one third of their original size [68].

13.2.5 Adverse Effects of Immunotherapy for Eyelid Tumors

As immunotherapies promote immune-mediated destruction of cancer cells, patients can experience "pseudoprogression" or an "immune flare." Pseudoprogression is a phenomenon in which it appears that the disease is getting worse shortly after treatment initiation, but it improves with continued use of the drug. An immune flare is an autoimmune response in which the apparent tumor burden increases but subsequently regresses with continued treatment [69]. Most common side effects of these therapies are immune-related pneumonitis, colitis, hepatitis, skin problems, nephritis, and endocrinopathies, and less commonly uveitis, conjunctivitis, iritis, and episcleritis [70]. The side effects are usually well tolerated and easily manageable with administration of steroids [57].

13.3 Conclusion

Emerging therapies including targeted and immunotherapies have altered the landscape of the treatment of advanced eyelid tumors. Either being used as a primary or an adjuvant therapy, they reduce the morbidity and increase the chance of globe-sparing surgeries. However, further studies showing the long time results of these emerging therapies as well as the determination of the best treatment regimens are needed.

References

1. Cook BE Jr, Bartley GB. Epidemiologic characteristics and clinical course of patients with malignant eyelid tumors in an incidence cohort in Olmsted County, Minnesota. Ophthalmology. 1999;106:746–50.
2. Deprez M, Uffer S. Clinicopathological features of eyelid skin tumors. A retrospective study of 5504 cases and review of literature. Am J Dermatopathol. 2009;31:256–62.
3. Silverman N, Shinder R. What's new in eyelid tumors. Asia Pac J Ophthalmol. 2017;6:143–52.
4. Sullivan TJ. Topical therapies for periorbital cutaneous malignancies: indications and treatment regimens. Curr Opin Ophthalmol. 2012;23:439–42.
5. Esmaeli B, Sagiv O. Targeted biological drugs and immune check point inhibitors for locally advanced or metastatic cancers of the conjunctiva, eyelid, and orbit. Int Ophthalmol Clin. 2019;59:13–26.
6. Baudino TA. Targeted cancer therapy: the next generation of cancer treatment. Curr Drug Discov Technol. 2015;12:3–20.
7. Saeed RF, Awan UA, Saeed S, Mumtaz S, Akhtar N, Aslam S. Targeted therapy and personalized medicine. Cancer Treat Res. 2023;185:177–205.
8. Kahana A, Bartley K, Meyer CS, Seetasith A, Lee J, McKenna E. Healthcare resource utilization and cost of care in patients with periocular basal cell carcinoma: a real-world study. Am J Ophthalmol. 2022;236:164–71.
9. Martel A, Lassalle S, Picard-Gauci A, et al. New targeted therapies and immunotherapies for locally advanced periocular malignant tumours: towards a new 'eye-sparing' paradigm? Cancer. 2021;13:2822.
10. Singalavanija T, Ceylanoglu KS, Juntipwong S, et al. Review of targeted therapy, vismodegib, for the treatment of periocular basal cell carcinoma. Ophthalmic Plast Reconstr Surg. 2023;40(1):1–10.
11. Skoda AM, Simovic D, Karin V, Kardum V, Vranic S, Serman L. The role of the Hedgehog signaling pathway in cancer: a comprehensive review. Bosn J Basic Med Sci. 2018;18:8–20.
12. Doheny D, Manore SG, Wong GL, Lo HW. Hedgehog signaling and truncated GLI1 in cancer. Cells. 2020;9:2114.
13. Danovi S. The story of vismodegib and skin cancer. Cancer Research UK - Cancer News. 2021. https://news.cancerresearchuk.org/2012/06/07/high-impact-science-hedgehogs-flies-and-skin-cancer-the-story-of-vismodegib/.
14. Sekulic A, Migden MR, Basset-Seguin N, et al. Long-term safety and efficacy of vismodegib in patients with advanced basal cell carcinoma: final update of the pivotal ERIVANCE BCC study. BMC Cancer. 2017;17:332.
15. Dummer R, Guminksi A, Gutzmer R, et al. Long-term efficacy and safety of sonidegib in patients with advanced basal cell carcinoma: 42-month analysis of the phase II randomized, double-blind BOLT study. Br J Dermatol. 2020;182:1369–78.
16. Lear JT, Migden MR, Lewis KD, et al. Long-term efficacy and safety of sonidegib in patients with locally advanced and metastatic basal cell carcinoma: 30-month analysis of the randomized phase 2 BOLT study. J Eur Acad Dermatol Venereol. 2018;32:372–81.
17. Demirci H, Worden F, Nelson CC, Elner VM, Kahana A. Efficacy of vismodegib (erivedge) for basal cell carcinoma involving the orbit and periocular area. Ophthalmic Plast Reconstr Surg. 2015;31:463–6.
18. Curragh DS, Huilgol SC, Selva D. Neoadjuvant vismodegib in the management of locally advanced periocular basal cell carcinoma. Eye. 2021;35:2740–5.
19. Kahana A, Unsworth SP, Andrews CA, et al. Vismodegib for preservation of visual function in patients with advanced periocular basal cell carcinoma: the VISORB trial. Oncologist. 2021;26:e1240–9.
20. Gonzalez AR, Etchichury D, Gil ME, Del Aguila R. Neoadjuvant vismodegib and mohs micrographic surgery for locally advanced periocular basal cell carcinoma. Ophthalmic Plast Reconstr Surg. 2019;35:56–61.
21. De Giorgi V, Trane L, Pieretti G, et al. Treatment of periocular advanced basal cell carcinoma with Hedgehog pathway inhibitors: a single-center study and a new dedicated therapeutic protocol. Dermatol Reports. 2021;13:9240.
22. Tiosano A, Ben-Ishai M, Fenig E, Ben Simon GJ, Yassur I. The initial rate of tumour response to vismodegib treatment, can predict a complete response outcome for periocular LA-BCC. Eye. 2023;37:531–6.
23. Sagiv O, Ding S, Ferrarotto R, et al. Impact of Food and Drug Administration approval of vismodegib on prevalence of orbital exenteration as a necessary surgical treatment for locally advanced periocular basal cell carcinoma. Ophthalmic Plast Reconstr Surg. 2019;35:350–3.
24. Dummer R, Ascierto PA, Basset-Seguin N, et al. Sonidegib and vismodegib in the treatment of patients with locally advanced basal cell carcinoma: a joint expert opinion. J Eur Acad Dermatol Venereol. 2020;34:1944–56.
25. Scalvenzi M, Cappello M, Costa C, Fabbrocini G, Luciano M, Villani A. Low-dose vismodegib as maintenance therapy after

locally advanced basal cell carcinoma complete remission: high efficacy with minimal toxicity. Dermatol Ther. 2020;10:465–8.
26. Ben Ishai M, Tiosano A, Fenig E, Ben Simon G, Yassur I. Outcomes of vismodegib for periocular locally advanced basal cell carcinoma from an open-label trial. JAMA Ophthalmol. 2020;138:749–55.
27. Tang JY, Mackay-Wiggan JM, Aszterbaum M, et al. Inhibiting the hedgehog pathway in patients with the basal-cell nevus syndrome. N Engl J Med. 2012;366:2180–8.
28. Wee P, Wang Z. Epidermal growth factor receptor cell proliferation signaling pathways. Cancer. 2017;9:52.
29. Yin VT, Merritt H, Esmaeli B. Targeting EGFR and sonic hedgehog pathways for locally advanced eyelid and periocular carcinomas. World J Clin Cases. 2014;2:432–8.
30. Toll A, Salgado R, Yebenes M, et al. Epidermal growth factor receptor gene numerical aberrations are frequent events in actinic keratoses and invasive cutaneous squamous cell carcinomas. Exp Dermatol. 2010;19:151–3.
31. Ivan D, Prieto VG, Esmaeli B, Wistuba II, Tang X, Lazar AJ. Epidermal growth factor receptor (EGFR) expression in periocular and extraocular sebaceous carcinoma. J Cutan Pathol. 2010;37:231–6.
32. Commandeur S, van Drongelen V, de Gruijl FR, El Ghalbzouri A. Epidermal growth factor receptor activation and inhibition in 3D in vitro models of normal skin and human cutaneous squamous cell carcinoma. Cancer Sci. 2012;103:2120–6.
33. Clark TJE, Harris GJ. Management of periocular cutaneous squamous cell carcinoma with perineural invasion: a case series and literature review. Orbit. 2022;41:34–43.
34. Lu SM, Lien WW. Concurrent radiotherapy with cetuximab or platinum-based chemotherapy for locally advanced cutaneous squamous cell carcinoma of the head and neck. Am J Clin Oncol. 2018;41:95–9.
35. Maubec E, Petrow P, Scheer-Senyarich I, et al. Phase II study of cetuximab as first-line single-drug therapy in patients with unresectable squamous cell carcinoma of the skin. J Clin Oncol. 2011;29:3419–26.
36. Moreira J, Tobias A, O'Brien MP, Agulnik M. Targeted therapy in head and neck cancer: an update on current clinical developments in epidermal growth factor receptor-targeted therapy and immunotherapies. Drugs. 2017;77:843–57.
37. El-Sawy T, Sabichi AL, Myers JN, et al. Epidermal growth factor receptor inhibitors for treatment of orbital squamous cell carcinoma. Arch Ophthalmol. 2012;130:1608–11.
38. Bonner JA, Harari PM, Giralt J, et al. Radiotherapy plus cetuximab for locoregionally advanced head and neck cancer: 5-year survival data from a phase 3 randomised trial, and relation between cetuximab-induced rash and survival. Lancet Oncol. 2010;11:21–8.
39. Saint-Jean A, Sainz de la Maza M, Morral M, et al. Ocular adverse events of systemic inhibitors of the epidermal growth factor receptor: report of 5 cases. Ophthalmology. 2012;119:1798–802.
40. Zeng Y, Hu C, Shu L, et al. Clinical treatment options for early-stage and advanced conjunctival melanoma. Surv Ophthalmol. 2021;66:461–70.
41. Pasquali S, Hadjinicolaou AV, Chiarion Sileni V, Rossi CR, Mocellin S. Systemic treatments for metastatic cutaneous melanoma. Cochrane Database Syst Rev. 2018;2:CD011123.
42. Demirci H, Demirci FY, Ciftci S, et al. Integrative exome and transcriptome analysis of conjunctival melanoma and its potential application for personalized therapy. JAMA Ophthalmol. 2019;137:1444–8.
43. Yin VT, Wiraszka TA, Tetzlaff M, Curry JL, Esmaeli B. Cutaneous eyelid neoplasms as a toxicity of vemurafenib therapy. Ophthalmic Plast Reconstr Surg. 2015;31:e112–5.
44. Bladen JC, Moosajee M, Tracey-White D, Beaconsfield M, O'Toole EA, Philpott MP. Analysis of hedgehog signaling in periocular sebaceous carcinoma. Graefes Arch Clin Exp Ophthalmol. 2018;256:853–60.
45. National Cancer Institute. Immune checkpoint inhibitors. 2022. https://www.cancer.gov/about-cancer/treatment/types/immunotherapy/checkpoint-inhibitors#:~:text=Immunotherapy%20drugs%20called%20immune%20checkpoint,checkpoint%20protein%20called%20CTLA%2D4.
46. Habib LA, Wolkow N, Freitag SK, Yoon MK. Advances in immunotherapy and periocular malignancy. Semin Ophthalmol. 2019;34:327–33.
47. Baksh K, Weber J. Immune checkpoint protein inhibition for cancer: preclinical justification for CTLA-4 and PD-1 blockade and new combinations. Semin Oncol. 2015;42:363–77.
48. Rudd CE, Taylor A, Schneider H. CD28 and CTLA-4 coreceptor expression and signal transduction. Immunol Rev. 2009;229:12–26.
49. Buchbinder E, Hodi FS. Cytotoxic T lymphocyte antigen-4 and immune checkpoint blockade. J Clin Invest. 2015;125:3377–83.
50. Balar AV, Weber JS. PD-1 and PD-L1 antibodies in cancer: current status and future directions. Cancer Immunol Immunother. 2017;66:551–64.
51. Centanni M, Moes D, Troconiz IF, Ciccolini J, van Hasselt JGC. Clinical pharmacokinetics and pharmacodynamics of immune checkpoint inhibitors. Clin Pharmacokinet. 2019;58:835–57.
52. Chen L, Han X. Anti-PD-1/PD-L1 therapy of human cancer: past, present, and future. J Clin Invest. 2015;125:3384–91.
53. Ediriwickrema LS, Liu CY, Kikkawa DO, Korn BS. Development of poliosis following checkpoint inhibitor treatment for cutaneous melanoma. Ophthalmic Plast Reconstr Surg. 2019;35:e121–2.
54. Shoji MK, Rong AJ. Ipilimumab and nivolumab for treatment of eyelid spindle cell melanoma. Am J Ophthalmol. 2023;250:e1–2.
55. Fan K, Waninger JJ, Yentz S, McLean S, Demirci H. Neoadjuvant immune checkpoint inhibition in metastatic conjunctival melanoma. Ophthalmic Plast Reconstr Surg. 2023;39:e152–5.
56. Emens LA, Middleton G. The interplay of immunotherapy and chemotherapy: harnessing potential synergies. Cancer Immunol Res. 2015;3:436–43.
57. Dhillon J, Li DQ, Burnier M, Shenouda G, Arthurs BP, El-Hadad C. Cemiplimab for metastatic squamous cell carcinoma of the orbit, periocular adnexa, and thigh. Orbit. 2022;43(2):258–64.
58. Conger JR, Grob SR, Tao J. Massive periocular squamous cell carcinoma with response to pembrolizumab (Keytruda). Ophthalmic Plast Reconstr Surg. 2019;35:e127.
59. Demirci H, Elner VM, Demirci FY, et al. Immunotherapy for conjunctival squamous cell carcinoma with orbital extension. Ophthalmology. 2021;128:801–4.
60. Falchook GS, Leidner R, Stankevich E, et al. Responses of metastatic basal cell and cutaneous squamous cell carcinomas to anti-PD1 monoclonal antibody REGN2810. J Immunother Cancer. 2016;4:70.
61. Mohan SV, Kuo KY, Chang AL. Incidental regression of an advanced basal cell carcinoma after ipilimumab exposure for metastatic melanoma. JAAD Case Rep. 2016;2:13–5.
62. Fischer S, Hasan Ali O, Jochum W, Kluckert T, Flatz L, Siano M. Anti-PD-1 therapy leads to near-complete remission in a patient with metastatic basal cell carcinoma. Oncol Res Treat. 2018;41:391–4.
63. Kandl TJ, Sagiv O, Curry JL, et al. High expression of PD-1 and PD-L1 in ocular adnexal sebaceous carcinoma. Onco Targets Ther. 2018;7:e1475874.
64. Wolkow N, Jakobiec FA, Afrogheh AH, Pai SI, Faquin WC. High expression of programmed death ligand 1 and programmed death ligand 2 in ophthalmic sebaceous carcinoma: the case for a clinical trial of checkpoint inhibitors. Am J Ophthalmol. 2020;220:128–39.

65. Xu S, Yu H, Fu G, Fan X, Jia R. Programmed death receptor Ligand 1 expression in eyelid sebaceous carcinoma: a consecutive case series of 41 patients. Acta Ophthalmol. 2019;97:e390–6.
66. Zhao P, Li L, Jiang X, Li Q. Mismatch repair deficiency/micro satellite instability-high as a predictor for anti-PD-1/PD-L1 im munotherapy efficacy. J Hematol Oncol. 2019;12(1):54.
67. Dany M. The DNA mismatch repair system in sebaceous tumors: an update on the genetics and workup of Muir-Torre syndrome. Cutis. 2020;105(3):E34–7.
68. Woods AD, Grushchak S, Williams KM, Tan A, Krunic AL. Combination treatment of bilateral periocular sebaceous carcinomas with microsatellite instability with neoadjuvant pembrolizumab and Mohs surgery. Australas J Dermatol. 2022;63:e345–9.
69. Ford J, Thuro BA, Thakar S, Hwu WJ, Richani K, Esmaeli B. Immune checkpoint inhibitors for treatment of metastatic melanoma of the orbit and ocular adnexa. Ophthalmic Plast Reconstr Surg. 2017;33:e82–5.
70. Schneider BJ, Naidoo J, Santomasso BD, et al. Management of immune-related adverse events in patients treated with immune checkpoint inhibitor therapy: ASCO guideline update. J Clin Oncol. 2021;39:4073–126.

Eyelid Tumors: Radiation Therapy

14

David Buchberger, Sheen Cherian, and Arun D. Singh

14.1 Introduction

Ophthalmic radiation therapy in several forms has been used with success to treat eyelid malignancies. As with other ocular tumors, the goal of radiation therapy is to eradicate tumor burden in a manner that maintains visual function and preserves surrounding sensitive ocular tissues. In the following chapter, the indications and outcomes of various modalities of radiation used to treat eyelid tumors like squamous cell carcinoma (SCC), basal cell carcinoma (BCC), sebaceous gland carcinoma, and melanoma are discussed. Radiation therapy of ocular adnexal lymphoma is reviewed with orbital tumors.

14.2 Squamous Cell Carcinoma

Moh's micrographic surgery (MMS) or wide excision with frozen section control is the primary treatment of choice for SCC of the eyelid (Chap. 6). Historically, the recurrence rate for MMS at 5 years has been under 4% [1, 2].

14.2.1 Indications

Advanced disease requiring substantial removal of tissue can result in poor cosmesis, extensive fibrosis, and loss of eyelid function. Radiation is an option for such patients and those who are unable to undergo extensive surgery due to other medical comorbidities. More recently, immunotherapy is being used with increasing frequency. After response rates close to 50% were demonstrated in early phase studies [3], a landmark trial investigating the use of PD-1 inhibitor cemiplimab in the treatment of stage II-IV (M0) cutaneous SCC prior to surgery was published showing a 51% pathological response rate and 68% objective response rate on imaging [4, 5]. In this setting, for inoperable patients and unresectable lesions immune-oncology (IO) offers an attractive first line option (Chap 13).

14.2.2 Techniques and Results

14.2.2.1 EBRT

In one series of 104 individuals with SCC of the eyelid treated with single (20–22.5 Gy) or fractionated EBRT at doses of 35 Gy/5 fx, the 5-year local tumor control rate was 93.3% with excellent cosmetic and functional outcomes [6]. Additional retrospective studies have reported favorable local control rates with EBRT ranging from 70% to 88% [7, 8]. Studies using proton therapy for the treatment of epithelial tumors of the orbit and ocular adnexa (including eyelid tumors) have also been published demonstrating the potential effectiveness of this approach with no local recurrences with a median follow-up of 27.1 months and favorable toxicity profile [9]. If treating with electrons, the use of eye shields can significantly improve vision and function preservation.

14.2.2.2 Brachytherapy

An alternative approach for radiation therapy of SCC of the eyelid is the use of high dose rate interstitial brachytherapy. Typically, this technique uses a plastic tubing system inserted into the tumor to cover the target area. In one series of ten patients with SCC of the eyelid treated with six fractions of 6.5 Gy over 6 days, a 90% 5-year disease-free survival was observed. No vision impairment was seen and cosmetic results were good and acceptable to patients [10]. Additional series reporting on outcomes of eyelid patient tumors treated with interstitial brachytherapy have continued to show excellent rates of local control at extended follow-up ranging from

D. Buchberger · S. Cherian (✉)
Department of Radiation Oncology, Taussig Cancer Center, Cleveland Clinic, Cleveland, OH, USA
e-mail: cherias@ccf.org

A. D. Singh
Cole Eye Institute, Cleveland Clinic, Cleveland, OH, USA
e-mail: singha@ccf.org

B. C. K. Patel et al. (eds.), *Clinical Ophthalmic Oncology*, https://doi.org/10.1007/978-3-031-72328-5_14

75% to greater than 95%, with acceptable toxicity and vision preservation [11–14].

14.3 Basal Cell Carcinoma

While BCC of the eyelid can be locally invasive and destructive, it does not frequently metastasize (Chap. 5). Surgical excision, MMS, and cryosurgery have been used to treat BCC with 5-year local control rates exceeding 90% with excellent preservation of vision, cosmesis and function [1, 2, 10]. In recent years, sonic hedgehog pathway inhibitors (vismodegib, sonidegib) are being used in situations where surgery is either not feasible or would result in significant morbidity. They are being used as definitive treatment, in the neoadjuvant setting to facilitate a more desirable surgery, and adjuvantly as consolidation. Objective response rates of 40–70% have been reported in the literature [15, 16]. The VISORB trial investigated the use of neoadjuvant vismodegib in preparation for surgery and found a 56% complete response rate on physical exam after vismodegib alone. Of the patients that had surgery, 67% had a pathological complete response (Chap. 13) [17].

14.3.1 Indications

For small and localized lesions, surgery is most frequently selected as primary therapy; however radiation therapy is an attractive option for cases when surgical excision will result in severe loss of function or unacceptable cosmesis. This is particularly relevant to lesions affecting the inner canthus and lower eyelid where surgical treatment may result in scarring or damage to the lacrimal apparatus. When the decision is made to perform exenteration in cases with orbital invasion by periocular BCC, radiation can be used as adjuvant therapy [18].

14.3.2 Techniques and Results

14.3.2.1 EBRT

Several large series have reported favorable local-control rates with primary radiation therapy for BCC of the eyelid. As a historical example, Fitzpatrick et al. reported excellent results using EBRT in the treatment of a large series of 1062 BCC of the eyelid. Depending on tumor size, patients were treated with single or fractionated exposures to doses of 20–60 Gy. Using this schedule, the five-year tumor control rate was 95% [6]. In the majority of these cases, a 5 day fractionated course of radiation to 35 Gy yielded excellent functional and cosmetic results. In the 5% of patients in whom recurrences developed, further radiation or surgery was effective in obtaining local tumor control [6]. A number of other studies since that time have continued to report local control rates of 90% or greater with primary external beam radiotherapy [19, 20]. Other investigators have cautioned against the use of radiation as primary therapy for periocular BCC. Recurrences, particularly those in the region of the midface, are difficult to treat by any modality and carry a high risk of mortality [21].

14.3.2.2 Brachytherapy

Historically, investigators have compared interstitial brachytherapy as well as other forms of radiation therapy to standard surgical excision for primary BCC of the face measuring less than 4 cm [22]. A study of 347 patients was conducted in which patients were either randomized to a surgery group or a radiation therapy group (55% were treated with interstitial brachytherapy, 33% with contact therapy, and 12% with conventional radiation therapy). The 4-year actuarial failure rate (95% CI) was 0.7% (0.1–3.9%) in the surgery group compared with 7.5% (4.2–13.1%) in the radiation therapy group. The cosmetic results were also assessed by independent observers and by the patients receiving treatment. In both cases, cosmesis was felt to be superior in those patients who underwent surgery. However, since this time, many series have been published documenting favorable results with brachytherapy for the treatment of eyelid tumors. Indeed, in many centers today, as with the treatment of SCC of the eyelid, high dose rate interstitial brachytherapy is used for the treatment of BCC of the eyelid. In two patients treated with six fractions of 6.5 Gy over 6 days, a 50% 5-year disease-free survival was observed [10]. Notably, the studies listed above referencing the treatment of SCC of the eyelid with interstitial brachytherapy also included BCC patients. As above, these studies showed excellent rates of local control at extended follow-up ranging from 75% to greater than 95%, with acceptable toxicity and vision preservation [11–14, 23, 24]. Brachytherapy can also be employed post-operatively in the setting of incomplete excision with promising local control in small institutional series [25]. It is to be noted that, brachytherapy is operator dependent and when done by a skilled and experienced brachytherapist the results could be superior.

14.4 Sebaceous Gland Carcinoma

Sebaceous gland carcinoma is an aggressive and rare cancer that can affect the eyelid. Updated guidelines on the management of sebaceous carcinoma were published in *Lancet Oncology* in 2019 and it guides management decisions [26]. Initial treatment is surgery, with radiotherapy reserved for inoperable and/or unresectable cases as well as unfavorable pathology including nodal involvement (Chap. 7). Historically, there has been some suggestion that these tumors are radioresistant [6] but more recent studies have shown local control rates of 90% or greater [27, 28], with doses above 55 Gy associated with increased control [29].

14.4.1 Indications

Per the 2019 guidelines, radiotherapy is not recommended as monotherapy in the treatment of sebaceous gland carcinoma and is reserved for medically inoperable/unresectable cases or tumors with nodal metastases that are also not resectable. Adjuvant (post-surgical) radiotherapy is also used in the setting of positive margins or perineural invasion (Figs. 14.1 and 14.2) [26]. Ultimately, reports related to the use of radiotherapy for the treatment of sebaceous gland carcinoma of the eyelid are limited. Radiotherapy decisions are best made in the multi-disciplinary setting at centers of expertise.

14.4.2 Techniques and Results

14.4.2.1 EBRT

The role of EBRT as curative therapy has been investigated by some groups [28]. In one series of 10 patients with sebaceous gland carcinoma of the ocular adnexa, four patients were treated definitively at a dose of 45–63 Gy over 4–7 weeks. The remaining six patients received post-operative radiation therapy to the parotid bed and ipsilateral cervical lymph node chain for parotid metastases, which developed within 36 months of initial surgical treatment. Local control was 90% after a follow-up ranging from 2 to 10 years, and overall disease specific actuarial survival was 96% at 5 years [28]. Hata et al. looked at 13 patients with sebaceous carcinoma of the eyelid treated with definitive radiotherapy (median dose 60 Gy) and found a 5-year local progression free survival rate of 100% and disease free survival rate of 89% [27]. A more recent series from Japan of 83 patients treated in both the definitive and adjuvant settings (median RT dose 60 Gy) found a 7-year local control rate of only 52% [30].

14.4.2.2 Brachytherapy

High dose rate interstitial brachytherapy has also been explored in some centers as a potential treatment of sebaceous gland carcinoma of the eyelid [10]. In one series of eight cases of sebaceous gland carcinoma treated with six fractions of 6.5 Gy over 6 days, a 5-year disease-free survival of 57% was observed [10]. In a systematic review of the use of brachytherapy in non-melanoma skin cancer of the eyelid, local control rates ranging from 57% to 100% were reported in various studies [24]. Longer-term follow-up with larger patient numbers is needed to confirm these results.

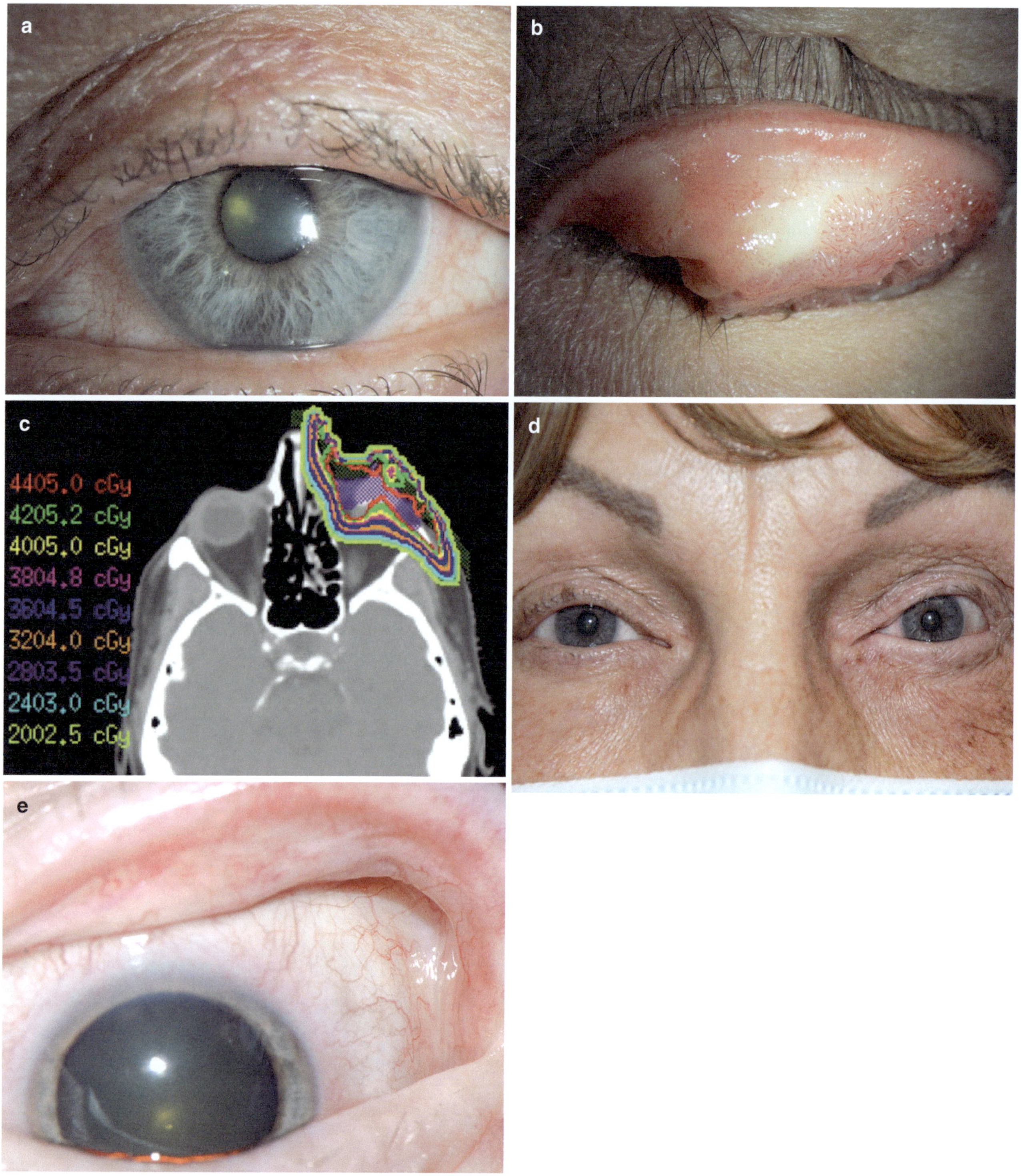

Fig. 14.1 A 45 year old woman with upper eyelid bump noted for approximately 2 years. The growth was not obvious on external examination (**a**) until the lid was everted (**b**) revealing papillomatous mass involving the upper lid up to the fornix and extending to eyelid margin laterally. The lesion was excised that confirmed sebaceous gland carcinoma with negative deep margin, but the lateral margin was positive. Adjuvant EBRT 40 Gy in 15 fractions was prescribed. 9 MeV electrons were delivered to the left eyelid using 5 mm bolus and a daily eye shield for posterior structure sparing with an En-Face technique to the total dose (**c**). Sentinel lymph node biopsy was negative. Other than mild dryness managed by artificial tears and a few episodes of trichiasis (epilated), at 4 year visit, patient remains recurrence free (**d**) without metastasis (negative CT neck soft tissues). The anterior segment examination was unremarkable mild radiation cataract causing visual acuity of 20/40 (**e**)

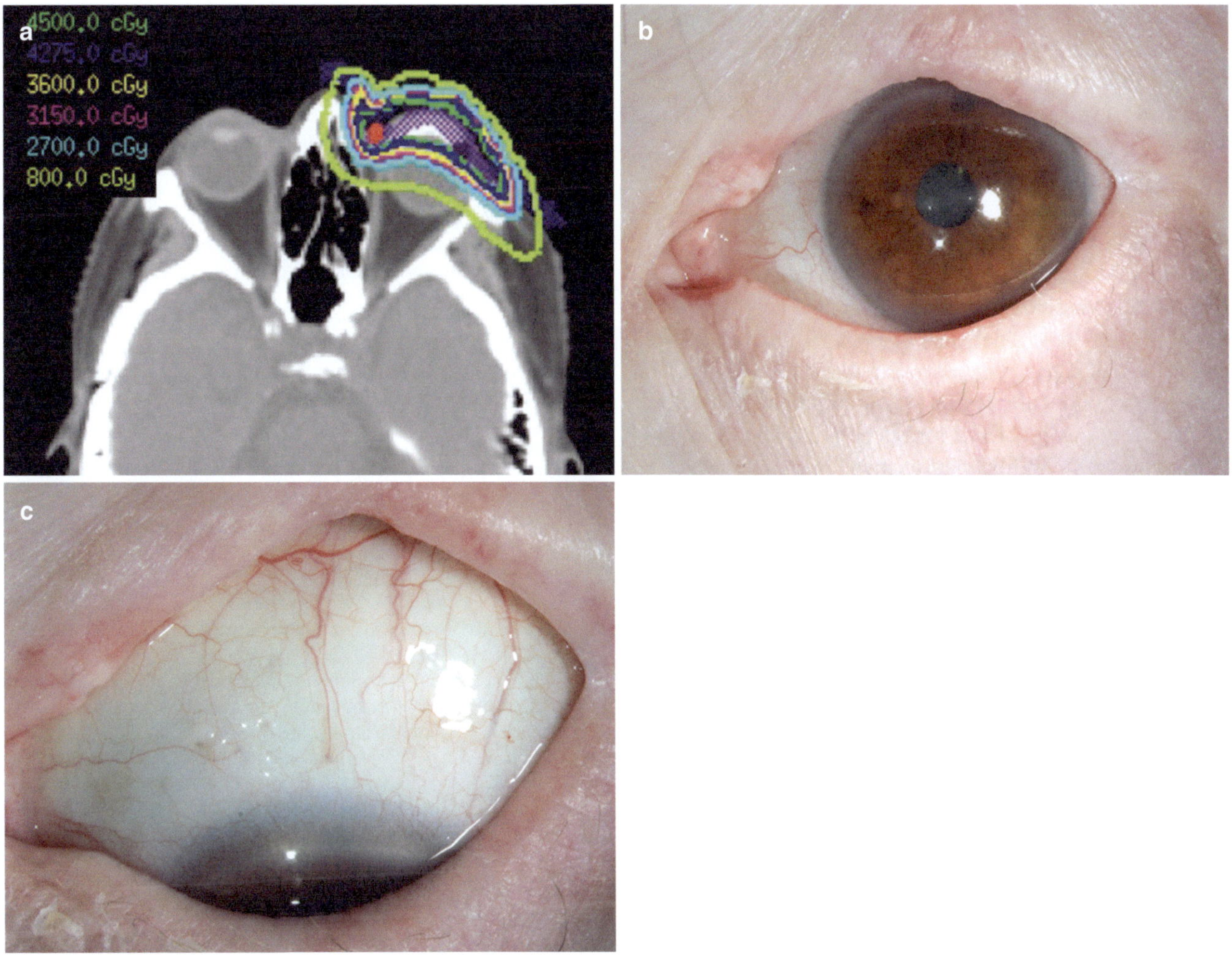

Fig. 14.2 A 65-year-old woman with invasive sebaceous carcinoma of the left upper eyelid resected with MOHS (positive margin) and followed by adjuvant EBRT 45 Gy in 25 fractions. 6 MeV electrons were delivered to the left eyelid using 5 mm bolus and a daily eye shield for posterior structure sparing with an En-Face technique to the total dose (**a**). Sentinel lymph node biopsy was negative. Subsequently had marginal recurrences (x2) that required excision about 2 and 2.9 years after radiation and conjunctival recurrence treated by excision and cryotherapy 3.4 years after radiation. Conjunctival map biopsies excluded widespread pagetoid extension. At 4 year post radiation, there was absence of local recurrence (**b**, **c**) and systemic metastasis (CT neck soft tissue). Patient was managing well with artificial tears and scleral contact lens for lid lag and dry eye

14.5 Eyelid Melanoma

For small, circumscribed malignant melanoma of the eyelid, surgical excision with wide margins is the recommended therapy (Chap. 8) [31]. This is generally followed by plastics repair and exenteration for large or diffuse neoplasms [32]. Immunotherapy plays an increasing role in the treatment of melanoma and may be preferred to radiotherapy in a variety of settings (Chap. 13).

14.5.1 Indications

Radiation therapy has been used following surgery in cases where residual disease is present at the margins of resection [33]. It has also been used as an alternative to exenteration in select cases [31].

14.5.2 Techniques and Results

14.5.2.1 EBRT

EBRT has been used in some centers when regional lymph node metastases are detected following wide local excision; however the small number of patients treated preclude meaningful analysis of outcomes [34].

14.5.2.2 Brachytherapy

In one series, 14 patients, all of whom had undergone previous debulking, incomplete resection, or recurrence following surgery, were treated with I-125 brachytherapy. A stainless steel pericorneal ring eye shield was used in combination with I-125 seeds in polythene tubes inserted into the eyelid. A median dose of 37 Gy (range, 17.3–67.6 Gy) was delivered over the course of 113 h (range, 47–190 h) to the outer surface of target tumor volume [31]. Local control was achieved in 13 patients after a median follow-up of 39 months. There were two recurrences at 8 and 13 months in one patient who received 17.3 Gy. Three patients subsequently died with metastatic disease at 44, 62, and 79 months following brachytherapy [31].

14.6 Eyelid Merkel Cell Carcinoma

Merkel cell carcinoma is a rare primary neuroendocrine tumor of the skin. Roughly half of all cases occur in the head and neck, and it has been estimated that 2.5–10% occur on the eyelid or periocular region [35]. It is a highly radiosensitive tumor with a proclivity for lymph node spread and distant metastases. Upfront management is surgery which is typically followed by EBRT (50–66 Gy) to the primary site and regional lymphatic basins with a growing role for sentinel lymph node biopsy and tailored lymphatic RT thereafter. While brachytherapy is not standard, there are case reports documenting its efficacy in treatment of Merkel cell carcinoma of the eyelid [36]. Recent retrospective data suggests that all Merkel cell carcinomas of the head and neck region should be considered high risk and treated with adjuvant radiotherapy after resection [37].

14.7 Conclusions

It is important to note that most experience using radiation to treat eyelid is based upon results from small case series. It is therefore difficult to assess overall efficacy and optimal treatment protocols for incorporating radiation into the treatment planning of these tumors. The rare nature of these tumors, varying tumor classification schemes, and confounding prognostic clinical factors such as tumor size and location contribute to the difficulty in analyzing outcomes following radiation. Eyelid tumors often need well curated radiation treatment plans and precision radiation delivery techniques, as they are generally surrounded by numerous critical structures, hence it's imperative they are treated at centers of excellence, by a skilled and experienced multidisciplinary team.

References

1. Mohs FE. Micrographic surgery for the microscopically controlled excision of eyelid cancers. Arch Ophthalmol. 1986;104(6):901–9.
2. Malhotra R, Huilgol SC, Huynh NT, Selva D. The Australian Mohs database: periocular squamous cell carcinoma. Ophthalmology. 2004;111(4):617–23.
3. Migden MR, Rischin D, Schmults CD, Guminski A, Hauschild A, Lewis KD, et al. PD-1 blockade with cemiplimab in advanced cutaneous squamous-cell carcinoma. N Engl J Med. 2018;379(4):341–51.
4. Gross ND, Miller DM, Khushalani NI, Divi V, Ruiz ES, Lipson EJ, et al. Neoadjuvant cemiplimab and surgery for stage II-IV cutaneous squamous-cell carcinoma: follow-up and survival outcomes of a single-arm, multicentre, phase 2 study. Lancet Oncol. 2023;24(11):1196–205.
5. Gross ND, Miller DM, Khushalani NI, Divi V, Ruiz ES, Lipson EJ, et al. Neoadjuvant cemiplimab for stage II to IV cutaneous squamous-cell carcinoma. N Engl J Med. 2022;387(17):1557–68.
6. Fitzpatrick PJ, Thompson GA, Easterbrook WM, Gallie BL, Payne DG. Basal and squamous cell carcinoma of the eyelids and their treatment by radiotherapy. Int J Radiat Oncol Biol Phys. 1984;10(4):449–54.
7. Petsuksiri J, Frank SJ, Garden AS, Ang KK, Morrison WH, Chao KS, et al. Outcomes after radiotherapy for squamous cell carcinoma of the eyelid. Cancer. 2008;112(1):111–8.
8. Inaba K, Ito Y, Suzuki S, Sekii S, Takahashi K, Kuroda Y, et al. Results of radical radiotherapy for squamous cell carcinoma of the eyelid. J Radiat Res. 2013;54(6):1131–7.
9. Holliday EB, Esmaeli B, Pinckard J, Garden AS, Rosenthal DI, Morrison WH, et al. A multidisciplinary orbit-sparing treatment approach that includes proton therapy for epithelial tumors of the orbit and ocular adnexa. Int J Radiat Oncol Biol Phys. 2016;95(1):344–52.
10. Azad S, Choudhary V. Treatment results of high dose rate interstitial brachytherapy in carcinoma of eye lid. J Cancer Res Ther. 2011;7(2):157–61.
11. Krengli M, Masini L, Comoli AM, Negri E, Deantonio L, Filomeno A, et al. Interstitial brachytherapy for eyelid carcinoma. Outcome analysis in 60 patients. Strahlenther Onkol. 2014;190(3):245–9.
12. Mareco V, Bujor L, Abrunhosa-Branquinho AN, Ferreira MR, Ribeiro T, Vasconcelos AL, et al. Interstitial high-dose-rate brachytherapy in eyelid cancer. Brachytherapy. 2015;14(4):554–64.
13. Pagliara MM, Tagliaferri L, Savino G, Fionda B, D'Aviero A, Lanza A, et al. High-dose-rate interstitial brachytherapy (interventional radiotherapy) for conjunctival melanoma with orbital extension. Ocul Oncol Pathol. 2021;7(3):199–205.
14. Cisek P, Kieszko D, Bilski M, Debicki R, Grywalska E, Hrynkiewicz R, et al. Interstitial HDR brachytherapy in the treatment of non-melanocytic skin cancers around the eye. Cancers (Basel). 2021;13:6.
15. Sekulic A, Migden MR, Basset-Seguin N, Garbe C, Gesierich A, Lao CD, et al. Long-term safety and efficacy of vismodegib in patients with advanced basal cell carcinoma: final update of the pivotal ERIVANCE BCC study. BMC Cancer. 2017;17(1):332.
16. Basset-Seguin N, Hauschild A, Grob JJ, Kunstfeld R, Dreno B, Mortier L, et al. Vismodegib in patients with advanced basal cell carcinoma (STEVIE): a pre-planned interim analysis of an international, open-label trial. Lancet Oncol. 2015;16(6):729–36.
17. Kahana A, Unsworth SP, Andrews CA, Chan MP, Bresler SC, Bichakjian CK, et al. Vismodegib for preservation of visual function in patients with advanced periocular basal cell carcinoma: the VISORB trial. Oncologist. 2021;26(7):e1240–e9.
18. Leibovitch I, McNab A, Sullivan T, Davis G, Selva D. Orbital invasion by periocular basal cell carcinoma. Ophthalmology. 2005;112(4):717–23.
19. Krema H, Herrmann E, Albert-Green A, Payne D, Laperriere N, Chung C. Orthovoltage radiotherapy in the management of medial canthal basal cell carcinoma. Br J Ophthalmol. 2013;97(6):730–4.
20. Garcia-Martin E, Gil-Arribas LM, Idoipe M, Alfaro J, Pueyo V, Pablo LE, et al. Comparison of imiquimod 5% cream versus radiotherapy as treatment for eyelid basal cell carcinoma. Br J Ophthalmol. 2011;95(10):1393–6.
21. Margo CE, Waltz K. Basal cell carcinoma of the eyelid and periocular skin. Surv Ophthalmol. 1993;38(2):169–92.
22. Avril MF, Auperin A, Margulis A, Gerbaulet A, Duvillard P, Benhamou E, et al. Basal cell carcinoma of the face: surgery

or radiotherapy? Results of a randomized study. Br J Cancer. 1997;76(1):100–6.
23. Caccialanza M, Piccinno R, Gaiani F, Contini D. Relevance of dermatologic radiotherapy in the therapeutic strategy of skin epithelial neoplasms: excellent results in the treatment of lesions localized on eyelids and skin overlying the cartilage of the nose. G Ital Dermatol Venereol. 2013;148(1):83–8.
24. Frakulli R, Galuppi A, Cammelli S, Macchia G, Cima S, Gambacorta MA, et al. Brachytherapy in non melanoma skin cancer of eyelid: a systematic review. J Contemp Brachytherapy. 2015;7(6):497–502.
25. Cuffaro G, Fionda B, Piccinni F, Pagliara MM, Sammarco MG, Blasi MA, et al. Post-operative interventional radiotherapy (brachytherapy) in advanced ocular surface and eyelid tumors as an alternative to surgical retreatment. Eur J Ophthalmol. 2023:11206721231215105.
26. Owen JL, Kibbi N, Worley B, Kelm RC, Wang JV, Barker CA, et al. Sebaceous carcinoma: evidence-based clinical practice guidelines. Lancet Oncol. 2019;20(12):e699–714.
27. Hata M, Koike I, Omura M, Maegawa J, Ogino I, Inoue T. Noninvasive and curative radiation therapy for sebaceous carcinoma of the eyelid. Int J Radiat Oncol Biol Phys. 2012;82(2):605–11.
28. Pardo FS, Borodic G. Long-term follow-up of patients undergoing definitive radiation therapy for sebaceous carcinoma of the ocular adnexae. Int J Radiat Oncol Biol Phys. 1996;34(5):1189–90.
29. Yen MT, Tse DT, Wu X, Wolfson AH. Radiation therapy for local control of eyelid sebaceous cell carcinoma: report of two cases and review of the literature. Ophthalmic Plast Reconstr Surg. 2000;16(3):211–5.
30. Takagawa Y, Tamaki W, Suzuki S, Inaba K, Murakami N, Takahashi K, et al. Radiotherapy for localized sebaceous carcinoma of the eyelid: a retrospective analysis of 83 patients. J Radiat Res. 2019;60(5):622–9.
31. Stannard CE, Sealy GR, Hering ER, Pereira SB, Knowles R, Hill JC. Malignant melanoma of the eyelid and palpebral conjunctiva treated with iodine-125 brachytherapy. Ophthalmology. 2000;107(5):951–8.
32. Hungerford JL. Management of ocular melanoma. Br Med Bull. 1995;51(3):694–716.
33. Lederman M. Radiotherapy of malignant melanomata of the eye. Br J Radiol. 1961;34:21–42.
34. Esmaeli B, Wang B, Deavers M, Gillenwater A, Goepfert H, Diaz E, et al. Prognostic factors for survival in malignant melanoma of the eyelid skin. Ophthalmic Plast Reconstr Surg. 2000;16(4):250–7.
35. Walsh NM, Cerroni L. Merkel cell carcinoma: a review. J Cutan Pathol. 2021;48(3):411–21.
36. Hao S, Zhao S, Bu X. Radioactive seed implantation in treatment of an eyelid primary Merkel cell carcinoma. Can J Ophthalmol. 2016;51(1):e31–3.
37. Bierma MM, Goff PH, Hippe DS, Lachance K, Schaub SK, Wallner K, et al. Postoperative radiation therapy is indicated for "low-risk" pathologic stage I Merkel cell carcinoma of the head and neck region but not for other locations. Adv Radiat Oncol. 2024;9(2):101364.

15 Eyelid Tumors: Systemic Associations

Nasrine Anais El Salloukh, Arun D. Singh, and Elias I. Traboulsi

Abbreviations

AVM	Arteriovenous malformation
BCC	Basal cell carcinoma
CHRPE	Congenital hypertrophy of retinal pigment epithelium
CM	Capillary malformations
CNC	Carney complex
CS	Cowden syndrome
FDA	Food Drug Administration
HNPCC	Hereditary nonpolyposis colorectal cancer
MRI	Magnetic resonance imaging
MTS	Muir-Torre syndrome
NBCCS	Nevoid basal cell carcinoma syndrome
NF1	Neurofibromatosis type 1
PDL	Pulsed dye laser
PDT	Photodynamic therapy
RPE	Retinal pigment epithelium
SWS	Sturge-Weber syndrome

15.1 Introduction

Patients with an inherited predisposition for tumors tend to develop these tumors at an early age, have multiple tumors with bilateral involvement, and may have a positive family history of similar lesions [1]. Most eyelid tumors in the setting of an inherited predisposition are benign, but some malignant tumors can have a syndromic association such as ones that occur (Table 15.1), in the setting of the Gorlin-Goltz syndrome. With eyelid tumors, one of the most important clues to the presence of an associated systemic disease is an unusual histopathologic feature. For example, tumors such as myxomas and sebaceous adenomas of the eyelid are unlikely to occur in the absence of a syndromic association. Eyelid tumors can also be metastatic, but such cases are rare and account for less than 1% of malignant eyelid tumors [2].

N. A. El Salloukh · E. I. Traboulsi (✉)
Department of Pediatric Ophthalmology and Strabismus, Center for Genetic Eye Diseases, Cole Eye Institute (i-32), Cleveland Clinic Foundation, Cleveland, OH, USA
e-mail: traboue@ccf.org

A. D. Singh
Cole Eye Institute, Cleveland Clinic, Cleveland, OH, USA

B. C. K. Patel et al. (eds.), *Clinical Ophthalmic Oncology*, https://doi.org/10.1007/978-3-031-72328-5_15

Table 15.1 Eyelid tumors that are markers of a syndromic association

Entity	Eyelid tumor	Associated features	Locus/gene
Neurofibromatosis type 1	Neurofibroma	Lisch nodules	17q
		Café au lait spots	*NF 1* gene
		Pheochromocytoma	
		Optic nerve glioma	
		Choroidal lesions	
Sturge-Weber Syndrome	Diffuse hemangioma	Leptomeningeal hemangioma	Sporadic
Gardner syndrome	Epidermoid cyst	Pigmented Ocular Fundus Lesions (POFLs)	5q21
	Fibroma	Colorectal polyps/carcinoma	*APC* gene
	Orbital osteoma		
Gorlin-Goltz syndrome	Basal cell carcinoma	Odontogenic cysts	9q 22
		Bifid ribs	*PTC* gene
		Palmar pits	
		Ovarian tumor	
Cowden syndrome	Trichilemmoma	Oral papilloma	10q23
		Breast tumor	*PTEN* gene
		Thyroid tumor	
Carney complex	Myxoma	Spotty mucocutaneous pigmentation	17q
		Schwannoma	*PRKAR1A* gene chromosome 2
		Endocrine overactivity	
		Testicular tumor	
Muir-Torre syndrome	Sebaceous adenoma	Keratoacanthoma	2p
		Basal cell carcinoma	*hMLH1, hMSH2*
		Colorectal adenocarcinoma	

15.2 Neurofibroma in Neurofibromatosis Type 1

Neurofibroma is the hallmark of neurofibromatosis type 1 (NF1). NF1 is inherited in an autosomal-dominant fashion in about 50% of patients and is sporadic in the remainder [3]. The disease affects 1 out of 3000 persons and is due to mutations in the *NF1* gene on chromosome 17q11.2, which encodes the protein neurofibromin [3].

Neurofibromas appear as discrete soft tumors on the face (including eyelids) (Fig. 15.1), hands, and trunk. Previously given different names, they are now designated as orbital-periorbital-plexiformal neurofibromas to include all the locations in which they appear [4]. Cutaneous neurofibromas arise from small nerves or nerve endings and protrude from the surface of the skin, while subcutaneous neurofibromas are firm nodules just below the surface of the skin [4]. They tend to be small and generally appear in the second decade of life, becoming more numerous as the patient ages, with no risk of malignant transformation. They rarely cause neurologic deficits [4]. In contrast, plexiform neurofibromas are complex nerve sheath tumors that follow multiple nerve branches, mainly diagnosed in early childhood [4]. They are more prone to cause functional and neurologic deficits, and there is a risk of malignant transformation [4]. In the eye and ocular adnexa, a plexiform pattern is more frequent [5]. These tumors are usually associated with other features of NF1. Solitary tumors are rare, but tumors masquerading as chalazia have been described

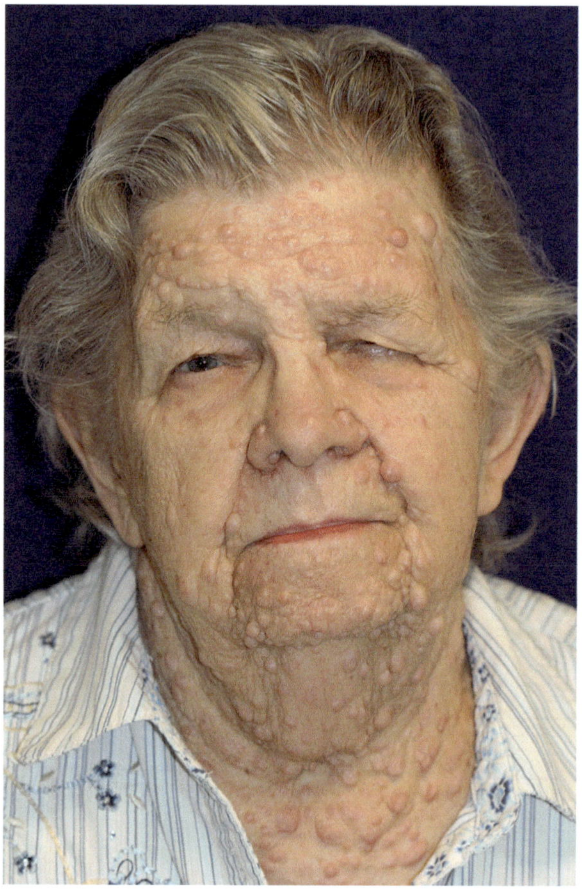

Fig. 15.1 Extensive facial neurofibromas. Courtesy of Bhupender C. Patel, MD Salt Lake City, Utah, USA

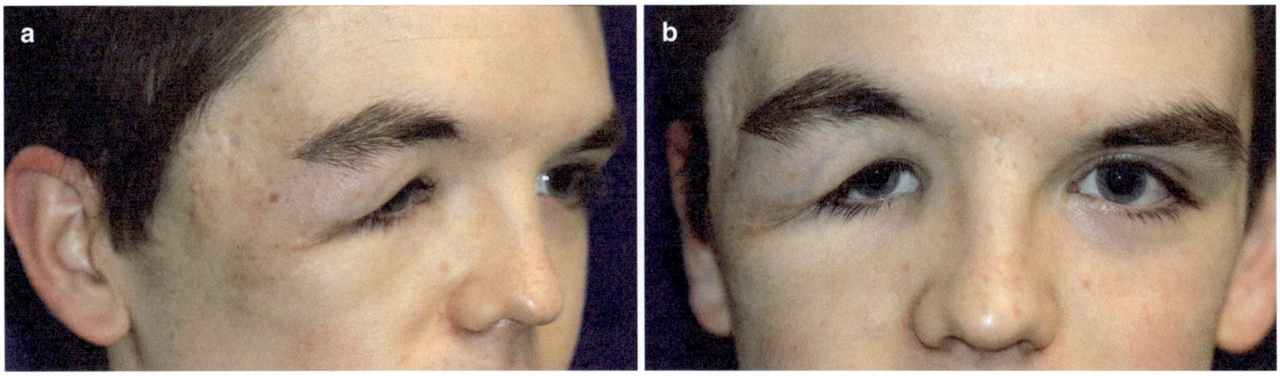

Fig. 15.2 (**a**, **b**) Plexiform neurofibroma S-shaped eyelid deformity. Courtesy of Bhupender C. Patel, MD Salt Lake City, Utah, USA

in the literature [6, 7]. Characteristics of plexiform neurofibromas of the eyelid are thickening of the upper lid, S-shaped eyelid deformity (Fig. 15.2a, b), "bag of worms"-like feel on palpation, and detachment of the lateral [8] or medial canthal ligaments [9]. The extent of a neurofibroma cannot be determined by clinical examination alone, so MRI is necessary [10].

Amblyopia can be caused by these lesions, mainly because of ptosis or anisometropia: a comprehensive ophthalmologic examination should be performed every 6 months throughout the period of visual development [11]. Debulking of the tumor mass, ptosis surgery, and canthal fixation are the surgical treatment modalities in cases of plexiform neurofibroma, to clear the visual axis and improve appearance [12]. Unfortunately, surgery can be challenging and associated with a high risk of complications and recurrences, because of the tumor's integration with the surrounding soft tissue (Figure 15.3a–d) [13]. With asymptomatic, non-progressive, and nonobstructive tumors, monitoring is an option, taking into consideration the fact that neurogenic tumors in NF1 carry a risk of approximately 10% for malignant transformation [14]. This risk is greater with atypical neurofibromas [15], whole-gene deletion [16], higher numbers of plexiform neurofibromas, larger whole body benign tumor volume, and younger age [17]. Selumetinib, a novel MEK inhibitor, did show durable tumor shrinkage and clinical benefit in inoperable plexiform neurofibroma in SPRINT, a phase 2 clinical trial, leading to its FDA approval for children older than 2 years with NFA and inoperable and symptomatic plexiform neurofibroma [18].

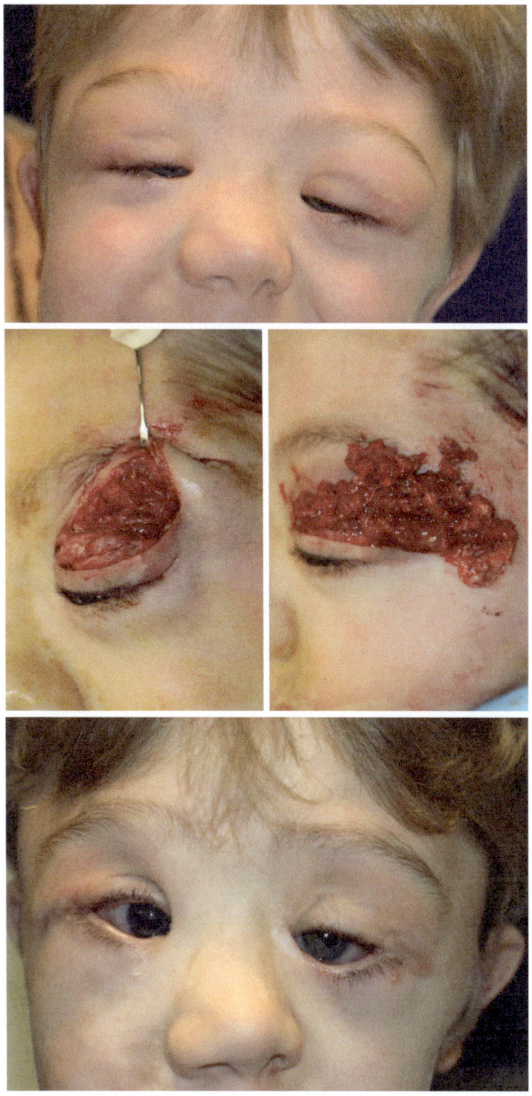

Fig. 15.3 Bilateral plexiform neurofibromas and orbital and facial neurofibromas (**a**). Surgical series showing how extensive these neurofibromas tend to be in the orbit, face and eyelids (**b**, **c**). Six months after bilateral eyelid and orbital debulking of neurofibromas and repair of ptosis and lower eyelid laxity (**d**). Courtesy of Bhupender C. Patel, MD Salt Lake City, Utah, USA

15.3 Nevus Flammeus

Nevus flammeus is also known as capillary malformation (CM) or port-wine stain and is the most common type of congenital vascular malformation. It is usually present at birth and persists throughout life, although its appearance or color may change [19]. It is initially flat and light red, or violaceous and affects the skin of the face in almost all cases (90%) (Fig. 15.4), followed by the neck, trunk, leg, arm, and hand. With an incidence of 0.3% in newborns, it usually occurs as a sporadic unifocal lesion, not associated with any underlying disease [19].

Recently proposed pathophysiologic mechanisms for tissue hypertrophy are a defect in the normal innervation to dermal blood vessels and genetic mutations causing dysregulation of angiogenesis [20]. Despite this, a definitive pathogenic mechanism is still not known. A somatic activating mutation in *GNAQ* has been identified as the cause of Sturge–Weber syndrome and apparently non-syndromic port-wine stains [21, 22]. Nevus flammeus associated with arteriovenous malformation subtypes have been found to result from dominant *RASA-1* gene mutations [22, 23].

Although multiple treatments are available, the gold standard for treatment of a facial nevus flammeus is the flash-lamp-pumped pulsed dye laser (PDL) treatment [24]. However, when there are hypertrophic skin changes, surgical intervention can achieve better results [24].

Nevus flammeus is sometimes associated with certain syndromes, such as Sturge-Weber syndrome, macrocephaly-CM syndrome, CM-arteriovenous malformation (AVM) syndrome, phacomatosis pigmentovascularis, and overgrowth syndromes such as Klippel-Trenaunay syndrome.

It is sometimes difficult to distinguish between different diseases. Doppler assessment may be helpful in differentiating nevus flammeus from AVMs [19]. It is also important to differentiate port-wine stain from other similar malformations such as infantile hemangiomas, which are associated with different syndromes such as PHACES (posterior fossa anomalies, hemangioma, arterial anomalies, cardiac anomalies and eye anomalies) [25]. A useful diagnostic clue is that the distribution is dermatomal in nevus flammeus and segmental in infantile hemangiomas [26]. Moreover, the endothelial cells of port-wine stains do not stain for GLUT-1, which is a specific marker for infantile hemangiomas [19].

In general, only about 10% of all patients with nevus flammeus or port-wine stain of the eyelid are associated with Sturge-Weber syndrome (SWS) (Fig. 15.5) [27]. SWS occurs in patients who have hemangiomas in the V1 or V2 areas of distribution of the trigeminal nerve. It is typically unilateral, present at birth, and does not change with age [28]. The size of the nevus flammeus in SWS has been found to be correlated with neurologic severity in patients more than 5 years old [29]. Bilateral port-wine stains of the eyelids have a higher likelihood of being associated with SWS than unilateral lesions [27]. In a study of 55 patients with SWS, glaucoma was the main ocular disease and was related to the extension of the nevus flammeus in the palpebral area [30]. If there is involvement of both upper and lower eyelids, the risk of glaucoma is as high as 50%. The glaucoma is almost always ipsilateral to the facial port-wine stain [28]. Diffuse choroidal hemangioma is present in about 40–50% of patients with SWS and is usually ipsilateral to the facial port-wine stain. Patients without nevus flammeus in the palpebral area do not develop glaucoma or choroidal hemangioma [30].

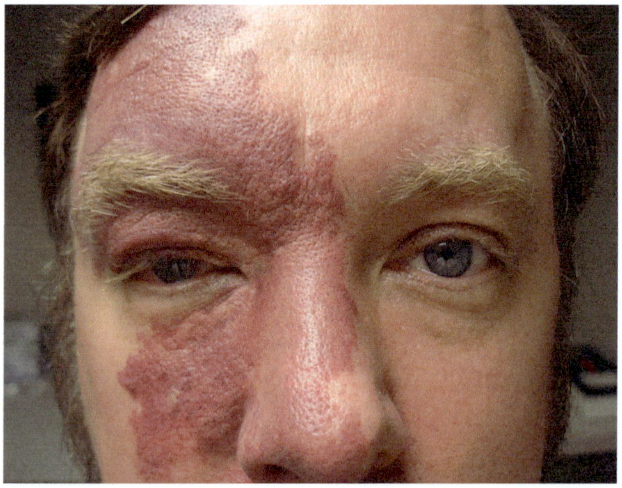

Fig. 15.4 Port-wine stain with associated ptosis. Courtesy of Bhupender C. Patel, MD Salt Lake City, Utah, USA

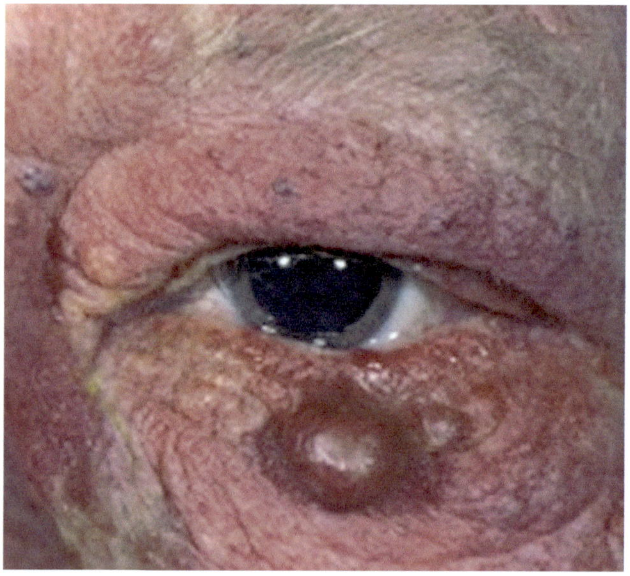

Fig. 15.5 Sturge-Weber syndrome. In addition to typical diffuse cutaneous involvement, note nodular hemangioma

In the setting of phakomatosis pigmentovascularis, port-wine stain can be associated with scleral and uveal hyperpigmentation, predisposing to uveal melanoma, similar to that observed in Nevus of Ota (Volume 5 Chap. 9).

Diagnosis of SWS is based on the typical clinical signs, facial appearance, and brain MRI with contrast findings [28]. In the absence of leptomeningeal involvement, patients should only be given a diagnosis of nevus flammeus, port-wine stain, or facial angioma to avoid the stigma associated with a diagnosis of SWS. In infants with nevus flammeus in the distribution of the trigeminal nerve, early referral to a pediatric neurologist is critical, considering that outcomes depend on prompt recognition of neurologic abnormalities and early seizure control [31]. There is no evidence that a pre-symptomatic Sturge-Weber syndrome diagnosis with magnetic resonance imaging results in better neurodevelopmental outcomes [31]. In SWS nevus flammeus, laser treatment should be performed early for better outcomes; however, its success depends on the location of the lesions. Lesions affecting the central forehead respond better than central facial lesions [32]. Unfortunately, lesions that are left untreated tend to thicken and get darker with time and, in some cases, become nodular [32].

15.4 Gardner Syndrome

Gardner syndrome was first described by Eldon J. Gardner in 1951 as a autosomal-dominant disorder characterized by the triad of multiple osteomas, colonic polyposis, and benign tumors of the skin and soft tissues [33]. Gardner syndrome is a variant of familial adenomatous polyposis caused by a mutation in the *APC* gene on chromosome 5q21 [33]. Extracolonic manifestations of Gardner syndrome include jaw anomalies, pigmented ocular fundus lesions that resemble congenital hypertrophy of the retinal pigment epithelium, soft tissue tumors, desmoid tumors, and other cancers [34, 35]. Orbital osteoma, soft tissue tumors of the brows or eyelids, and epidermoid cysts of the eyelid may also occur [36–38].

15.5 Nevoid Basal Cell Carcinoma Syndrome (Gorlin-Goltz Syndrome)

Nevoid basal cell carcinoma syndrome (NBCCS) is also referred to as basal cell nevus syndrome, Gorlin syndrome, or Gorlin-Goltz syndrome [39, 40]. Its incidence is estimated at 1 in 50,000 with no sex predilection. The median age at diagnosis is 23 years in sporadic cases and 12 years in familial cases [41].

NBCCS is inherited in an autosomal-dominant fashion with complete penetrance and variable expressivity; however, about 30% of probands have a de novo mutation [40]. The mutation is in the *PTCH* gene on chromosome 9q22.3 [42, 43]. *PTCH* sequence alterations can be detected in about 60–85% of cases that meet clinical diagnostic criteria for NBCCS [43]. Studies have shown that the *PTCH* gene may be inactivated by haploinsufficiency or through dominant-negative isoforms [44]. To date, approximately 448 unique *PTCH1* mutations are known [45]. Furthermore, mutations in the *SUFU* and *PTCH2* genes have been detected in patients with signs and symptoms of Gorlin syndrome and no *PTCH1* mutations [46, 47].

NBCCS is characterized by the classic clinical triad of multiple basal cell carcinomas, keratocystic odontogenic tumors and bifid ribs; however cutaneous, ophthalmic, and neurological abnormalities may also be present [48]. Associated neoplasms are medulloblastoma, astrocytoma, meningioma, and ovarian fibroma [48].

Although basal cell nevi may occur in early childhood, it is the risk for multiple basal cell carcinoma and developmental anomalies that characterizes NBCCS [49]. The tumors tend to be multiple (>5 in a lifetime) and occur before the age of 30 years. They may arise from preexisting basal cell nevi or de novo. In general, about 0.5% of patients with basal cell carcinoma have underlying NBCCS [50]. The proportion is much higher (22%) in patients with basal cell carcinoma developing before the age of 20 years [51]. White race, age, sun exposure, and radiation therapy are major risk factors for inducing basal cell carcinoma [52].

Jaw keratocysts and calcification of the falx cerebri are some of the most frequent (90%) manifestations of the NBCCS (Fig. 15.6) [49, 53]. Patients could be characterized by typical facial features that include forehead bossing and macrocephaly [53].

A wide variety of ophthalmic manifestations may be present in 26% of patients with NBCCS [49]. Periocular basal cell carcinoma [54, 55], hypertelorism, strabismus [56, 57], nystagmus, and cataracts are some of the common features (Fig. 11.2) [49, 54]. The occurrence of microphthalmia [58], coloboma, combined retinal and RPE hamartoma [59], and vitreoretinal abnormalities [60] in the setting of NBCCS implicates the *PTCH1* gene in ocular development [58, 60]. Other less common features include subconjunctival epidermoid cysts [61], congenital orbital teratoma [62], epiretinal membrane and myelinated nerve fibers [63], bilateral macular holes [64], orbital cysts, and congenital blindness [48].

Diagnosis is difficult because of the great phenotypic variation of this disease, with over 100 clinical manifestations in many major organs. Diagnosis is based on the presence of major and minor clinical and radiological criteria (Table 15.2) and confirmed by DNA analysis [49]. If there are no *PTCH1* mutations, testing of *SUFU* and *PTCH2* should be considered [41]. The best approach in the diagnosis and management of patients with NBCCS is multidisciplinary, in order to achieve a diagnosis and to optimize care.

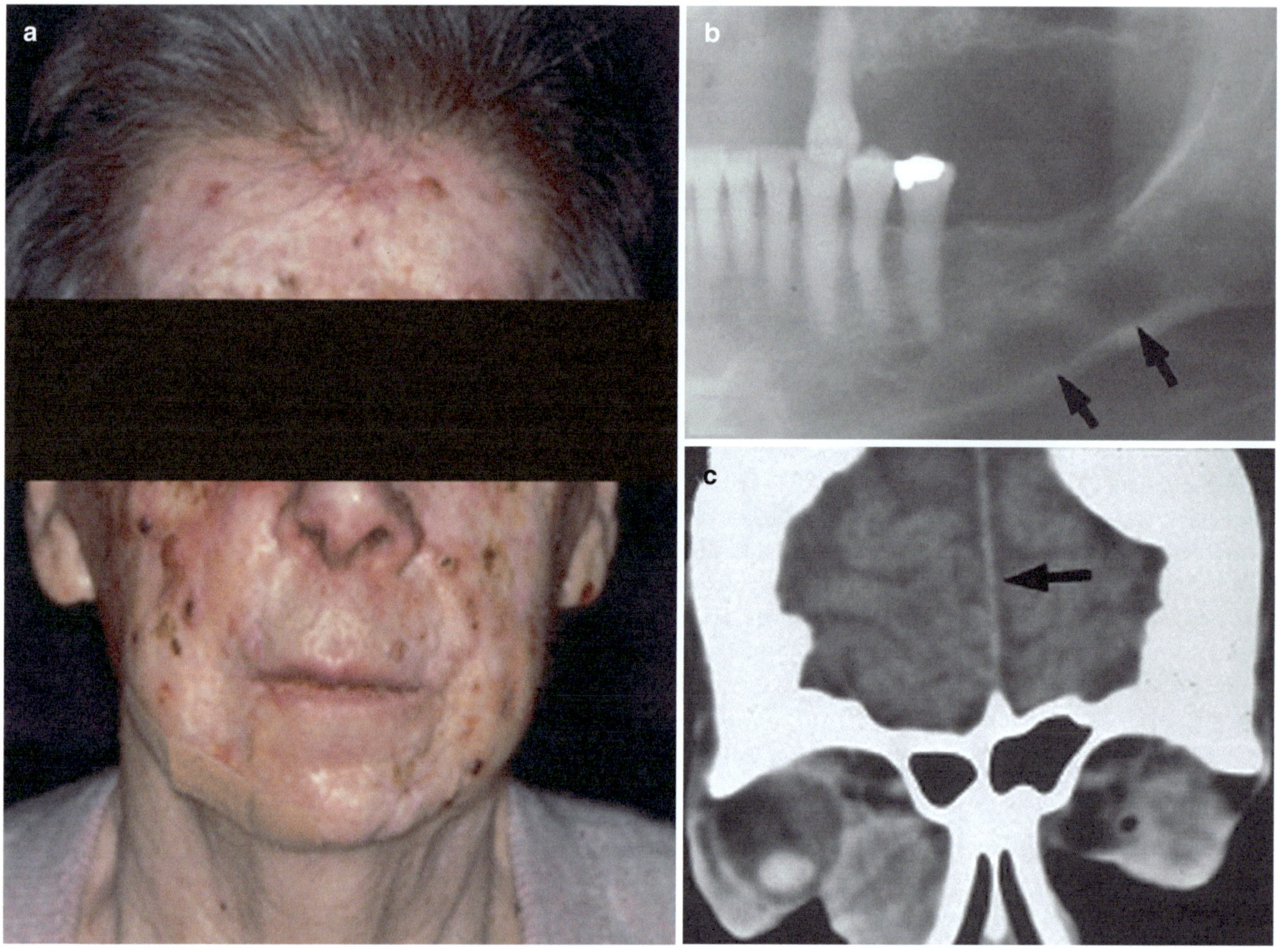

Fig. 15.6 External photograph showing multiple facial basal cell carcinoma (**a**). Orthopantomograph of the right mandible shows odontogenic keratocysts seen as *round*, well-circumscribed radiolucent areas (**b**, *arrows*). Coronal noncontrast computed tomography scan of the skull showing calcification of falx cerebri (*arrows*) and large diffuse lesion in the medial orbit (**c**). (Reprinted from Honavar et al. [54]. With permission from Elsevier)

Table 15.2 Clinical diagnostic criteria for nevoid basal cell nevus syndrome

Major criteria	≥2 major and ≥ 1 minor criteria	Jaw keratocyst
		Falx cerebri calcification
		Palmar or plantar pits
		Basal cell carcinoma >5 in a lifetime or before the age of 30 years
		Affected first-degree relative
Minor criteria	≥1 major and ≥3 minor criteria	Craniofacial anomalies
		Medulloblastoma
		Lympho-mesenteric or pleural cysts
		Cleft lip/palate
		Vertebral/rib anomalies
		Polydactyly
		Ovarian/cardiac fibromas
		Ocular anomalies

Based on data from Ref. [49]

Basal cell carcinoma is usually treated by surgical excision, with an overall success rate of 94–98% [65]. Other therapies are PDT, cryosurgery, and electrocauterization [66]. A recent alternative therapy is Vismodegib, a small-molecule inhibitor of the Hedgehog pathway. It is approved by the United States Food and Drug Administration (FDA) for the treatment of metastatic, and locally advanced basal cell carcinomas [67]. Treatment with Vismodegib reduces the tumor burden and prevents new basal cell carcinomas [67]. Sonidegib is another Hedgehog pathway inhibitor with FDA approval for use in adults with locally advanced recurrent basal cell carcinomas after radiation or surgery, and patients who cannot undergo surgery or radiation therapy [68]. Chemoprevention with isotretinoin can be used when existing lesions have been controlled [69].

Patients with NBCCS can have a normal life span if they have adequate multidisciplinary monitoring to check for medulloblastoma and invasive or metastatic BCC, which are the most common, albeit rare, causes of early mortality [70].

15.6 Multiple Hamartoma Syndrome (Cowden Syndrome)

Cowden syndrome was first described in 1963 [71]. Initially considered a predominantly dermatologic disease, the phenotypic spectrum has broadened to include increased cancer risk as well as neurodevelopmental disorders [72].

Cowden syndrome is inherited as an autosomal-dominant trait with 90–99% penetrance by the age of 30 years. Ten to 50% of individuals with Cowden syndrome have an affected parent [73]. It has generally been reported that 80% of patients with Cowden syndrome have detectable *PTEN* (*p*hosphatase and *ten*sin homolog) missense mutations [74]; however, in large cohorts, actual mutation rates are reported to occur in 30–35% of patients [75].

PTEN is a tumor suppressor gene located on chromosome 10 that codes for a lipid phosphatase in the PI3K/Akt pathway to arrest the cell in G1 phase and promote apoptosis, also acting as a protein phosphatase in the MAPK pathway that regulates cell survival [76]. *PTEN* has been hypothesized to play a role in cell migration and adhesion due to its homology to focal adhesion molecules such as tensin and auxilin [76]. As *PTEN* mutations are also present in closely related clinical entities, Cowden syndrome is now considered to be within the spectrum of the *PTEN* hamartoma tumor syndrome, which includes Bannayan-Riley-Ruvalcaba syndrome, Proteus syndrome, and Proteus-like syndrome [77].

As most tumors in this syndrome are hamartomatous malformations, it has also been referred to as multiple hamartoma syndrome [78].

Patients have greatly increased lifetime risks for breast, thyroid, renal, and endometrial cancers and slightly elevated risks for colorectal cancers and melanoma, without any recognized genotype-phenotype correlations [79].

Eyelid trichilemmomas are hallmark manifestation of Cowden syndrome (Fig. 15.7).

The tumors appear as multiple flesh-colored papular lesions of the eyelid [80]. One study found that complete PTEN loss, as determined by immunohistochemistry, occurs in 83% of trichilemmomas associated with Cowden syndrome, but only in 3% of sporadic trichilemmomas [81].

Several other ophthalmic features associated with Cowden syndrome and PTEN mutations have been described, such as anterior stromal and epithelial alterations in the cornea [82], iris mammillations [83], uveal ganglioneuroma [84], cataract [85], retinal angioma [86], choroidal pigmented schwannoma [87], proliferative retinopathy [88], and optic nerve head drusen [89].

In addition to the ophthalmic features, mucocutaneous lesions such as trichilemmomas, papillomatous papules, acral keratoses, and plantar keratoses are most striking manifestations of Cowden syndrome. More significantly, this syndrome has been found to be associated with a lifetime increased risk for breast tumors (benign 67%, malignant 25–50%) [90], thyroid tumors (benign 75%, malignant 10%) [91], and uterine tumors (benign fibroids and malignant 10%). Other uncommon hamartomatous manifestations include gastrointestinal polyps and cerebellar dysplastic gangliocytoma (Lhermitte-Duclos disease) [77].

The National Comprehensive Cancer Network (NCCN) propose clinical diagnostic criteria for Cowden syndrome/PTEN Hamartoma Tumor Syndrome (PHTS) based on Pilarski et al. criteria (Table 15.3) [75], with a substantial improvement in the specificity of these criteria. Thanks to the Cleveland Clinic PTEN Risk Calculation tool, it is now possible to calculate the percentage risk for PTEN mutation

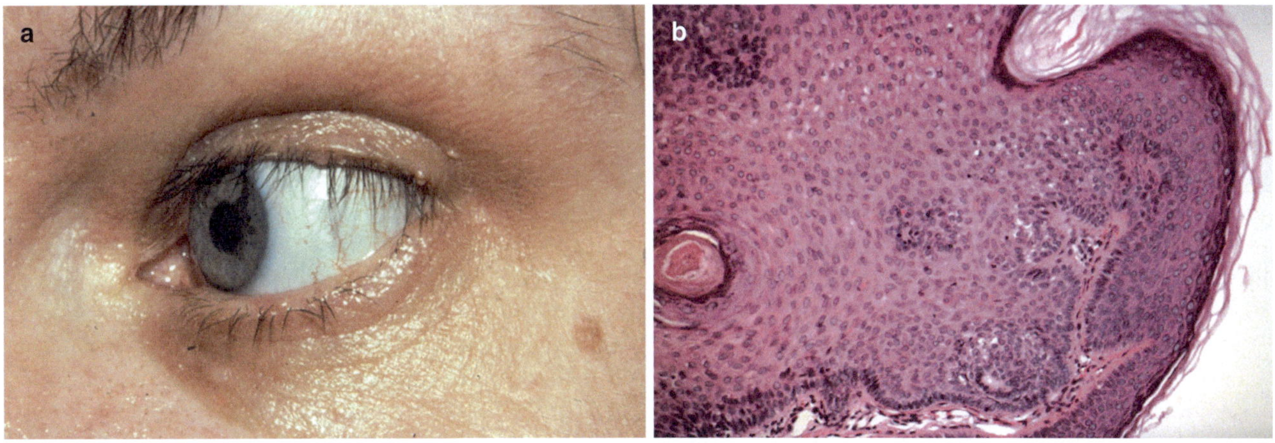

Fig. 15.7 Clinical photograph of flesh-colored papular lesions at the eyelid margin (**a**). High-power photomicrograph of trichilemmoma with basal palisading and bland-looking cells with more cytoplasm than basal cell carcinoma cells (**b**, H&E original magnification ×200). (Reprinted from Bardenstein et al. [80]. With permission from Elsevier)

Table 15.3 Revised PTENhamartomatumor syndrome clinical diagnostic criteria

Operational diagnosis in an individual (either of the following) 1. Three or more major criteria, but one must include macrocephaly, Lhermitte-Duclos disease, or gastrointestinal hamartomas 2. Two major and three minor criteria	
Operational diagnosis in a family where one individual meets revised PTEN hamartoma tumor syndrome clinical diagnostic criteria or has a PTEN mutation: 1. Any two major criteria with or without minor criteria 2. One major and two minor criteria 3. Three minor criteria	
Major	Breast cancer
	Endometrial cancer (epithelial)
	Thyroid cancer (follicular)
	Multiple gastrointestinal hamartomas or ganglioneuromas
	Lhermitte-Duclos disease (adult)
	Macrocephaly (≥58 cm in adult women, ≥60 cm in adult men)
	Macular pigmentation of the glans penis
	Mucocutaneous lesions (any of the following): Multiple trichilemmomas (≥3, at least one biopsy proven) Acral keratoses (≥3 palmoplantar keratotic pits and/or acral hyperkeratotic papules) Mucocutaneous neuromas (≥3) Oral papillomas (particularly on the tongue and gingiva), multiple (≥3) OR biopsy proben OR dermatologist diagnosed
Minor	Autism spectrum disorder
	Colon cancer
	Esophageal glycogenic acanthosis (≥3)
	Lipomas (≥3)
	Intellectual disability (i.e., IQ ≤ 75)
	Renal cell carcinoma
	Testicular lipomatosis
	Thyroid cancer (papillary or follicular variant of papillary)
	Thyroid structural lesions (e.g., adenoma, multinodular goiter)
	Vascular anomalies (including multiple intracranial developmental venous anomalies)

Based on data from Ref. [75]

and then decide whether or not to refer the patient for PTEN testing/genetics [92]. This tool is freely available online at http://www.lerner.ccf.org/gmi/ccscore/. It weights score for each patient's characteristic in order to help decide whether to recommend a genetic test.

The presence of three or more trichilemmomas, among other mucocutaneous manifestations, should raise a strong suspicion of Cowden syndrome [75].

The management of Cowden syndrome consists of surveillance for early cancer detection and treatment in the hope of improving survival. All patients should undergo an annual thyroid ultrasound scan and dermatologic evaluation. Women should receive an annual mammogram and breast MRI from the age of 30 years, along with annual transvaginal ultrasound and blind suction endometrial biopsies, while prophylactic mastectomy or prophylactic hysterectomy may also be considered after appropriate counseling. All adults with CS should have a colonoscopy beginning at the age of 35 years and renal imaging every 2 years, beginning at the age of 40 years [93].

15.7 Carney Complex

Carney complex (CNC) is a multiple neoplasia syndrome characterized by cutaneous pigmentary abnormalities, myxomas, endocrine tumors, and schwannomas [94, 95]. It has also been designated by descriptive acronyms such as NAME syndrome (nevi, atrial myxomas, ephelides) and LAMB syndrome (lentigines, atrial myxoma, blue nevi). Carney complex should be differentiated from a completely unrelated entity "Carney triad," which refers to gastric leiomyosarcoma, pulmonary chondroma, and extra-adrenal paraganglioma [96].

Carney complex is inherited as an autosomal-dominant trait [97]. In about 30% of patients, the disease is due to de novo mutations. It is a genetically heterogeneous disease, with >70% patients with CNC carrying mutations of the *PRKAR1A* gene [98], which encodes the 1-α regulatory subunit of the cAMP-dependent protein kinase A and functions as a tumor suppressor gene [99]. Pathogenic *PRKAR1A* mutations include single base substitutions, small (≤15bp) deletions/insertions, combined rearrangements, and large deletions [100]. One hundred forty different *PRKAR1A* gene mutations have been registered at the CNC consortium database; however, linking genotype to phenotype has been challenging [101]. Although previous studies have demonstrated associations between specific mutations and CNC manifestations, only 3 pathogenic variants (c.82C>T, c.491_492delTG, and c.709–2_709–7 delATTTTT) have been identified in >3 unrelated pedigrees [98]. The other mutations are unique (i.e., present in a single kindred) [102]. Mutations in *PRKAR1A* appear to be the most common cause of CNC. Patients carrying *PRKAR1A* mutations have more severe disease, with earlier presentation and higher frequency of myxomas, thyroid, and gonadal tumors, schwannomas, and lentigines compared with *PRKAR1A*-negative patients [98]. However, in most cases, genotype cannot predict phenotype or penetrance [102].

Periocular involvement is frequent, both by pigmentary changes [103] and myxomas [104]. In a study of 63 patients, facial and eyelid lentigines were observed in 70%, conjunctival andcaruncular pigmentation in 27%, and eyelid myxomas in 16% of the patients (Fig. 15.8) [104]. Other ocular lesions seen are conjunctival myxoma [105], Also, uveal melanoma associated with CNC were reported [106]. Lentigines typically involve the centrofacial area, including

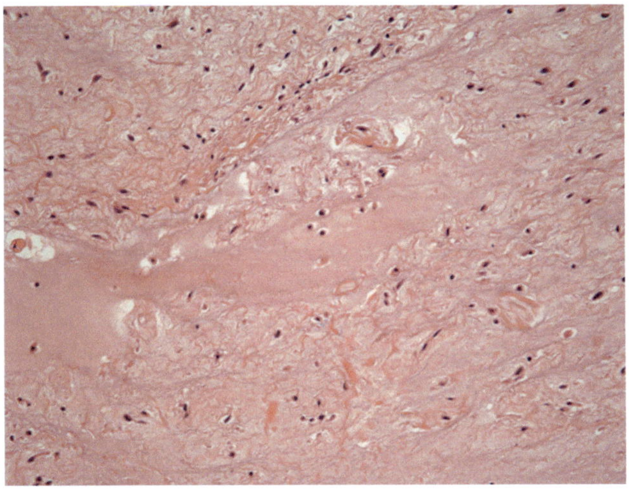

Fig. 15.8 Eyelid myxoma in a patient with Carney complex. Hypocellular myxomatous mass composed of ground substance and collagen fibers (H&E original magnification ×200). (Courtesy of Ralph C. Eagle Jr., MD)

the lips, and the conjunctiva [107]. Cutaneous myxomas are usually less than 1 cm in diameter and often affect the eyelids, ears, and nipples but can also be seen on other areas of the face, ears, trunk, and perineum [107]. Myxomas are typically diagnosed during the teenage years and appear as sessile, small papules and large, fingerlike, pedunculated lesions [107].

The median age at diagnosis is 20 years. Cutaneous pigmentary abnormalities are the most common presenting feature. The brown or black lentigines may be present anywhere in the body and become prominent during puberty. The most common non-cutaneous lesions in CNC are cardiac myxomas (affecting 20–40% of patients), which are responsible for >50% of CNC-related mortality [108]. Although cardiac myxomas are typical, myxomas may occur in the skin and other sites. Endocrine tumors and hormonal hypersecretion may manifest as thyroid adenoma (75%), Sertoli cell tumors (33%) in males, Cushing syndrome (25%), and acromegaly (10%) [95]. Psammomatous melanotic schwannoma, a rare variant of schwannoma, is also a manifestation of Carney complex [109].

The diagnosis of CNC is made if two of the main manifestations of the syndrome are present (Table 15.4); these need to be confirmed by histology, biochemical testing, or imaging; alternatively, the diagnosis is made when one of the criteria is present and the patient is a carrier of a known inactivating mutation of the *PRKAR1A* gene [95]. Clinical and biochemical screening for CNC remain the gold standard for the diagnosis of CNC. Molecular testing for *PRKAR1A* mutations is not recommended at present for all patients with CNC, but in families with known mutations may be useful for detecting affected patients and avoiding unnecessary medical surveillance of non-carriers [110].

Table 15.4 Clinical diagnostic criteria for Carney complex

Disease manifestation	Any ≥2 present	Spotty skin pigmentation with a typical distribution (lips, conjunctiva and inner or outer canthi, vaginal and penile mucosa)
		Myxoma (cutaneous and mucosal)
		Cardiac myxoma
		Breast myxomatosis or fat-suppressed magnetic resonance imaging findings suggestive of this diagnosis
		Primary pigmented nodular adrenocortical disease or paradoxical positive response of urinary glucocorticosteroids to dexamethasone administration during Liddle's test
		Acromegaly due to growth hormone-producing adenoma
		Large-cell calcifying Sertoli cell tumor or characteristic calcification on testicular ultrasonography
		Thyroid carcinoma or multiple, hypoechoic nodules on thyroid ultrasonography
		Psammomatous melanotic schwannoma
		Blue nevus, epithelioid blue nevus (multiple)
		Breast ductal adenoma (multiple)
		Osteochondromyxoma of bone
Supplemental manifestation	≥1 Disease manifestation	Affected first-degree relative
	≥1 Disease manifestation	Inactivating mutation of the PRKAR1A gene

Based on data from Ref. [95]

Considering that Carney reported that more than 50% of patients have a significant embolic event in their lifetime related to cardiac myxomas and that the ophthalmic manifestations have been shown to precede embolic events, early identification of ocular myxomas and subsequent screening and monitoring for cardiac myxoma is recommended [111].

15.8 Muir-Torre Syndrome

Muir-Torre syndrome is a rare cancer-predisposition syndrome characterized by unusual cutaneous tumors and internal malignancy [112]. It is considered to be a subset of the hereditary nonpolyposis colorectal cancer (HNPCC) or Lynch syndrome [113]. The cutaneous tumors associated with Muir-Torre syndrome include mainly sebaceous gland neoplasms (sebaceous adenoma and sebaceous carcinoma), keratoacanthoma, and basal cell carcinoma [114]. The internal malignancies include upper gastrointestinal, colorectal, endometrial, and urological tumors [115], but in rare cases glioblastoma multiforme has been described [116].

MTS is seen in about 9% of individuals with HNPCC, mainly in Caucasian and men [117]. Malignant tumors appear between 23 and 89 years of age [118]. Although Muir-Torre syndrome is characterized by autosomal-dominant inheritance, sporadic cases do occur.

Similar to HNPCC, the majority of MTS cases result from highly penetrant but variably expressed germline mutations in the *MSH2* and *MLH1* genes, though a disease variant without mismatch repair (*MMR*) gene defects has also been described [119]. Ninety percent of MTS patients have mutations in *MSH2*, but rare cases with mutations in *MSH6*, *PMS22*, or *MLH3* have been described [117].

Sebaceous neoplasms, such as adenomas, epitheliomas, and carcinomas, are reported to be so rare that finding one of these tumors should alert the clinician to the possibility of Muir–Torre syndrome [120]. Solitary or multiple sebaceous adenomas are uncommon. They are benign, yellow flesh-colored nodular tumors, approximately 0.5 cm in diameter, which occasionally ulcerate or bleed, and which grow slowly in older individuals, typically on the face (Fig. 15.9) [114, 121]. The Meibomian and Zeis glands of the eyelids are modified sebaceous glands and can also be the site of origin of sebaceous adenomas [122]. Cystic change within a sebaceous adenoma is indicative of Muir-Torre syndrome because sporadic sebaceous adenomas do not exhibit this feature [123].

Sebaceous epitheliomas are benign, yellowish papulonodules, usually present on the face and scalp, with similar appearance, localization, and age incidence as basal cell carcinomas [121]. They grow slowly and tend not to recur after treatment [121].

Sebaceous carcinomas, occasionally associated with MTS, may arise in the ocular adnexa or at extraocular sites. They clinically appear as painful red nodules, often on the upper eyelid, and may be mistaken for an inflammatory condition, such as chalazion or blepharoconjunctivitis, resulting in a delay in diagnosis [124]. Tumors occurring in the ocular adnexa are more common and account for 1% of all eyelid neoplasms, while extraocular tumors are uncommon and usually located in the head-and-neck region [121]. Although sebaceous gland carcinomas of the eyelid and extraocular sites [125] have been reported in patients with Muir-Torre syndrome, such patients also had sebaceous adenomas [126].

Rarely, keratoacanthomas may be associated with MTS. They are flesh-colored, rapidly growing, dome-shaped nodules with a central keratin plug. They may cause local destruction, especially if they are on the eyelids, and they tend to involute spontaneously after several months [121]. One case of intraductal papilloma of a meibomian gland possibly associated with MSH6 subtype has been reported [127].

In a review of 120 patients with Muir-Torre syndrome, sebaceous tumors were diagnosed prior to the internal malignancy in almost 40% of patients [114]. Almost half of the patients with Muir-Torre syndrome develop colorectal adenocarcinoma and one-fourth develop genitourinary tumors. Adenocarcinoma of the colon in the setting of Muir-Torre syndrome tends to be multifocal and occurs almost a decade earlier than in sporadic cases [114]. In addition, the proximal colon is more often affected as compared with unifocal involvement of the distal colon in sporadic cases [128]. There are significant variations in the phenotypic manifestations of Muir-Torre syndrome, which in some individuals may resemble those of hereditary nonpolyposis colorectal carcinoma [129].

MTS is rarely encountered by ophthalmologists, who may not consider the systemic implications of certain periocular skin tumors. Importantly, these tumors present commonly on the face, and ophthalmologists may receive referrals of patients with these lesions in the periocular region [121]. Of the defining skin lesions, sebaceous adenomas and epitheliomas are the most sensitive markers of the syndrome, whereas sebaceous carcinomas and keratoacanthomas are much less frequently associated [121].

The clinical diagnostic criteria are known as Amsterdam criteria and the Bethesda guidelines, the latter being more sensitive; these are used also for the diagnosis of hereditary non-polyposis colorectal cancer [130, 131]. Additional microsatellite instability testing or germline mutation analysis is recommended if all of the Amsterdam criteria or one of the Bethesda guidelines is met [130, 131]. The Mayo MTS risk scoring algorithm may be used to identify patients who should undergo further germline genetic testing [132]. Management is based on screening recommendations and a surveillance program of patients with MTS and their first-degree relatives (Table 15.5) [133].

Managing cutaneous MTS is challenging because patients present with multiple and disfiguring tumors. Aggressive surgical treatment usually provides a good outcome with prolonged survival, even in the presence of metastases [124]. Sebaceous adenomas and sebaceous epitheliomas are either excised or treated with cryotherapy. Sebaceous carcinomas should be widely excised. Keratoacanthomas are best treated with excision [121]. Radiation can be considered for recurrence or local metastasis, as can 5-fluorouracil and cisplatin combination chemotherapy [134].

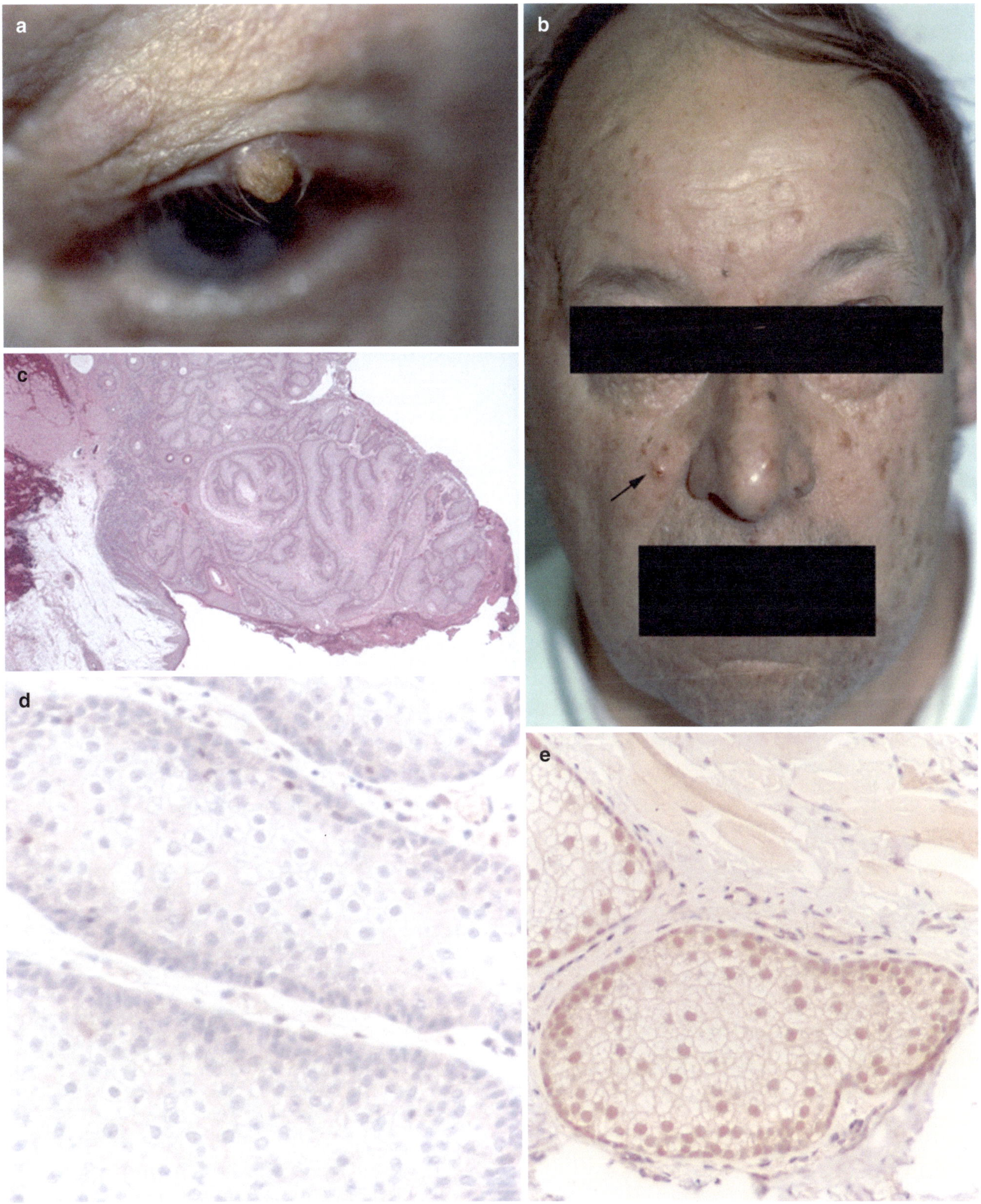

Fig. 15.9 Sebaceous adenomas on the face in a patient with Muir-Torre syndrome. Note a *yellowish pink* warty growth arising from anterior lamella of the left upper eyelid (**a**). Multiple *yellow* nodular lesions involving the central forehead, nose, and adjacent cheek area (**b**). Both eyelid and facial biopsies revealed sebaceous adenomas (**c**, original magnification ×10). Immunohistochemical staining with an antibody to MSH-2 protein was absent in the sebaceous adenoma (**d**, magnification ×50). Normal positive nuclear staining of sebaceous lobules adjacent to the sebaceous adenoma serves as an internal control (**e**, magnification ×50). (Reprinted from Singh et al. [122]. With permission from American Medical Association)

Table 15.5 Screening recommendations for patients with Muir-Torre syndrome and their first-degree relatives

Physical examination yearly including breast examination in women, testicular and prostate examination in men, and laboratory tests including full blood cell count, carbohydrate antigen 125, carcinoembryonic antigen, fecal occult blood, and urinalysis
Colonoscopy every 1–2 years from age 25 years or at 5 years before the youngest age at diagnosis of colorectal cancer in family and annually from age 40 years
Pelvic examination annually in women with transvaginal ultrasonographic scan and endometrial biopsy in patients with a gene mutation, from age 25 years
Consider prophylactic colectomy in patients with a gene mutation
Consider gastroscopy every 1–2 years in families with a history of gastric cancer
Consider renal ultrasonographic scan every 1–2 years in families with a history of renal tract cancer

Based on data from Ref. [133]

References

1. Ponder B. Inherited cancer syndromes. In: Carney D, Sikora K, editors. Genes and cancer, vol. 99. New York: John Wiley & Sons; 1990. p. 106.
2. Bianciotto C, Demirci H, Shields CL, Eagle RC, Shields JA. Metastatic tumors to the eyelid: report of 20 cases and review of the literature. Arch Ophthalmol. 2009;127(8):999–1005.
3. Boyd KP, Korf BR, Theos A. Neurofibromatosis type 1. J Am Acad Dermatol. 2009;61(1):1–14.
4. Avery RA, Katowitz JA, Fisher MJ, Heidary G, Dombi E, Packer RJ. Orbital/periorbital plexiform neurofibromas in children with neurofibromatosis type 1: multidisciplinary recommendations for care. Ophthalmology. 2017;124(1):123–32.
5. Zhang ML, Suarez MJ, Bosley TM, Rodriguez FJ. Clinicopathological features of peripheral nerve sheath tumors involving the eye and ocular adnexa. Hum Pathol. 2017;63:70–8.
6. Pai HV, Abbagani S, Jaishankar PP. Isolated neurofibroma of the eyelid mimicking recurrent chalazion. Indian J Ophthalmol. 2018;66(3):451–3.
7. Chen N, Hsu Y-H, Lee Y-C. Solitary neurofibroma of eyelid masquerading as chalazion. Int Med Case Rep J. 2017;10:177–9.
8. Savar A, Cestari DM. Neurofibromatosis type I: genetics and clinical manifestations. Semin Ophthalmol. 2008;23(1):45–51.
9. Jain G, Jain VK, Sharma IK, Sharma R, Saraswat N. Neurofibromatosis type 1 presenting with ophthalmic features: a case series. J Clin Diagn Res. 2016;10(11):SR01–3.
10. Hirbe AC, Gutmann DH. Neurofibromatosis type 1: a multidisciplinary approach to care. Lancet Neurol. 2014;13(8):834–43.
11. Avery RA, Dombi E, Hutcheson KA, Acosta MT, Baldwin AM, Madigan WP. Visual outcomes in children with neurofibromatosis type 1 and orbitotemporal plexiform neurofibromas. Am J Ophthalmol. 2013;155(6):1089–94.e1
12. Altan-Yaycioglu R, Hintschich C. Clinical features and surgical management of orbitotemporal neurofibromatosis: a retrospective interventional case series. Orbit. 2010;29(5):232–8.
13. Gandhi NG. Treatment of neuro-ophthalmic and orbitofacial manifestations of neurofibromatosis type 1. Curr Opin Ophthalmol. 2013;24(5):506–11.
14. Rasmussen SA, Yang Q, Friedman JM. Mortality in neurofibromatosis 1: an analysis using U.S. death certificates. Am J Hum Genet. 2001;68(5):1110–8.
15. Higham CS, Dombi E, Rogiers A, et al. The characteristics of 76 atypical neurofibromas as precursors to neurofibromatosis 1 associated malignant peripheral nerve sheath tumors. Neuro-Oncology. 2018;20:818–25.
16. Kehrer-Sawatzki H, Vogt J, Mußotter T, Kluwe L, Cooper DN, Mautner V-F. Dissecting the clinical phenotype associated with mosaic type-2 NF1 microdeletions. Neurogenetics. 2012;13(3):229–36.
17. Nguyen R, Jett K, Harris GJ, Cai W, Friedman JM, Mautner V-F. Benign whole body tumor volume is a risk factor for malignant peripheral nerve sheath tumors in neurofibromatosis type 1. J Neuro-Oncol. 2014;116(2):307–13.
18. Gross AM, Wolters PL, Eva D, Andrea B, Patricia W, Fisher MJ, Brian W, AeRang K, Miriam B, Shah AC, Staci M, Roderick MC, Pichard DC, Amanda C, Paul SM, Janet T, Oxana K, Kara H, Wade CD, Chi Z, Peer CJ, Figg WD, Malcolm S, John G, Blakeley JO, Steinberg SM, Venzon DJ, Austin DL, Widemann BC. Selumetinib in children with inoperable plexiform neurofibromas. N Engl J Med. 382(15):1430–42. https://doi.org/10.1056/NEJMoa1912735.
19. Lee JW, Chung HY. Capillary malformations (Portwine stains) of the head and neck. Otolaryngol Clin N Am. 2018;51(1):197–211.
20. Vi N, Marcelo H, Mihm MC, Stuart NJ, Wenbin T. The pathogenesis of port wine stain and Sturge weber syndrome: complex interactions between genetic alterations and aberrant MAPK and PI3K activation. Int J Mol Sci. 2019;20(9):2243. https://doi.org/10.3390/ijms20092243.
21. Shirley MD, Tang H, Gallione CJ, Baugher JD, Frelin LP, Cohen B. Sturge–Weber syndrome and port-wine stains caused by somatic mutation in *GNAQ*. N Engl J Med. 2013;368(21):1971–9.
22. Frigerio A, Wright K, Wooderchak-Donahue W, Tan OT, Margraf R, Stevenson DA. Genetic variants associated with port-wine stains. Rieux-Laucat F, editor. PLoS One. 2015;10(7):e0133158.
23. Yadav P, De Castro DK, Waner M, Meyer L, Fay A. Vascular anomalies of the head and neck: a review of genetics. Semin Ophthalmol. 2013;28(5–6) 257, 266
24. Sivarajan V, Maclaren WM, Mackay IR. The effect of varying pulse duration, wavelength, spot size, and fluence on the response of previously treated capillary vascular malformations to pulsed-dye laser treatment. Ann Plast Surg. 2006;57(1):25–32.
25. Thomson J, Greig A, Lloyd C, Morrison D, Flohr C. PHACE syndrome misdiagnosed as a port-wine stain. BMJ Case Rep. 2015, 2015:bcr2015209889.
26. Haggstrom AN, Lammer EJ, Schneider RA, Marcucio R, Frieden IJ. Patterns of infantile hemangiomas: new clues to hemangioma pathogenesis and embryonic facial development. Pediatrics. 2006;117(3):698–703.
27. Tallman B, Tan OT, Morelli JG, Piepenbrink J, Stafford TJ, Trainor S. Location of port-wine stains and the likelihood of ophthalmic and/or central nervous system complications. Pediatrics. 1991;87(3):323–7.
28. Singh AK, Keenaghan M. Sturge-Weber syndrome. [updated 2018 Oct 27]. In: StatPearls [internet]. Treasure Island, FL: StatPearls Publishing; 2018. Available from: https://www.ncbi.nlm.nih.gov/books/NBK459163/.
29. Dymerska M, Kirkorian AY, Offermann EA, Lin DD, Comi AM, Cohen BA. Size of facial port-wine birthmark may predict neurologic outcome in Sturge-weber syndrome. J Pediatr. 2017;188:205.e1–9.e1.
30. Pascual-Castroviejo I, Pascual-Pascual S-I, Velazquez-Fragua R, Viaño J. Sturge-weber syndrome: study of 55 patients. Can J Neurol Sci. 2008;35(3):301–7.
31. Zallmann M, Leventer RJ, Mackay MT, Ditchfield M, Bekhor PS, Su JC. Screening for Sturge-weber syndrome: a state-of-the-art review. Pediatr Dermatol. 2018;35(1):30–42.
32. Abdolrahimzadeh S, Scavella V, Felli L, Cruciani F, Contestabile MT, Recupero SM. Ophthalmic alterations in the Sturge-weber syndrome, Klippel-Trenaunay syndrome, and the Phakomatosis

Pigmentovascularis: an independent Group of Conditions? Biomed Res Int. 2015;2015:786519.
33. Panjwani S, Bagewadi A, Keluskar V, Arora S. Gardner's syndrome. J Clin Imaging Sci. 2011;1(1):65.
34. Blair NP, Trempe CL. Hypertrophy of the retinal pigment epithelium associated with Gardner's syndrome. Am J Ophthalmol. 1980;90(5):661–7.
35. Gardner EJ, Richards RC. Multiple cutaneous and subcutaneous lesions occurring simultaneously with hereditary polyposis and osteomatosis. Am J Hum Genet. 1953;5(2):139–47. Available from: http://www.ncbi.nlm.nih.gov/pmc/articles/PMC1716470/
36. Gardner EJ. Follow-up study of a family group exhibiting dominant inheritance for a syndrome including intestinal polyps, osteomas, fibromas and epidermal cysts. Am J Hum Genet. 1962;14(376):390.
37. Whitson WE, Orcutt JC, Walkinshaw MD. Orbital osteoma in Gardner's syndrome. Am J Ophthalmol. 1986;101(2):236–41.
38. Lewis RA, Crowder WE, Eierman LA, Nussbaum RL, Ferrell RE. The Gardner syndrome. Significance of ocular features. Ophthalmology. 1984;91(8):916–25.
39. Gorlin RJ, Goltz RW. Multiple nevoid basal-cell epithelioma, jaw cysts and bifid rib. N Engl J Med. 1960;262(18):908–12.
40. Gorlin RJ. Nevoid basal cell carcinoma (Gorlin) syndrome. Genet Med. 2004;6(6):530–9.
41. Akbari DMDM, Chen H, Guo G, et al. Basal cell nevus syndrome (Gorlin syndrome): genetic insights, diagnostic challenges, and unmet milestones. Pathophysiology. 2017;25:77–82.
42. Farndon PA, Mastro Del RG, Evans DG, Kilpatrick MW. Location of gene for Gorlin syndrome. Lancet. 1992;339(8793):581–2.
43. Hahn H, Wicking C, Zaphiropoulous PG, Gailani MR, Shanley S, Chidambaram A. Mutations of the human homolog of drosophila patched in the nevoid basal cell carcinoma syndrome. Cell. 1996;85(6):841–51.
44. Pan S, Dong Q, Sun L-S, Li T-J. Mechanisms of inactivation of PTCH1 gene in nevoid basal cell carcinoma syndrome: modification of the two-hit hypothesis. Clin Cancer Res. 2010;16(2):442–50.
45. Reinders MG, van Hout AF, Cosgun B, Paulussen AD, Leter EM, Steijlen PM. New mutations and an updated database for the patched-1 (*PTCH1*) gene. Mol Genet Genomic Med. 2018;6:409–15.
46. Fan Z, Li J, Du J, Zhang H, Shen Y, Wang C-Y. A missense mutation in PTCH2 underlies dominantly inherited NBCCS in a Chinese family. J Med Genet. 2008;45(5):303–8.
47. Pastorino L, Ghiorzo P, Nasti S, Battistuzzi L, Cusano R, Marzocchi C. Identification of a *SUFU* germline mutation in a family with Gorlin syndrome. Am J Med Genet A. 2009;149A(7):1539–43.
48. Rouhani B, Ramasubramanian A. Pediatric genetic ocular tumors. J Pediatr Genet. 2014;3(259):–269.
49. Evans DG, Ladusans EJ, Rimmer S, Burnell LD, Thakker N, Farndon PA. Complications of the naevoid basal cell carcinoma syndrome: results of a population based study. J Med Genet. 1993;30(6):460–4.
50. Springate JE. The nevoid basal cell carcinoma syndrome. J Pediatr Surg. 1986;21(10):908–10.
51. Rahbari H, Mehregan AH. Basal cell epithelioma (carcinoma) in children and teenagers. Cancer. 1982;49(2):350–3.
52. Solis DC, Kwon GP, Ransohoff KJ, Li S, Chahal HS, Ally MS. Risk factors for basal cell carcinoma among patients with basal cell nevus syndrome. JAMA Dermatol. 2017;153(2):189.
53. Shanley S, Ratcliffe J, Hockey A, Haan E, Oley C, Ravine D. Nevoid basal cell carcinoma syndrome: review of 118 affected individuals. Am J Med Genet. 1994;50(3):282–90.
54. Honavar SG, Shields JA, Shields CL, Eagle RC, Demirci H, Mahmood EZ. Basal cell carcinoma of the eyelid associated with Gorlin-Goltz syndrome. Ophthalmology. 2001;108(6):1115–23.
55. Nerad JA, Whitaker DC. Periocular basal cell carcinoma in adults 35 years of age and younger. Am J Ophthalmol. 1988;106(6):723–9.
56. Knowlton PB, Mawn LA, Atkinson JB, Donahue SP. Strabismus resulting from an anomalous extraocular muscle in Gorlin syndrome. J AAPOS. 2014;18(5):495–8.
57. Shripadh C, Jineet P, Shravan R, Christopher L, Jennifer R, Kayla K, Kimberly S, Natario C. Nevoid basal cell carcinoma syndrome: a case report and literature review. Ophthalmic Genet. 43(1):27–35. https://doi.org/10.1080/13816810.2021.1983847.
58. Ragge NK, Salt A, Collin JRO, Michalski A, Farndon PA. Gorlin syndrome: the PTCH gene links ocular developmental defects and tumour formation. Br J Ophthalmol. 2005;89(8):988–91.
59. Sánchez-Vicente JL, Contreras-Díaz M, Rueda T, Rodríguez E, de la Rúa-Franch FE, Molina-Socola, Vital-Berral C. Combined hamartoma of the retina and retinal pigment epithelium in a patient with Gorlin syndrome: spontaneous partial resolution of traction caused by epiretinal membrane. Case Rep Ophthalmol Med. 2016;2016(1):5.
60. Black GCM, Mazerolle CJ, Wang Y, Campsall KD, Petrin D, Leonard BC. Abnormalities of the vitreoretinal interface caused by dysregulated hedgehog signaling during retinal development. Hum Mol Genet. 2003;12(24):3269–76.
61. Craene De S, Batteauw A, Lint Van M, Claerhout I, Decock C. Subconjunctival epidermoid cysts in Gorlin-Goltz syndrome. Orbit. 2014;33(4):280–2.
62. Rodrigues AL, Carvalho A, Cabral R, Carneiro V, Gilardi P, Duarte CP. Case report multiple nevoid basal cell carcinoma syndrome associated with congenital orbital teratoma, caused by a PTCH1 frameshift mutation. Genet Mol Res. 2014;13(3):5654–63.
63. Farley ND, Sassalos TM, Ober MD. Basal cell nevus syndrome presenting as epiretinal membrane and myelinated nerve fiber layer. Retin Cases Brief Rep. 2017;11:S151–4.
64. Romano M, Lacovello D, Cascone NC, Contestabile MT. Identification of a novel mutation in the PTCH gene in a patient with Gorlin-Goltz syndrome with unusual ocular disorders. Eur J Ophthalmol. 2011;21(4):516–9.
65. Yin VT, Pfeiffer ML, Esmaeli B. Targeted therapy for orbital and periocular basal cell carcinoma and squamous cell carcinoma. Ophthalmic Plast Reconstr Surg. 2013;29(2):87–92.
66. Chen JJ, Sartori J, Aakalu VK, Setabutr P. Review of ocular manifestations of nevoid basal cell carcinoma syndrome: what an ophthalmologist needs to know. Middle East Afr J Ophthalmol. 2015;22(4):421–7.
67. Tang JY, Ally MS, Chanana AM, Mackay-Wiggan JM, Aszterbaum M, Lindgren JA. Inhibition of the hedgehog pathway in patients with basal-cell nevus syndrome: final results from the multicentre, randomised, double-blind, placebo-controlled, phase 2 trial. Lancet Oncol. 2016;17(12):1720–31.
68. Jain S, Song R, Xie J. Sonidegib: mechanism of action, pharmacology, and clinical utility for advanced basal cell carcinomas. Onco Targets Ther. 2017;10:1645–53.
69. Bettoli V, Zauli S, Virgili A. Retinoids in the chemoprevention of non-melanoma skin cancers: why, when and how. J Dermatolog Treat. 2013;24(3):235–7.
70. Figueira JA, de Batista FRS, Rosso K, Veltrini VC, Pavan AJ. Delayed diagnosis of Gorlin–Goltz syndrome. J Craniofac Surg. 2018;29:e530.
71. Lloyd KM, Dennis M. Cowden's disease. A possible new symptom complex with multiple system involvement. Ann Intern Med. 1963;58(136):142.
72. Mester J, Eng C. Cowden syndrome: recognizing and managing a not-so-rare hereditary cancer syndrome. J Surg Oncol. 2015;111(1):125–30.
73. Schrager CA, Schneider D, Gruener AC, Tsou HC, Peacocke M. Clinical and pathological features of breast disease in Cowden's

syndrome: an underrecognized syndrome with an increased risk of breast cancer. Hum Pathol. 1998;29(1):47–53.
74. Liaw D, Marsh DJ, Li J, Dahia PLM, Wang SI, Zheng Z. Germline mutations of the PTEN gene in Cowden disease, an inherited breast and thyroid cancer syndrome. Nat Genet. 1997;16(1):64–7.
75. Pilarski R, Burt R, Kohlman W, Pho L, Shannon KM, Swisher E. Cowden syndrome and the PTEN hamartoma tumor syndrome: systematic review and revised diagnostic criteria. J Natl Cancer Inst. 2013;105(21):1607–16.
76. Pilarski R. Cowden syndrome: a critical review of the clinical literature. J Genet Couns. 2009;18(1):13–27.
77. Zhou X-P, Marsh DJ, Morrison CD, Chaudhury AR, Maxwell M, Reifenberger G. Germline inactivation of PTEN and dysregulation of the phosphoinositol-3-kinase/Akt pathway cause human Lhermitte-Duclos disease in adults. Am J Hum Genet. 2003;73(5):1191–8.
78. Weary PE, Gorlin RJ, Gentry WC, Comer JE, Greer KE. Multiple hamartoma syndrome (Cowden's disease). Arch Dermatol. 1972;106(5):682–90.
79. Tan M-H, Mester JL, Ngeow J, Rybicki LA, Orloff MS, Eng C. Lifetime cancer risks in individuals with germline PTEN mutations. Clin Cancer Res. 2012;18(2):400–7.
80. Bardenstein DS, McLean IW, Nerney J, Boatwright RS. Cowden's disease. Ophthalmology. 1988;95(8):1038–41.
81. Al-Zaid T, Ditelberg JS, Prieto VG, Lev D, Luthra R, Davies MA. Trichilemmomas show loss of PTEN in Cowden syndrome but only rarely in sporadic tumors. J Cutan Pathol. 2012;39(5):493–9.
82. Sbordone S, Savastano A, Savastano MC, Romano V, Bifani M, Savastano S. Corneal confocal microscopy anomalies associated with Cowden syndrome: a case report. Case Rep Ophthalmol. 2013;4(2):76–80.
83. Suaiti L, Al-Haseni A, Lee H, Sahni D. Iris mammillations in a pair of twins with Cowden syndrome. JAAD Case Rep. 2016;2(4):323–5.
84. DeParis SW, Bloomer M, Han Y, Vagefi MR, Shieh JTC, Solomon DA. Uveal ganglioneuroma due to germline PTEN mutation (Cowden syndrome) presenting as unilateral infantile glaucoma. Ocul Oncol Pathol. 2017;3(2):122–8.
85. Sellitto C, Li L, Gao J, Robinson ML, Lin RZ, Mathias RT. AKT activation promotes PTEN hamartoma tumor syndrome–associated cataract development. J Clin Invest. 2013;123(12):5401–9.
86. Gicquel J-J, Vabres P, Bonneau D, Mercié M, Handiri L, Dighiero P. Retinal angioma in a patient with Cowden disease. Am J Ophthalmol. 2003;135(3):400–2.
87. Venturini G, Moulin AP, Deprez M, Uffer S, Bottani A, Zografos L. Clinicopathologic and molecular analysis of a choroidal pigmented schwannoma in the context of a PTEN hamartoma tumor syndrome. Ophthalmology. 2012;119(4):857–64.
88. Mansoor Q, Steel DHW. Proliferative retinopathy in Cowden syndrome. Case Rep. 2012;2012:bcr1120115273.
89. Gama I, Almeida L. Optic nerve head drusen as a rare manifestation of Cowden syndrome: multimodal imaging. Ophthalmology. 2017;124(8):1164.
90. Brownstein MH, Wolf M, Bikowski JB. Cowden's disease: a cutaneous marker of breast cancer. Cancer. 1978;41(6):2393–8.
91. Harach HR, Soubeyran I, Brown A, Bonneau D, Longy M. Thyroid pathologic findings in patients with Cowden disease. Ann Diagn Pathol. 1999;3(6):331–40.
92. Tan M-H, Mester J, Peterson C, Yang Y, Chen J-L, Rybicki LA. A clinical scoring system for selection of patients for PTEN mutation testing is proposed on the basis of a prospective study of 3042 probands. Am J Hum Genet. 2011;88(1):42–56.
93. Gosein MA, Narinesingh D, Nixon CA-AC, Goli SR, Maharaj P, Sinanan A. Multi-organ benign and malignant tumors: recognizing Cowden syndrome: a case report and review of the literature. BMC Res Notes. 2016;9:388.
94. Carney JA, Gordon H, Carpenter PC, Shenoy BV, Go VL. The complex of myxomas, spotty pigmentation, and endocrine overactivity. Medicine (Baltimore). 1985;64(4):270–83.
95. Stratakis CA, Kirschner LS, Carney JA. Clinical and molecular features of the Carney complex: diagnostic criteria and recommendations for patient evaluation. J Clin Endocrinol Metab. 2001;86(9):4041–6.
96. Carney JA. The triad of gastric epithelioid leiomyosarcoma, pulmonary chondroma, and functioning extra-adrenal paraganglioma: a five-year review. Medicine (Baltimore). 1983;62(3):159–69.
97. Carney JA, Hruska LS, Beauchamp GD, Gordon H. Dominant inheritance of the complex of myxomas, spotty pigmentation, and endocrine overactivity. Mayo Clin Proc. 1986;61(3):165–72.
98. Bertherat J, Horvath A, Groussin L, Grabar S, Boikos S, Cazabat L. Mutations in regulatory subunit type 1A of cyclic adenosine 5′-monophosphate-dependent protein kinase (PRKAR1A): phenotype analysis in 353 patients and 80 different genotypes. J Clin Endocrinol Metab. 2009;94(6):2085–91.
99. Stratakis CA, Kirschner LS, Carney JA, Pack SD, Taymans SE, Giatzakis C. Mutations of the gene encoding the protein kinase A type I-alpha regulatory subunit in patients with the Carney complex. Nat Genet. 2000;26(1):89–92.
100. Salpea P, Horvath A, London E, Faucz FR, Vetro A, Levy I. Deletions of the PRKAR1A locus at 17q24.2-q24.3 in Carney complex: genotype-phenotype correlations and implications for genetic testing. J Clin Endocrinol Metab. 2014;99(1):E183–8.
101. Anselmo J, Medeiros S, Carneiro V, Greene E, Levy I, Nesterova M. A large family with carney complex caused by the S147G PRKAR1A mutation shows a unique spectrum of disease including adrenocortical cancer. J Clin Endocrinol Metab. 2012;97(2):351–9.
102. Liu Q, Tong D, Liu G, Yi Y, Zhang D, Zhang J. Carney complex with PRKAR1A gene mutation: a case report and literature review. Medicine (Baltimore). 2017;96(50):e8999.
103. Cohen C, Turner ML, Stratakis CA. Pigmented lesions of the conjunctiva in Carney's complex. J Am Acad Dermatol. 2000;42(1 Pt 1):145.
104. Kennedy RH, Waller RR, Carney JA. Ocular pigmented spots and eyelid myxomas. Am J Ophthalmol. 1987;104(5):533–8.
105. Tatyana M, Salomao Diva R, Ida Cristiane M, Capiz Correa Daniel R, Grossniklaus Hans E, Qiang Z, Hamershock Rose A, Carol S, Shields Jerry A, Irving R, Rapuano Christopher J, Ravi P, Eagle Ralph C. Conjunctival Myxoid Lesions: Clinical-Pathologic Multiparametric Analysis, Including Molecular Genetics (An American Ophthalmological Society Thesis). Am J Ophthalmol. 205(115):131. https://doi.org/10.1016/j.ajo.2019.04.027.
106. Salomão DR, Ida CM, Greipp PT, Aidan CJ. Case report with review of the literature: uveal melanoma in a patient with Carney complex—another rare component of the syndrome? Ocul Oncol Pathol. 2020;6(5):311–7. https://doi.org/10.1159/000506205.
107. Horvath A, Stratakis CA. Carney complex and lentiginosis. Pigment Cell Melanoma Res. 2009;22(5):580–7.
108. Boikos SA, Stratakis CA. Carney complex: the first 20 years. Curr Opin Oncol. 2007;19(1):24–9.
109. Carney JA. Psammomatous melanotic schwannoma. A distinctive, heritable tumor with special associations, including cardiac myxoma and the Cushing syndrome. Am J Surg Pathol. 1990;14(3):206–22.
110. Stratakis CA. Carney complex: a familial lentiginosis predisposing to a variety of tumors. Rev Endocr Metab Disord. 2016;17(3):367–71.
111. Carney JA. Carney complex: the complex of myxomas, spotty pigmentation, endocrine overactivity, and schwannomas. Semin Dermatol. 1995;14(2):90–8.

112. Muir EG, Bell AJ, Barlow KA. Multiple primary carcinomata of the colon, duodenum, and larynx associated with kerato-acanthomata of the face. Br J Surg. 1967;54(3):191–5.
113. Hampel H, Peltomaki P. Hereditary colorectal cancer: risk assessment and management. Clin Genet. 2000;58(2):89–97.
114. Cohen PR, Kohn SR, Kurzrock R. Association of sebaceous gland tumors and internal malignancy: the Muir-Torre syndrome. Am J Med. 1991;90(5):606–13.
115. Ponti G, de Leon MP. Muir-Torre syndrome. Lancet Oncol. 2005;6(12):980–7.
116. Lehrer MD, Lynch H, Glembocki DJ, Patel NB. Glioblastoma multiforme as initial internal malignancy in Muir-Torre syndrome (MTS). JAAD Case Rep. 2015;1(6):381–3.
117. South CD, Hampel H, Comeras I, Westman JA, Frankel WL, de la Chapelle A. The frequency of Muir-Torre syndrome among Lynch syndrome families. J Natl Cancer Inst. 2008;100(4):277–81.
118. Ponti G, Pellacani G, Seidenari S, Pollio A, Muscatello U, Tomasi A. Cancer-associated genodermatoses: skin neoplasms as clues to hereditary tumor syndromes. Crit Rev Oncol Hematol. 2013;85(3):239–56.
119. John AM, Schwartz RA. Muir-Torre syndrome (MTS): an update and approach to diagnosis and management. J Am Acad Dermatol. 2016;74(3):558–66.
120. Coldron J, Reid I. Muir-Torre syndrome. J R Coll Surg Edinb. 2001;46(3):178–9.
121. Tay E, Schofield JB, Rowell NP, Jones CA. Ophthalmic presentation of the Muir Torre syndrome. Ophthalmic Plast Reconstr Surg. 2003;19(5):402–4.
122. Singh AD, Mudhar HS, Bhola R, Rundle PA, Rennie IG. Sebaceous adenoma of the eyelid in Muir-Torre syndrome. Arch Ophthalmol. 2005;123(4):562–5.
123. Burgdorf WH, Pitha J, Fahmy A. Muir-Torre syndrome. Histologic spectrum of sebaceous proliferations. Am J Dermatopathol. 1986;8(3):202–8.
124. Gauthier A-S, Campolmi N, Tumahai P, Kantelip B, Delbosc B. Sebaceous carcinoma of the eyelid and Muir-Torre syndrome. JAMA Ophthalmol. 2014;132(8):1025.
125. Propeck PA, Warner T, Scanlan KA. Sebaceous carcinoma of the breast in a patient with Muir-Torre syndrome. AJR Am J Roentgenol. 2000;174(2):541–2.
126. Mencía-Gutiérrez E, Gutiérrez-Díaz E, Santos-Briz A, Madero-García S. Sebaceous gland carcinoma of the eyelid and palpebral conjunctiva in a patient with Muir-Torre syndrome. Br J Ophthalmol. 2000;84(11):1325–6.
127. Jakobiec FA, Paula CB, Lefebvre Daniel R, Tatyana M. Intraductal sebaceous papilloma of a meibomian gland: a new entity possibly associated with the MSH6 subtype of the Muir-Torre syndrome. Surv Ophthalmol. 65(2):227–38. https://doi.org/10.1016/j.survophthal.2019.09.002.
128. Rustgi AK. Hereditary gastrointestinal polyposis and nonpolyposis syndromes. N Engl J Med. 1994;331(25):1694–702.
129. Kruse R, Rütten A, Lamberti C, Hosseiny-Malayeri HR, Wang Y, Ruelfs C. Muir-Torre phenotype has a frequency of DNA mismatch-repair-gene mutations similar to that in hereditary nonpolyposis colorectal cancer families defined by the Amsterdam criteria. Am J Hum Genet. 1998;63(1):63–70.
130. Umar A, Risinger JI, Hawk ET, Barrett JC. Testing guidelines for hereditary non-polyposis colorectal cancer. Nat Rev Cancer. 2004;4(2):153–8.
131. Umar A, Boland CR, Terdiman JP, Syngal S, de la Chapelle A, Ruschoff J. Revised Bethesda guidelines for hereditary nonpolyposis colorectal cancer (Lynch syndrome) and microsatellite instability. J Natl Cancer Inst. 2004;96(4):261–8.
132. Roberts ME, Riegert-Johnson DL, Thomas BC, Rumilla KM, Thomas CS, Heckman MG. A clinical scoring system to identify patients with sebaceous neoplasms at risk for the Muir–Torre variant of Lynch syndrome. Genet Med. 2014;16(9):711–6.
133. Jones B, Oh C, Mangold E, Egan CA. Muir-Torre syndrome: diagnostic and screening guidelines. Australas J Dermatol. 2006;47(4):266–9.
134. Le S, Ansari U, Mumtaz A, et al. Lynch syndrome and Muir-Torre syndrome: an update and review on the genetics, epidemiology, and management of two related disorders. Dermatol Online J. 2017;23:11.

Index

B. C. K. Patel et al. (eds.), *Clinical Ophthalmic Oncology*, https://doi.org/10.1007/978-3-031-72328-5

T

MIX
Papier aus verantwortungsvollen Quellen
Paper from responsible sources
FSC® C105338
FSC
www.fsc.org

If you have any concerns about our products,
you can contact us on
ProductSafety@springernature.com

In case Publisher is established outside the EU,
the EU authorized representative is:
Springer Nature Customer Service Center GmbH
Europaplatz 3, 69115 Heidelberg, Germany

Printed by Libri Plureos GmbH
in Hamburg, Germany